S0-BMG-669

VITAMINS AND HORMONES

VOLUME 43

Editorial Board

VITAMINS AND HORMONES

ADVANCES IN RESEARCH AND APPLICATIONS

Editor-in-Chief

G. D. AURBACH
Metabolic Diseases Branch
National Institute of Arthritis,
Diabetes, and Digestive and Kidney Diseases
National Institutes of Health
Bethesda, Maryland

Editor

DONALD B. MCCORMICK
Department of Biochemistry
Emory University School of Medicine
Atlanta, Georgia

Volume 43
1986

ACADEMIC PRESS, INC. **Harcourt Brace Jovanovich, Publishers**
Orlando San Diego New York Austin
Boston London Sydney Tokyo Toronto

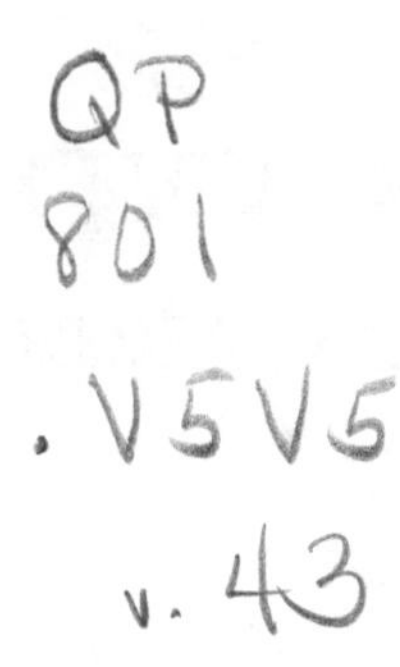

ACADEMIC PRESS, INC.
Orlando, Florida 32887

United Kingdom Edition published by
ACADEMIC PRESS INC. (LONDON) LTD.
24–28 Oval Road, London NW1 7DX

LIBRARY OF CONGRESS CATALOG CARD NUMBER: 43-10535

ISBN 0–12–709843–7 (alk. paper)

PRINTED IN THE UNITED STATES OF AMERICA

86 87 88 89 9 8 7 6 5 4 3 2 1

Contents

The Hormonal Regulation of Prolactin Gene Expression: An Examination of Mechanisms Controlling Prolactin Synthesis and the Possible Relationship of Estrogen to These Mechanisms

James D. Shull and Jack Gorski

Hormonal Regulation in *In Vitro* Fertilization

Gary D. Hodgen

Intracellular Processing and Secretion of Parathyroid Gland Proteins

David V. Cohn, Ramasamy Kumarasamy, and Warren K. Ramp

Preface

Volume 43 of *Vitamins and Hormones* provides further informative reviews for researchers and scholars in endocrinology and nutrition. Several of the discussions are of considerable health and social significance. G. Hodgen's article describes the potential and biology of *in vitro* fertilization and the endocrine manipulations favoring success with the method. Ongoing work with this system provides a remarkable opportunity to study processes controlling fertilization and gestation, but engender, as well, profound social and ethical responsibilities. E. Sims has developed a monumental work on energy balance in normal and pathophysiologic states. Obesity may represent the result of metabolic and satiety patterns at one time important for survival. At least in some types of obesity, impairments in ability to adapt to excessive caloric intake have been identified.

L. Elsas and D. McCormick discuss genetic variations in vitamin and nutrient requirements. Such variations imply that what is satisfactory intake for some subjects is inadequate for others of differing genetic makeup. This article relates to fat-soluble vitamins; an article in the subsequent issue will deal with water-soluble vitamins.

F. George and J. Wilson review the hormonal control of sexual development. The classical postulate of Jost appears to stand the test of time—chromosomal sex dictates gonadal sex which in turn governs phenotypic sex. Multiple hormones and many genes, not simply those of the sex chromosomes alone, are involved in sexual differentiation in man.

J. Shull and J. Gorski provide an analysis of mechanisms involved in the control of prolactin synthesis. *In vitro* regulation by estrogen is entirely at the transcriptional level. *In vivo* regulation is not yet so completely characterized.

D. Cohn, R. Kumarasamy, and W. Ramp review biosynthetic processing and secretory processes in the elaboration of products from the parathyroid gland. A particularly challenging problem persists—unraveling the role of PSP (chromogranin) protein in the secretory processes of many endocrine cells.

To the staff of Academic Press, we convey our thanks for expert help in preparing this volume.

G. D. Aurbach
Donald B. McCormick

VITAMINS AND HORMONES, VOL. 43

Energy Balance in Human Beings: The Problems of Plenitude

ETHAN A. H. SIMS

Metabolic Unit, Department of Medicine,
College of Medicine, University of Vermont,
Burlington, Vermont 05405

They came to the old philosopher and asked "Why in our country are so many so sadly augmented in weight?"
He replied "Charge them not, for there are many demons within and without."

From the *Lost Sayings of Ching Chang Chung,* Eleventh Century B.C.

I. Introduction

In addressing the Western Hemisphere Nutrition Congress VII in 1983, the Honorable Billie Miller, Minister of Education of the Barbados, emphasized that the problems of overnutrition are not limited to the affluent countries. In her not very rich country when rural workers gave up the hard physical work of farming to take up urban employment, the commercial promotion of food, the use of labor-saving devices, and the change in dietary patterns and in physical activity often led to obesity. The problems of this imported plenitude have led to a documented increase in type II diabetes and hypertension in areas such as the Caribbean as well as in our own (Sims, 1984). It is urgent that we gain an understanding of man's defenses against overnutrition and its physiologic effects.

Until relatively recently, one assumed that energy in man followed relatively simple rules in which the fire of life burned quite steadily and a given caloric intake could be expected to give a predictable surfeit or deficit of stored energy, depending upon the amount of energy expended on the environment. It has long been evident that to withstand extreme cold, there must be mechanisms whereby isothermic animals and man can increase heat production. It has been less evident that there must be adaptation to changes in the supply of food. For survival, mechanisms must exist to preserve the leanness and agility of the hunter or in different circumstances, well-padded energy reserves to withstand famine. These two goals may be in conflict and changing circumstances may make one or the other conflicting or inappropriate. This is particularly apparent in our changing and affluent society. We are in an exciting period of learning that many factors can affect the rate of thermogenesis. We live in a world in which overnutrition with its associated major problems may exist side by side with undernutrition and its attendant problems.

One might expect that man has retained or developed one or more adaptations for control of thermogenesis. Extraordinary adaptations can be seen among plants and animals. The skunk cabbage, for example raises its temperature above ambient to waft its scent more effectively (Knutson, 1974). The elephant beetle turns on endogenous warmers on a particularly chilly day (Morgan and Bartholamew, 1982). The bombadier beetle can form and cleave hydrogen peroxide to generate steam to blast its enemies with a toxic vapor in a manner so spectacular it was taken by the Creationists as proof against evolution. The bumble bee indulges in a substrate cycle between fructose 6-phosphate and fructose 1,6-phosphate to warm his wing muscles before takeoff (Clark *et al.,* 1973a). The rat disposes of extra calories as heat when it has overindulged in a cafeteria diet (Rothwell and Stock, 1983). The blue whale lives for many months entirely on her blubber when she leaves the krill of the antarctic to bear and nurse her young in tropic waters (Rice and Wolman, 1971).

In this review I discuss the mechanisms of energy balance in normals and later in the overweight with emphasis on those which may either increase or diminish thermogenesis. I will not attempt a comprehensive review of this huge subject, but will emphasize recent developments and particularly the problems of overnutrition. It is in this area that our laboratory has had most experience. A critical inspection of abdominal contours of our fellow man and woman, and perhaps our own, indicates that this is a major problem. It is one closely linked to the epidemic of diabetes, hypertension, and hyperlipidemia in this and other more privileged countries (Sims, 1984). Possible adaptive mechanisms for disposal of excess calories from food through facultative increases in thermogenesis will be explored. Recent research has produced a wealth of contradictory results regarding mechanisms of energy balance and possible derangements in the overweight. One of the objectives of this review is to examine these studies in the hope of identifying the sources of such disagreement. Obesity is not a simple matter of gluttony; there are many subtypes of obesity differing in mechanism and in optimal management. Adaptive mechanisms may be blunted in some of these subtypes. Further research in this field must take these subtypes into consideration.

A classic work in this field is the book by Garrow (1974) and its 1978 update. Others include a definitive and very completely referenced book on obesity by Bray published in 1976, and the recent volume edited by Girardier and Stock (1983), in which mammalian thermogenesis is reviewed. Recent symposia bearing on thermogenesis in man include that of the Fourth International Congress on Obesity (Hirsch and Van Itallie, 1985) and its satellite (Horton *et al.*, 1985). A symposium at Harrow (Garrow and Halliday, 1984) gave particular emphasis to protein turnover, and another at Marseille gave emphasis to the importance of the distribution of body fat (Vague and Björntorp, 1985).

II. Elements of Normal Energy Balance

A. In Search of a Common Terminology

The elements of energy expenditure are diagrammed in Fig. 1. They may be defined as follows. The *resting metabolic rate* (RMR) includes the endothermic component, plus the additional energy production as measured under resting conditions to qualify us as homoiothermous

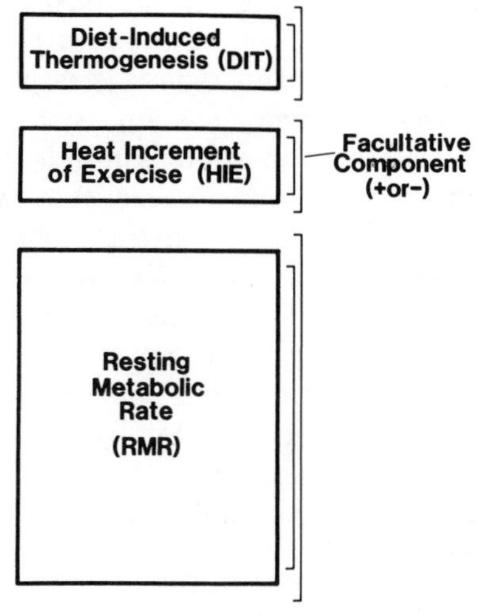

Fig. 1. The components of thermogenesis. Diet-induced thermogenesis is the thermic response above the resting metabolic rate and represents the obligatory component. Intravenous substrates may provoke a comparable response. The heat increment of exercise is also referred to as the thermic effect of exercise (TEE). The resting metabolic rate includes the basal metabolic rate, the RMR measured under defined conditions of complete rest. The light brackets indicate that each of the three components may be increased to a limited extent under various conditions.

animals. The clinical term *basal metabolic rate* (BMR) refers to the RMR measured under defined conditions of rest after a night's sleep. The *heat increment of exercise* (HIE) or *thermic effect of exercise* (TEE), not to be confused with total energy expenditure, refers to the additional energy expenditure associated with the physical activity above basal conditions. The metabolic efficiency of exercise is somewhat variable and is usually less than 30% of the increased heat which is dissipated. For relatively affluent and sedentary Americans living in a world of labor-saving appliances, the RMR accounts for perhaps 65–75% of the daily energy expenditure. The *thermic effect of food* (TEF) refers to the obligatory energy utilization associated with breakdown, absorption, net resynthesis, and storage of food, and is usually expressed as the expenditure above baseline. The additional bracketed areas indicate the variable amounts of *facultative thermogenesis,* which has also been called adaptive thermogenesis, and which may be associated with any one of the three main elements. It represents expended energy that yields heat, but no work or net synthesis, and is that portion of an increase in RMR not attributable to changes in the respiring mass. The other commonly used term, *diet-induced thermogenesis* (DIT), may include both the obligatory and facultative components of TEF. Note that facultative thermogenesis may be either positive, as when induced by cold, protein undernutrition, or overfeeding, or negative, as in caloric undernutrition. It is predominantly under control of the sympathetic nervous system, with a permissive role of thyroid hormone and at least in small animals a contribution from stimulation of nonshivering thermogenesis in brown fat.

A major component of the RMR and the body temperature under varying ambient temperature is the *essential heat* required for minimal metabolic activity and renewal of tissues at complete rest. Under usual conditions this is inadequate to maintain body temperature at the characteristic set level. Additional *obligate heat* is required, and this is modulated on a long-term basis by thyroid hormone. The essential as well as the obligate heat may be affected by insulin both through effects on the flow of body fuels and by direct action on cellular ion pumping (see Section II,E,2,d).

B. The Relation of Basal or Resting Metabolic Rate to the Fat-Free Mass

It is commonly assumed that the basal or resting metabolic rate in man bears a fixed relationship to the fat-free mass (FFM). Webb (1981) found that energy expenditure, measured by direct calorimetry with his "space suit," correlated highly ($r = 0.95$, $p < 0.001$) with fat-free mass in 15 men and women of ages 22–55. Neither age nor sex affected the relationship. Also, Dore *et al.* (1982) found that in women who had undergone marked weight reduction the same relationship was maintained in both the initial and the reduced state.

Keys *et al.* (1973), anticipating recent work in their discussion of their studies of metabolic rate and aging, stated that "so far no references proposed explain more than a small part of the total variance in BMR."

C. Bogardus *et al.* (personal communication) have studied the relation of RMR to fat-free mass derived from body density by underwater weighing, with simultaneous measurement of residual lung volume in 94 Pima Indians. In the group as a whole, the FFM explained 85% of the variance of RMR. The sample included 39 families with two to four siblings. The variance of RMR among families was significantly less than the variance among the entire group. When the family component was added, the variance was very much smaller. Plots of results for a given family fell consistently above or below the regression line for the group as a whole. This certainly suggests that there is a variation in the relationship between RMR and fat-free mass which may be genetically determined. Supporting this conclusion are the results of Fontaine *et al.* (1985), who studied the resting metabolic rate in relation to fat-free mass in 20 monozygotic and 19 dizygotic healthy male twin pairs. The intraclass coefficient ($r = 0.45$) was significant for the monozygotic pairs, but not for the dizygotic, which again strongly suggests a genetic component. Differences in RMR/FFM between individuals may be real and should not be attributed to analytical error. Some populations, such as the day laborers subsisting on a low caloric intake studied by Shetty (1984), may have a lower ratio of RMR to FFM (see Section IV).

C. Energy Storage and Balance in the Various Stages and Activities of Man

1. *Neonatal Period*

When thrust into a cold world at birth, the neonate comes equipped with a security blanket of brown fat capable of warming his neck, the great vessels, and vital organs such as the heart and kidney. The degree to which this is preserved in adult years is discussed below (Section II,E,3,a).

2. *Childhood and the Determination of Adipocyte Number*

In animals and in man the period up to adolescence was believed to mark the accumulation of one's final complement of adipocytes. Until quite recently it was considered that the cell number did not increase in later years and that enlargement of the adipose mass was effected through hypertrophy alone. It is now evident that overloading of adipocytes with lipid (over 1 μg/cell) prompts development of new cells by recruitment of preadipocytes (Hirsch and Batchelor, 1976). On the other hand, there is no evidence to date that excess cells formed in youth can regress in number, although there are no long-term studies to substantiate this. Brook *et al.* (1972) have suggested that preadolescence is particularly critical for development of adipocyte hyperplasia and later development of obesity. However, the obese child does not necessarily become an obese adult (Abraham and Nordseik, 1960). We need to learn more about the subtypes of obesity that may run in families in order to predict which children are at greatest risk and most in need of early help.

Cellular hyperplasia of in the obese is not limited to adipocytes. Naeye and Roode (1970) measured cell size and estimated total cell number of various organs in young obese subjects at autopsy and found a marked increase in liver, spleen, heart, and pancreas. Thus the fat-free mass shares in the hyperplasia.

3. *Menstruation*

In a marathon 92-day laboratory study of six young women in Callaway's laboratory metabolic rate was found to decrease at the time of menstruation, being at its lowest point approximately 1 week prior to ovulation (Solomon *et al.*, 1982). There was a subsequent slow rise until the time of the next period. Activity and dietary intake were controlled in the study and weight changes were small. The rise in RMR is coincident with the increase in aldosterone secretory rate, but since this merely compensates for the natriuretic effect of increased progesterone, it is doubtful that the rise in RMR is related to aldosterone-stimulated Na–K pump activity. Bisdee *et al.* (1986) studied energy expenditure during repeated 36-hour whole-body calorimetry and hormonal changes in women maintaining a constant dietary intake and activity over 6 weeks. There were significant increases in sleeping metabolic rate during the latter half of the menstrual cycle, which coincided with peak urinary and salivary progesterone concentrations, but did not correlate with their degree. The early luteal rise of body temperature did not correlate directly with the rise in sleeping metabolic rate.

4. *Pregnancy and Lactation*

Blackburn and Calloway's laboratory (1976a) also reported an increase in basal metabolic rate in the latter half of pregnancy. The change is out of proportion to the increase in body mass. The actual excess energy requirements for pregnancy vary depending upon the initial level of activity and the demands for physical activity. Estimates for net cost have varied from 23,000 to 80,000 kcal, and it seems futile to try to generalize. Blackburn and Calloway (1976b) estimated the cost in energy during lactation to be approximately 675 kcal per day. A portion of this is normally drawn from endogenous sources, acquired in part during pregnancy. The high cost of lactation is advantageous to a breast-feeding mother striving to return to prepartum weight. Certain women gain exorbitantly during pregnancy and escalate weight gain during successive pregnancies. Identifying those at risk and learning more about the permissible level of caloric restriction in pregnancy should be given priority.

5. *Advancing Age*

The variable relation of resting metabolic rate to fat-free mass and the problems of measurement were discussed above in Section II,B. Lean body mass also may decline with age, especially when there is decreased physical activity. Thus a decline in the RMR may not necessarily be a concomitant of age per se, but may reflect the reduction in fat-free mass. Keys *et al.* (1973) have shown that the BMR per lean body mass in the elderly declines only slowly (possibly 1% per decade); BMR per body weight declines more rapidly. It is thus difficult to say how much of the apparent decline may be due to "normal" aging and how much may be a reflection of our current life-style and environmental factors. To accept a marked decline, at least before the Judgment Day and its inevitable abrupt decline in RMR, may be to accept an inappropriate standard of normality.

There is, however, one possible pitfall in relating RMR to lean body mass as currently estimated. If there were a significant degree of skeletal demineralization from any cause, the respiring mass would be underestimated and the RMR relative to fat-free mass would be apparently increased. Nevertheless the life-style and degree of preservation of muscle mass are apparently critical factors. It seems more logical in studies of thermogenesis to match subjects for fat-free mass rather than for age, although admittedly this is not ideal.

Minaker *et al.* (1982) reported a decline with age in the response of the sympathetic nervous system to stimulation by intravenous insulin with the concentration of glucose maintained constant by the clamp procedure. In a well-controlled study Golay *et al.* (1982) concluded that age contributed to the reduced thermic response to oral glucose of those with insulin resistance. This contrasts with the earlier finding of the same group that the sympathetic response to oral glucose is greater in the elderly. Again, it is difficult to say how much of these changes are an inevitable consequence of age per se.

6. *Energy Storage in Catastrophic Illness. The Role of Cachectin*

In severe infection and with malignancies mammals may undergo rapid wasting of energy stores in spite of continued caloric intake (Jeejeebhoy, 1985). A factor named *cachectin* is apparently produced by macrophages upon stimulation with endotoxin and this in turn inhibits enzymes of lipogenesis in adipocytes. The molecular basis of its formation has recently been reported by Torti *et al.* (1985). Passive immunization against cachectin protects mice against the lethal effect of endotoxin (Beutler *et al.,* 1985).

7. *The Effect of High Altitude on Energy Balance*

On expeditions to high mountains (over 18,000 ft) mountaineers characteristically lose considerable weight; conventional wisdom attributes this to altitude hypoxia. Since living conditions are harsh on great mountains, food spartan and often unappetizing, and adequate water difficult to obtain, some question whether the weight loss is due to these factors rather than to hypoxia alone. Dr. Charles S. Houston has shared preliminary findings of a recent collaborative study employing the decompression chamber at the United States Army Institute of Environmental Research at Natick, Massachusetts. Ample fluids and appetizing foods were available yet all eight subjects lost weight as altitude increased. During the first 10 days of gradual ascent to 18,000 ft the average loss was 4.4 lb (range, 1–7.6 lb). During the next 30 days with gradual ascent to 25,000 ft and above, the average loss was 7.6 lb (range, 1–13 lb). The subjects were highly trained competitive athletes. During the first 2 weeks they exercised strenuously on cycle ergometer and treadmill; above 25,000 ft they exercised much less. Though they all ate 2600–3600 kcal a day during the first week, in the final 2 weeks intake fell to less than half this amount. It appeared that anorexia induced by altitude hypoxia plus confinement decreased their caloric intake more than their desire to exercise and thus led to weight loss, despite comfortable living conditions and ample, appetizing meals. There is a possibility that the experience may have induced a catecholamine response and also that increased substrate cycling may have increased the rate of thermogenesis. Detailed reports from this study will be of great interest.

8. *The Effect of Higher Altitude on Energy Balance: Weightlessness of Space Flight*

It has long been known that immobilization or prolonged bed rest impair carbohydrate metabolism and retention of calcium in the body. A new concern is the effect of total weightlessness during space flight. Leonard *et al.* (1983) have reported the effect on body composition of crew members in Skylab missions lasting 29–84 days. Total body weight loss was 2.7 ± 0.3 kg, with 56% derived from lean body mass, and the remainder from fat. The loss appeared to plateau after 1 month.

D. Factors Affecting Intake of Food

Factors affecting appetite and hunger are considered at length in the book edited by Novin *et al.* (1976) and in the recent reviews by Kissileff and Van Itallie (1982) and by Castonguay *et al.* (1984). Additional mechanisms of control and the effect of drugs upon them were considered in a recent symposium edited by Sullivan and Garattini (1984). Both psychological and physiological factors are involved, but only the latter will be discussed here.

1. *Hormonal Factors*

a. Adrenal Hormones. Bray (1986) has recently published an innovative review of the symphony of factors which control and integrate energy intake and expenditure. Emphasis is placed on the importance of the glucocorticoid hormones. The role of the adrenal hormones is well documented in animals, but except in frank Cushing's disease, it is not clear whether they play a facilitative or more primary role in all humans or perhaps only in some subtypes of obesity (see Section II,E,2,e).

b. Brain Peptides. Hormones other than glucocorticoids are involved. In one of her last reviews, Dorothy Krieger (1984) considered the brain peptides and their possible role in feeding behavior in the preceding volume of this series. The endogenous peptides, the endorphins and enkephalins, are prominent in the reaction to stress, and also stimulate food intake (Morley and Levine, 1980). Intraventricular injection in rats increases food intake (McKay *et al.,* 1981), while the receptor blocker naloxone and its analogs reduced food intake. In feeding experiments it is important to distinguish whether a particular agent simply makes an animal feel poorly, or specifically inhibits appetite or hunger. It is more convincing if an effect is independent of any effect on intake of water. Naloxone, the opioid antagonist, reduces food intake in humans (Cohen *et al.*, 1985) and an analog, naloxodone, acts similarly in obese subjects (Wolkowitz *et al.*, 1985). Fantino *et al.* (1986) found that the orally active opioid antagonist naltrexone affects taste perception, reducing the preference for solutions sweetened with sucrose. (For studies on brain peptides in obesity, see Section V,B, 5.)

c. Gut Hormones. Since the discovery by Gibbs and co-workers that cholecystokinin decreases food intake in rats, the hypothesis that the gut hormones serve as satiety signals and inhibit feeding has been intensively investigated. Such signals would act before the metabolic effects of feeding can be fully established and terminate feeding before an excess is consumed. Over 10 years later this is still somewhat uncertain (Smith, 1984). A number of gut hormones other than cholecystokinin produce satiety (Smith and Gibbs, 1984). These include bombesin (Gibbs *et al.*, 1979), glucagon (Geary and Smith, 1982), and somatostatin (Lotter *et al.*, 1981). It is not certain whether these function as normal physiological regulators, but several show pharmacological actions in inhibiting food intake in normal and obese humans (Kissileff *et al.*, 1981; Pi-Sunyer *et al.*, 1982; Smith, 1984).

d. Insulin. There is evidence in animals that insulin itself may affect feeding behavior through an effect on hypothalamic centers. Insulin-specific binding sites exist in the hypothalamus and olfactory bulb. Glucoreceptor neurons are found in the ventromedial hypothalamus and the lateral hypothalamus and affect pancreatic vagal activity. Oomura and Kita (1981) have reviewed the complicated functional interrelationships of this system. It has been known for some time that the mere sight of food in the obese provokes a cephalic stimulation of insulin release (see also following section). Sjöstrom *et al.* (1980) found a significant increase in the area under the insulin response curve following exposure to food-related stimuli in a large number of control and obese women. There was, however, much individual variation. Blockade by atropine showed that the response was mediated via the vagus nerve. Basal insulin concentrations are also related to the size of the body's energy store. Woods *et al.* (1981) have summarized the evidence that insulin may provide a signal to the CNS regarding the state of body energy stores. Rodin, with the collaboration of DeFronzo's group at Yale (1985), recently studied the relationship of perceived intensity and pleasantness of sucrose solutions while plasma glucose and insulin were independently varied. Even under the unnatural conditions of the clamp procedure, increasing plasma insulin to 100 μU/ml clearly increased appreciation of sweetness.

e. Prolactin. The significance of prolactin in affecting food intake in man is uncertain. In animals, however, it is important in the orchestra of regulatory hormones affecting food intake (Meier, 1976, 1977). It regulates energy stores on a seasonal basis in the killifish and topminnow, the green anole lizard, and the migratory white-throated sparrow. The latter nearly quadruples its body fat in the 10 days prior to migration. In pigeons injected with bovine prolactin, weight gain is associated with an increase in release of fatty acids from the liver (Goodridge and Ball, 1970). During lactation in the rat, inhibition by prolactin of lipoprotein lipase in fat depots and stimulation in mammary tissue provide a supply of fatty acids for milk production (Zinder *et al.*, 1974). Joseph and Meier (1974) have shown that in the hamster fattening and reproductive effects are also dependent upon circadian adrenal cortical rhythms. Cincotta and Meier (1984) found that there is a circadian rhythm of sensitivity of the liver to insulin, which is maximal during the 6–8 hours of the day when the animals do 80% of their feeding. The increased sensitivity corresponds to the number of active hepatic receptor sites for insulin, and the increased sensitivity is found as long as 3 days in cultured cells. A rise in serum prolactin precedes the rise in insulin by approximately 20 hours and appears to entrain the increased sensitivity. This can be blocked by bromocryptine, which inhibits prolactin release from the pituitary, and prolactin by injection can mimic the natural sequence. This may be of considerable importance in the obese golden hamster, since Meier's group found that obese individuals or strains have a high circadian rise in prolactin, while the lean have a lesser rise. Gerardo *et al.* (1985) found that in rats made hyperprolactinemic by ectopic pituitary transplants food intake increased, white fat depots increased, and thermogenesis in brown fat was depressed, as indicated by decreased GDP binding in this tissue.

In view of the evidence that prolactin may regulate energy storage in animals one might expect prolactin to be involved in the storage of fat and development of obesity in man. There is, however, no convincing evidence to date. Some years ago Molitsch looked for a correlation between body mass index and serum prolactin in 52 patients with prolactin-secreting pituitary adenomas. The probability of an association was $p < 0.05$, but only 12% of the variance was explained (M. Molitsch, personal communication).

f. Catecholamines. Stricker and Zigmond (1984) concluded that brain catecholamines nonspecifically influence feeding behavior by affecting sensitivity to specific stimuli of eating and drinking. Rats with central lesions affecting dopaminergic activity maintain their body weight at a lower level than that of controls.

2. *Responses to Changes in the Quality, Route of Administration, and Composition of the Diet*

It is now apparent that normal subjects react physiologically to the mere sight of food, to the taste, to the route of administration, as well as to the content of protein, fat, and carbohydrate, and to their relative proportions.

a. The Look. Overweight adolescents respond with a striking increase in serum insulin on the mere sight of an appetizing breakfast (Parra-Covarrubias *et al.*, 1971). Adults have a similar cephalic response (Fisher *et al.*, 1972; Louis-Sylvestre, 1976; Porikos and Van Itallie, 1984; Rolls and Rowe, 1981), which may affect eating some hours after a meal. See also the discussion on insulin in the previous section. Salivation also increases at the sight of food (Powers *et al.*, 1982).

b. Gourmet Quality. The ease of provoking gluttony in a laboratory rat by feeding a "cafeteria diet" containing a variety of snack foods is well known. The same influences apply to man. In a simple and ingenious experiment LeBlanc and Brondel (1985) found that the thermogenic response was significantly greater when subjects were given a mixed meal than when they were given the same constituents homogenized and compressed into a biscuit (20 versus 12% increase in oxygen consumption). The rise in insulin and catecholamine concentrations was also greater. Many research protocols have employed liquid feedings containing crude constituents mixed with little culinary expertise for prolonged periods, up to 92 days in one study. One wonders whether the use of such meals, for perhaps long periods, may not produce distortion in the findings, such as in the insulin or catecholamine response.

c. The Route. In LeBlanc's laboratory (LeBlanc *et al.*, 1984) it was shown that identical foodstuffs administered by gavage provoke a lesser thermogenic response than those taken in the conventional manner.

d. Other Changes. Other changes in the composition of the diet by limiting the concentration of an essential nutrient or providing an abundance of one element such as fat can greatly stimulate intake (see Section II,E,1,b below).

When normal subjects are given preload meals of varying caloric content but disguised to appear similar, they adjust rather imprecisely (Spiegel, 1973; Kissileff and Van Itallie, 1982). Durrant *et al.* (1982) found that subjects corrected only about a third of a 600-kcal deficit within 3 days. Duncan *et al.* (1983) also showed that the caloric density of meals is important as well. Reduction of density to half by dilution with fresh fruits, vegetables, and dried beans produced satiety in experimental subjects with virtually half the original caloric intake, even though effort was made to make each diet equally attractive. The result is difficult to interpret, however, since in this study fat content was higher in the concentrated diets and Drewnowski has shown in an elegant series of studies that addition of fat adds to the pleasurable taste of carbohydrate (Drewnowski and Greenwood, 1983; Drewnowski, 1984; Drewnowski *et al.,* 1985).

E. Mechanisms and Regulation of Heat Production and Factors Affecting Storage of Energy

The goal of this section is to outline factors, mechanisms, and sites of action involved in thermogenic control and storage of energy. This is to serve as background information concerning problems of over- and undernutrition.

1. *The Cost of Metabolism of Foods*

a. Obligatory Costs. Garrow and Hawes (1972) showed that the so-called "specific dynamic action" of protein was not simply related to urea synthesis and amino acid degradation and suggested that protein synthesis was of more importance. Flatt (1978, 1985) has provided valuable detailed analyses of the biochemistry of energy expenditure. For each mole of ATP consumed he estimates an energy expenditure of 20 kcal. Carbohydrate storage as glycogen requires expenditure of 4% of the calories in the process. This increases to at least 20% if stored as fat, but we now know that direct storage of the carbons of glucose as fat is negligible under usual conditions. The direct cost of oxidation of glucose is less than 1%. The cost for ingested fat can be as low as 2% if oxidized and 4% if stored in adipose tissue.

Using the euglycemic–hyperinsulinemic clamp technique combined with indirect calorimetry, Thiebaud *et al.* (1983) found that throughout a wide range of hyperinsulinemia there is a close relationship between energy expenditure and glucose storage, with a cost of 0.45 kcal per gram of glucose stored. If, however, all the glucose is stored as glycogen, the theoretical cost can account for only 45–63% of the total expenditure. It is this increment, which is variable and may be reduced in subjects with obesity and other disorders, that is referred to as facultative or adaptive thermogenesis (see Section III,A,2). Recent work in McGarry's laboratory employing specifically labeled glucose in fasted rats indicates, however, that only a third of administered glucose goes via the direct pathway to glycogen and that a larger portion of glycogen is formed via conversion of glucose to three-carbon intermediates such as lactate. This pathway is energetically more costly. Similar findings were reported by Shulman *et al.* (1985) at Yale using nuclear magnetic resonance. They found that the direct pathway accounted for only a third of hepatic glycogen formation in fasted rats, and that only half of the total glycogen synthesis could be accounted for by the pathway involving conversion of glucose to triose phosphates and back to glycogen, via gluconeogenesis from alanine/lactate, or by the direct pathway. In his recent studies at Lausanne employing the glucose clamp technique in man, E. Danforth and others (personal commmunication) found the cost of the nonoxidative disposal of glucose was double that predicted from direct conversion to glycogen. The degree of the apparent facultative component varied with the increase in the appearance rate of norepinephrine as indicated by kinetic studies (see Section III,A,3,d). If the degree of catecholamine response does indeed directly affect the route and cost of glucose disposal, this may help to explain the variation in the facultative thermogenic response between individuals and in the various disease states discussed later in this review.

Protein provokes the greatest obligatory metabolic response, 25% of ingested calories, due to the high cost of peptide bond synthesis, and because of the high cost of gluconeogenesis and ureogenesis, regardless of whether the amino acids are oxidized or reused for synthesis. Flatt (1978, 1985) pointed out the importance of the composition of the substrates metabolized in comparison with that of the diet. He proposed considering the "food quotient" (FQ) which describes the ratio of CO_2 to O_2 during the combustion of the dietary mixture. When a usual fat intake of 40% is taken, the overnight fasting resting quotient (RQ) is barely below the FQ, and it may be difficult to achieve a total daily RQ as low as the FQ. He suggested that types of physical activity involving endurance, which favor a low RQ, be increased when weight loss is desired.

Heymsfield and associates in DiGirolamo's laboratory at Emory University (1985) have developed a method whereby each of the components of nitrogen and energy balance can be modeled mathematically with considerable accuracy. A dietary formula is continuously infused for long enough (up to 3 days) for equilibrium to develop. All excreta are collected and analyzed, and heat losses are measured by direct gradient layer and indirect calorimetry. Activity is calibrated by indirect calorimetry and logged. The procedure cannot take into account such factors as the response to orogastric stimulation and effects of circadian rhythms, but it does lend itself to many applications in the study of energy balance.

b. The Effect of Change in Composition of Isocaloric Diets on Both Storage and Expenditure of Energy. i. The protein content. The world of nutrition was shaken by the results of Miller and Payne's (1968) studies on two piglets, one of which was given a diet containing inadequate protein (2.6%) for 40 days. The pig taking the low-protein diet ate five times as much as a litter mate taking a diet with 26% protein but fed in such restricted quantities that it gained little above its weanling weight. This observation was all the more remarkable since activity, urinary and fecal losses, and weight were similar for both pigs. The protein-restricted piglet, apparently striving for its fair share of protein, took in 47,500 kcal as opposed to 9750 kcal taken in by its sibling. This study stimulated an experiment of similar design in rats (Stirling and Stock, 1968) in which animals fed a diet low in protein apparently overate to obtain adequate protein and appeared to waste calories. A series of further experiments in rats showed that stimulation of brown fat accounts for much of the loss of energy as heat. This adaptation is obviously advantageous for survival. The original Miller and Payne experiments have been criticized on several counts. They have been put in perspective by the recent studies of Gurr *et al.* (1980) in Rothwell and Stock's laboratory in London. Small (6 kg) and larger (20 kg) pigs were fed high- and low-protein diets (2 and 26%) for 6 weeks. As in the original experiments, both groups taking the low-protein diet overate. However, the small pigs showed markedly inefficient weight gain and the heavier pigs deposited the excess calories as fat. In the smaller pigs serum triiodothyronine and the lipolytic response to norepinephrine were increased. Adult, but not young, pigs apparently lack brown fat, but, as in rats, there was an increase in hepatic α-glycerol-phosphate dehydrogenase activity, producing a decrease in the P : O ratio and yield of ATP. This helps to explain the slow rate of gain in animals taking the low-protein diet. More recent studies in rats by Rothwell *et al.* (1983a) demonstrated that the uncoupling of mitochondrial oxidation in brown fat is of much greater importance in this response (see Section II,E,3,a). Miller and Mumford (1967a) reported similar effects, but to a much lesser degree, on weight gain in human subjects given low-protein diets ad lib. However, the experimental conditions of forced feeding were quite different.

ii. The content of carbohydrate and of fat. Schwartz *et al.* (1985), while working in our laboratory, compared the response over a 6-hour period to 800-kcal liquid "meals," each containing 15% of calories as protein and the remainder as either carbohydrate or fat, plus a bit of flavoring. In spite of the unappealing quality, the thermic response to the formula high in carbohydrate was twice as great as to the formula high in fat. There was no evident relationship between the response of plasma glucose, insulin, epinephrine, or norepinephrine in these normal subjects to the composition of the meals. Sharief and Macdonald (1982) found that sucrose given as a drink to normal subjects provokes a greater thermic response than an equal weight of glucose. However, the study was terminated after 3 hours when the thermic response was still at its peak, so that the full thermogenic response could not be evaluated.

The situation with respect to fat is somewhat more complicated, and has been reviewed recently by Danforth (1985). It has been generally assumed that storage of potential energy in adipose tissue simply represents the net of caloric intake minus energy expended. This must, of course, be true, but the assumption that if the proportion of fat in an isocaloric diet is increased, utilization of carbohydrate and protein for energy will be "spared" is no longer tenable. Oscai and associates (1984) expected that a group of rats given a diet for a prolonged period in which 42–60% of calories were derived from fat would develop hyperphagia and become obese in contrast to a control group eating laboratory chow low in fat. The rats did become obese, but fortuitously the estimated caloric intake through the 60-week period was apparently similar for both groups. Those taking the high-fat diets developed 51% body fat, in contrast to 30% body fat for those eating the chow. Thus, severe obesity developed without obvious hyperphagia. The metabolizable energy of the unfortified laboratory commercial chow was only based on estimates of the supplier, so that it will be important to repeat the experiment with pair feeding.

Björntorp and Sjöström (1971) originally concluded that human lipogenesis from a single generous mixed meal may be less than 1%, although recent tracer studies employing adipose tissue biopsy and isotopically labeled glucose after 100 g of glucose taken orally suggest that this is nearer 5% (Marin *et al.*, 1985). Acheson *et al.* (1982) have challenged the popular belief about excess carbohydrate consumption, "One moment on the lips; forever on the hips." In subjects given a meal equivalent to 480 g of starch, they estimated from prolonged indirect calorimetry that there was a net synthesis of only 9 g of fat. They calculated that as much as 346 g of glycogen were formed. In further studies extending over 24 hours they again noted the effect on net lipogenesis from carbohydrate and the theromogenic response to the large meal (Acheson *et al.*, 1984a). Carbohydrate oxidation and conversion to fat were largest (approximately 9 g) after 3 days of a diet calculated to maximize glycogen stores and lowest when glycogen stores were depleted by taking a diet high in fat. The lipogenesis was inadequate to compensate for ongoing fat oxidation. The increase in *de novo* synthesis of fat is at a greater obligatory cost (25% of the calories from the carbohydrate) than is incurred from depositing dietary fatty acids as triglyceride. As the antecedent carbohydrate intake was increased in this study, the thermic effect of the meal also increased.

In a third study at the Lausanne laboratory (Flatt *et al.*, 1985) the effect over 9 hours of supplementing mixed meals with fat was studied. The same amounts of protein and carbohydrate were oxidized under each condition, regardless of whether fat was added to the meal. The fat metabolized was drawn from body reserves when the intake of fat was low, and from dietary fat when fat supplements were given. Thus fat balance was negative when no fat supplement was given, while carbohydrate and protein balance was maintained regardless of fat supplementation. Flatt pointed out that a state of equilibrium can be reached only when the rates of oxidation of carbohydrate and of fat correspond to their proportion in the diet. This may take considerable time and may be regarded as a compensatory mechanism. Thus it is the fat content of the diet rather than the total caloric intake that influences the level where weight will plateau; total energy content alone is not the critical factor.

The effect of increased dietary fat is of concern, as Danforth has emphasized (1985), since the average content of dietary fat in the United States was 44% in 1984, as opposed to 27% in 1910, and this increased consumption may be contributing to the current epidemic of obesity. A more recent countertrend may be setting in, however. Per capita consumption of beef has dropped from a high of 94 lb in 1976 to 75 lb in 1985, while that of chicken rose from 43 to 70 lb over the same period. Limitation of dietary fat is difficult, however, since, as noted above (Section II,D,2), addition of fat in appropriate proportions increases the hedonic ratio of a food, or in plain English, makes it taste better (Drewnowski and Greenwood, 1983). However, satiety may be achieved sooner and for longer periods as fat content is increased.

c. Effects of Caloric Intake above and below Maintenance. See Sections III,A,2 and IV).

2. *Control of the Rate and Efficiency of Thermogenesis*

a. Hypothalamic Control. Recent authoritative reviews include the book by Girardier and Stock (1983) and papers by Danforth (1983) and by Landsberg and Young (1984). The "High Command" is located in the hypothalamus. Work by Perkins *et al.* (1983) indicates that electrical stimulation of the ventromedial nucleus in rats inhibits energy intake and stimulates energy output, both through sympathetic stimulation. Thyroid-stimulating hormone from the pituitary presumably modulates the long-term effect of thyroid hormones in adjusting the endothermic component of the RMR.

The concentration of several neurotransmitters in the central nervous system which are involved in feeding behavior is modulated by the ability of their precursor amino acids to cross the blood–brain barrier. Wurtman and co-workers at the Massachusetts Institute of Technology have enthusiastically stressed the relation of the amount of these precursors to a number of disorders, as recently reviewed (Wurtman *et al.,* 1981).

b. Sympathoadrenal Pathway and Catecholamines. The rate of thermogenesis can be modulated in the short term by sympathoadrenal stimulation (Landsberg *et al.,* 1984). This is closely interrelated with the action of both thyroid hormones and insulin and is subject to a number of modulating factors, as described below.

c. Thyroid Hormones and Sodium Ion Pumping. Thyroid hormones and the sympathetic nervous system work synergistically in modulating energy expenditure in the long term. Their role in modulating thermogenesis in over- and underfeeding is discussed in Sections III,A,3 and IV).

d. Insulin. Insulin is prominent among the factors controlling energy balance and can either promote energy storage or its dissipation (Landsberg and Young, 1985a; Danforth and Sims, 1983). As already noted (Section II,D,1 and 2), there is a cephalic phase of insulin release triggered either by the sight of palatable food or by orogastric stimulation.

Chronic administration of insulin increases fat deposition by a direct effect on lipid storage as well as by stimulating appetite. Torbay and others in Hashim's laboratory (1985) have shown in rats given small daily doses of protamine zinc insulin that fat deposition increases at the expense of protein and water, independent of any change in caloric intake or physical activity. The activity of lipoprotein lipase, which promotes lipogenesis, also increases in white adipose tissue (Brunzell *et al.,* 1981).

Insulin can directly *increase* energy expenditure in several ways. One is by stimulating Na^+–K^+ pumping across the cell membrane (Moore, 1981) and by stimulating the sympathetic nervous system (Rowe *et al.,* 1981). Increased sodium pumping activity has been demonstrated in muscle (Zierler, 1964; Clausen and Kohn, 1977; Landsberg and Young, 1985). Rothwell and Stock (1985) assigned greater importance to the role of insulin as a link between dietary intake and activity of the sympathetic nervous system. It is known that under conditions of diminished glucose metabolism, sympathetic activity is blunted. Moreover, during the euglycemic–hyperinsulinemic clamp procedure, variation in insulin concentration leads to a dose-dependent change in concentration of plasma norepinephrine without change in plasma glucose (Rowe *et al.,* 1981). Again, β-adrenergic blockade blunts this thermic effect. Prior exercise may greatly enhance the thermogenic effect of physiological amounts of insulin, at least in the perfused hind portions of the rat (Balon *et al.,* 1984). This effect is independent of glucose uptake by muscle and can only partially be explained by increased synthesis of glycogen.

Fasting causes a decrease in both plasma glucose and insulin. Lilavathana *et al.* (1978) dissociated the two effects by measuring the insulin response with or without glucose infusion adequate to maintain plasma glucose concentration. Fasting lowered plasma insulin equally under either condition.

Christin *et al.* (1985), in Acheson's laboratory at Lausanne, have probed the role of insulin per se in the thermic response to insulin and glucose infusions. In a series of clamp studies utilizing somatostatin to block insulin secretion, they showed that stepwise increases in glucose uptake alone, with insulin constant, caused an increase in thermic expenditure comparable to that found when plasma insulin was allowed to rise. On the other hand, when insulin was increased without change in glucose uptake, plasma catecholamines increased, and this increase correlated with increase in energy expenditure. Thus either of two mechanisms can increase thermogenesis, the former obligatory and the latter facultative.

e. Adrenal Steroids and Sex Hormones and the Relation to Truncal Obesity. Glucocorticoid hormones undoubtedly are important in energy balance. In the fatty rat there is evidence of increased sensitivity to corticosterone, with perhaps a secondary effect upon appetite (Yukimura *et al.,* 1978). The central distribution of obesity of Cushing's syndrome and the leanness of the Addisonian are well known. Lesser derangements of corticoid secretion, not diagnosable by our relatively crude tests for adrenal hyperfunction, may be important in subtypes of human obesity (Esanu *et al.,* 1972) (see Section V,B,9,a). The truncal or central form of human obesity is associated in women with increase in plasma androgens (Evans *et al.,* 1983) and is strongly associated with diabetes, hypertension, and hyperlipidemia (Kalkhoff *et al.,* 1983; Kissebah *et al.,* 1984; Evans *et al.,* 1984). Fat tissue is an important reservoir for steroid hormones as well as a site of interconversion (Deslypere *et al.,* 1985). Both androgens and estrogens can be concentrated, and estradiol to estrogen conversion can take place at this site. Obesity from simple overeating, as in our Vermont Study of experimental obesity (Sims *et al.*, 1973), is associated with increased turnover of corticosteroids, but with no increase in free cortisol of plasma or urine (O'Connell *et al.*, 1973). Consistent with this was our finding that the deposition of fat over this relatively short period of about 3 months was generalized rather than confined to central depots (Salans *et al.*, 1971). More research is needed to define subtypes of obesity for which disturbances of steroid metabolism may be important.

3. *Possible Sites and Mechanisms of Facultative Thermogenesis*

a. The Contribution of Brown Adipose Tissue and of Skeletal Muscle. i. In animals. A mass of evidence has accumulated in small animals that brown adipose tissue (BAT) is the major site of nonshivering thermogenesis in the cold and the site of diet-associated adaptive increase in heat production when food of poor quality is taken in large amounts. This adaptation may enable animals to obtain adequate amounts of an essential nutrient without incurring the penalty of obesity. A diet low is protein provokes such a response in rats (Stirling and Stock, 1968; Tulp, 1981; Rothwell *et al.*, 1983a). Samonds and Hegsted (1979) found that young cebus monkeys given a diet low in protein also react with a striking increase in thermogenesis. Recent work on BAT is reviewed by Himms-Hagen (1985) and in the book edited by Girardier and Stock (1983).

BAT is laden with fat in small globules with increased surface area. Mitochondria are extremely abundant and under sympathetic stimulation can metabolize fatty acid substrates to produce heat and less than the usual number of ATP molecules. The reduced efficiency of metabolism may be the result of several mechanisms, either by change in substrate or by an uncoupling mechanism. Twenty years ago Chaffee and co-workers (1964) showed increased respiratory rates in cold-adapted hamsters with either β-hydroxybutyrate or α-glycerol phosphate. The latter is formed from dihydroxyacetone and NADH, shuttles across the mitochondrial membrane, and is then oxidized by a flavoprotein, yielding a less efficient formation of ATP. The activity of the dehydrogenase concerned is increased by thyroid hormone (Oppenheimer, 1979) or by low-protein diets (Tyzbir *et al.*, 1981). Stirling and Stock (1968) have found an increase in this enzyme in the livers of rats given a diet low in protein. The other important mechanism of dissipation of heat in BAT is brought about through an uncoupling mechanism unique to this tissue via the mitochondrial proton conductance pathway (Nichols and Locke, 1983). This is effected by a 32,000-Da protein, and the degree of uncoupling can be estimated by measuring tritiated guanosine diphosphate (GDP) binding.

Activation of BAT is dependent on activation of the sympathetic nervous system. This activation is dependent upon intact or increased thyroidal activity, and the thyroid status regulates the response to catecholamines (Sundin *et al.,* 1984). In rats the adaptive thermogenic response can be evoked equally well by isocaloric diets high in fat as by control diets fed at 2.5 times above maintenance, but the effect is masked by the greater efficiency of triglyceride deposition from dietary fat (Rothwell *et al.,* 1985a).

ii. In man. As mentioned earlier, the newborn infant is well supplied with brown fat adjacent to the great vessels, better to enable him or her to survive on precipitation into a cold world. These gross and obvious accumulations disappear in early childhood, and it is somewhat uncertain just how much of this built-in "head-bolt heater" persists to adulthood (Himms-Hagen, 1985). On the basis of histologic appearance, Heaton (1972) has reported a wide distribution in the first decade, with restriction to the kidneys, suprarenals, aortic region, and neck during adult years. Lean and James (1983) and Bouillard *et al.* (1983) found brown adipose tissue in adult man by using specific antiserum to the 32,000 M_r uncoupling protein of mitochondria.

Stimulation produces hypertrophy of this tissue, as in animals. Finnish lumberjacks exposed to cold show an increase in brown fat not shared by sedentary indoor workers (Huttunen *et al.,* 1981), and I suspect that the same is true of Vermonters at the end of a long winter. A celebrated photograph in *Nature* (Rothwell and Stock, 1978) showed an increase in infrared radiation attributed to brown fat in areas of the back of one of the investigators after infusion of norepinephrine. However, in similar experiments using ephedrine, Astrup *et al.* (1984) could find no evidence of brown adipose tissue on biopsy of such "hot" areas, and they attributed the change in skin temperature to increased blood flow and decreased insulation by fat in these areas. They further (1986) found in tissue from 87 medicolegal autopsies of lean, relatively young subjects that BAT was more prominent in the perirenal, pericardial, and cervical areas. They studied the thermic response to ephedrine by continuous monitoring of local temperature and blood flow by the xenon-133 clearance method for the perirenal area and by monitoring arterial and venous temperature and blood flow in the leg. Assuming a generous 700 g of BAT, they calculated that this tissue could account for only 25% of the observed increase in oxygen uptake, while whole-body skeletal muscle could account for approximately 50%, thus assigning the major role to skeletal muscle. In small animals with a relatively large surface area the BAT mechanism for dissipation of heat to avoid crippling obesity or to provide heat on exposure to cold is apparently essential; in larger animals such as man, becoming hot between the shoulder blades (and under the collar) is less essential. It is of particular importance, therefore, to consider other mechanisms for heat production.

b. Substrate Cycles Once Known as "Futile." Postulating "futile" processes may seem intemperate yet such do seem to exist. These include cycling of fructose 6-phosphate to fructose 1,6-phosphate and return, and synthesis and degradation of glycogen, protein, and triglyceride. All require hydrolysis of ATP and liberation of heat. Even though no net synthesis is accomplished, this is far from futile.

Newsholme (1976, 1980) presented a compelling argument that these cycles can provide extremely sensitive regulators for the flow of body fuels through the sequences of metabolic pathways, provided key enzymes control the direction of cycling in each direction. He suggested that they may have evolved initially for this purpose and only later have become sources of heat production and a means of moderating weight gain. A small change in the concentration of regulators can cause a marked increase in net flux. The higher the rate of cycling in relation to the rate of flux through a pathway, the greater the increase in sensitivity. As an example he suggested that such an increase in substrate cycling prepares a sprinter tensely awaiting the starting gun for the acute increase in aerobic glycolysis required during a short race. He suggests that epinephrine, glucagon and adrenal corticoids, norepinephrine, or possibly prostaglandins released locally in muscle from sympathetic stimulation greatly increase the rate of substrate cycling. The latter mechanism, which can operate acutely, seems the more likely. Activation of phosphofructokinase by various regulators, of which reduction in creatine phosphate and ATP seem the most important, produces a greater response than possible at the slow resting rate of cycling. Since the period of racing the motor prior to the start is relatively brief, minimal heat is lost as a result of "futile" cycling. For a thermodynamic explanation of the increase in sensitivity, see the above references. Newsholme also suggested that a more chronic stimulation of the substrate cycling may be a factor in control of body weight.

Apparently it is the fructose 1-phosphate to fructose 1,6-phosphate cycle that enables the bumble bee to take flight with a burst of energy, once having warmed its wing muscles by increased cycling (M. G. Clark *et al.,* 1973a). D. G. Clark *et al.* (1973b) reported similar cycling in the liver of the rat, but Hue and Hers (1973) did not find this, using double isotopic labeling of glucose in fed mice.

4. *Interrelationships between Food Intake and Physical Activity, Physical Training, and Thermogenesis*

In this mechanized age the level of physical activity may account for only 12–15% of total energy expenditure in humans (Brownell and Stunkard, 1980). More important relationships may be the effect of exercise on resting metabolic rate, the effect of exercise on the thermic response to meals, and conversely, the effect of antecedent meals on the energy cost of exercise. The psychological effects may be equally important.

Energy intake and activity were the topics of a recent international conference (Pollitt and Amante, 1984), and exercise, nutrition, and energy balance in the normal, the obese, and the diabetic are the subjects of a multiauthored book now in preparation (Horton and Terjung, 1986).

Brownell and Stunkard (1980) have reviewed evidence for the theory originally advanced by Jean Mayer that increasing activity in the sedentary decreases food intake and body weight, whereas increasing activity in the more active range leads to increased food intake and stable body weight. A recent well-controlled study was that of Woo *et al.* (1982), working in Garrow's laboratory in England. Obese women, unaware of the objective of the experiment and given free access to food, were assigned a program of exercise. They initially ate an amount that maintained body weight when sedentary. When mild or moderate treadmill exercise was added to their regimen in periods of 19 days, they did not spontaneously alter their intake. This phenomenon was tested recently in a similar study by Woo in which normal women were assigned a program of physical activity and were also given free access to food (Woo *et al.*, 1985). In contrast to obese women, they appropriately increased intake to maintain their usual weight.

Resting metabolic rate and the thermic response to food are increased for a period after strenuous exercise. Beilinski *et al.* (1985) measured energy expenditure for a 42-hour period in the chamber at Lausanne. Eighteen hours after a 3-hour period of exercise at 50% V_{max} the RMR was still 4.7% elevated. A mixed meal given 4 hours after exercise induced a greater fraction of lipid oxidation and persisted to the following day. Devlin and Horton (1985) measured the thermic response to infused insulin at two concentrations using the euglycemic clamp procedure in normal untrained subjects 12–16 hours after exercise to exhaustion. These lean subjects showed a significant 3–7% increase in basal energy expenditure; lipid oxidation was also increased, while that of glucose was reduced. The thermic effect of insulin at either physiological or elevated concentrations was potentiated.

In contrast, LeBlanc *et al.* (1984) reported that highly physically trained women show a reduced diet-induced response to a meal than moderately active or sedentary persons. They attributed this both to reduced sympathetic nervous responses to eating and to enhanced formation of glycogen rather than flux through more costly metabolic routes. Later studies (LeBlanc *et al.*, 1984) indicated that supertrained subjects show reduced insulin and catecholamine responses compared to those of sedentary subjects. Direct comparison is limited by the short, 2-hour period of measurement for oxygen uptake, but one would expect these differences to be significant for longer periods, and the conclusion was independent of whether the RMR was related to body weight or to lean body mass or taken at the actual value per minute.

Segal and Gutin (1983) have reported that when food is taken before a bout of exercise, the thermic response to the exercise is increased above that of the exercise alone. In their studies the amount of exercise was matched to the so-called aerobic threshold. In a similar series of studies they compared the reaction to exercise with or without an antecedent meal in men matched for age, weight, and height, but differing in percentage body fat (10 versus 30%) (Segal *et al.*, 1985). The two groups were comparable in resting oxygen uptake related to lean body mass, but due to greater lean body mass, the lean showed 15–17% greater uptake, either total or in relation to body weight. These findings contrasted sharply with those of the LeBlanc study of supertrained women. The thermic responses to a meal alone among the lean increased above the responses of the obese, and presumably, sedentary subjects. The thermic response to exercise after a 750-kcal meal was also considerably greater in the lean, either during or following 30 minutes of exercise. The one important variable between these studies may be the type of physical training, aerobic by the avid runners, skiers, and cyclists versus anaerobic in the iron pumpers. The types of people who select these contrasting activities may also condition the results. A study of matched twins taking up contrasting types of training would be of no interest. The increased thermic response to exercise in the postprandial state suggests that more rapid shuttling across the substrate cycles emphasized by Newsholme (1976, 1978, 1980) may also explain the results of the latest study by Segal.

The β-endorphin response to exercise may account in part for the differences between the lean and the obese in the effect on intake of food. Endorphins stimulate intake of food, apparently by a central action in both man and animals, and there is apparently a difference in response to the opioids in the lean and obese. The opioid antagonist naloxone reduced intake of food in normals (Cohen *et al.,* 1985), while in a carefully controlled study using comparable doses of the antagonist naltrexone, Malcolm *et al.* (1985) found no effect in the obese. Exercise increases opioids in the plasma of normal subjects (Kelso *et al.,* 1984), but as discussed in Section V,B,5, hyperendorphinemia is markedly elevated in young obese persons (Genazzani *et al.,* 1986). Whether there is less relative change in the opioid concentrations in the obese has not been established, but if there were such, it could explain the different effect of exercise on appetite in the obese.

The Effects of Physical Training on Plasma Norepinephrine Concentrations. Studies of the interrelationship between catecholamines and physical activity based upon plasma concentrations have given inconsistent results. Schwartz (1985) recently used the tritiated nonepinephrine technique of Essler to study the effects of a 3-month walk/jog program in eight normal young subjects. There was a positive correlation between both norepinephrine release and clearance, and hence of turnover, with the change in V_{O_2max}.

An ingenious experiment recently reported by Woo *et al.* (1985) does much to clarify the mechanism of diet-induced thermogenesis. To estimate whether energy balance or change in substrate traffic is the more important factor, a comparison was made between the response of six subjects taking, in random order for 6-day periods, either a maintenance diet, a diet increased in caloric content by 50% with sufficient exercise added to maintain basal weight, or the high-caloric diet without added exercise. Both overfed groups showed a significant increase in resting metabolic rate, but only those taking excess food alone showed a significant increase in free T_3 and insulin. Norepinephrine in the plasma was not significantly increased during either period of overfeeding, but this is difficult to interpret, since kinetic studies were not included. Thus increases in RMR can occur without changes in thyroid hormones or insulin, and a high level of substrate turnover with increased nitrogen metabolism may produce the increase in thermogenesis.

5. *"Set Points" for Body Weight and Body Fat*

In any discussion of energy balance the term *set point,* which takes on an aura of immutable biological law, is likely to appear. In writing for the lay public it is currently popular to emphasize the hopelessness of fighting one's habitual weight (Bennett and Gorin, 1982). Mrosovsky and Powley (1977) reviewed the several concepts of set point and concluded "the term can be valuable in the descriptive, the functional, and the control system sense, but is liable to confuse issues, if it is not made clear in which sense it is used." Wirtshafter and Davis (1977a) argued that constancy of body weight may be controlled by a simple feedback control model rather than a neural system containing a reference point. Keesey (1980) recently reviewed the mechanisms whereby animals and man can maintain body weight within narrow limits. He pointed out that nothing appears to be wrong with the systems for regulation of body weight in lean animals with lesions of the lateral hypothalamus or in obese Zucker rats, but they do defend different weights. Their energy expenditure increases or decreases depending upon whether weight is forced above or below habitual weight, but intake and expenditure are appropriate for "metabolic body size." Kleiber (1975) concluded that this metabolic body size is equal to the body weight raised to the 0.75 power. Keesey suggested that human beings appear to regulate weight around values that differ as much between individuals as between many species. Rapid regain of weight by the obese after dieting is all too frequent.

6. *Genetic and Familial Factors in the Control of Body Weight*

Leanness and obesity clearly run in families, but the unresolved question is the relative importance of environmental versus genetic factors. Even studies designed with monozygotic twins, raised together or apart, or adopted children have failed to give clear-cut answers (Greenwood and Turkenkopf, 1983). A genetic factor is clear, but at times this can be overridden by strong environmental factors. Very recently Poehlman *et al.* (1986) found in a series of six pairs of monozygotic twins large individual variations in diet-induced thermogenesis, but strong concordance within twin pairs in the magnitude of responses to a single meal. Hormonal responses showed a weaker genotype dependency. Consistent with Poehlman's findings, DeLuise and Flier (1985) just recently found that there is much interindividual variation in the sodium–potassium pump density, estimated by a test of ouabain sensitivity, ^{86}Rb uptake, and cell sodium concentration in erythrocytes and lymphocytes, but, again, marked concordance was found among twins. One problem with the twin studies, however, is that the pairs have shared the same habits of diet and energy expenditure. Garn *et al.* (1979) have shown that genetically unrelated individuals living together may display considerable similarities in such parameters as stature, fatness, and long-term change in fatness, thus making genetic analysis difficult.

We were impressed with the variation in weight gain response to overfeeding in the Vermont Study of experimental obesity in man (Sims *et al.*, 1976). Essentially identical studies of the thermogenic response to norepinephrine yielded quite different results in Pima Indians (Kush *et al.*, 1986) as opposed to those in Caucasians (Katzeff *et al.*, 1986), but as the studies were carried out in different regions (Arizona and Vermont), environmental factors could be equally important.

7. *Factors Affecting Loss of Body Heat*

Jequier *et al.* (1974) have studied extensively the effect of body fat thickness in modifying heat loss and its function in development and perpetuation of obesity. Quaade (1963) has also evaluated the diminished reponse of the obese to cold exposure.

III. Increased Facultative Thermogenesis in Normal Man

There is controversy whether there exists a facultative or adaptive response to overfeeding comparable to those responses brought about by other stimuli such as cold. The closely related question of whether a defect in any such mechanism may be important in at least some subtypes of obesity in man is considered in Section V,B.

A. Response to Physiological States and Environmental Stress

1. *Nonshivering Thermogenesis in Response to Cold*

In their monumental review in 1962 Smith and Hoijer summarized knowledge of cellular mechanisms for increasing heat production in the face of cold by nonshivering thermogenesis. Current knowledge is summarized in the recent book by Girardier and Stock (1983). The mechanisms involved have been discussed in the previous section. Dr. Jean Himms-Hagen has called my attention to a relevant quotation from Walter Cannon (1932):

> We must recognize that among civilized people the physiological devices for the maintenance of constant temperature may have little opportunity to function. In wintry weather we spend our days in heated houses and offices and travel about in heated cars. Encased in warm clothing we carry with us everywhere a temperate climate. Thus only few occasions arise which demand either the conservation of the heat always being produced by the organism, or the development of extra heat by bodily activity. And in summer, likewise, mechanically operated fans, cold drinks, ice cream and refrigerated rooms lessen the use of the natural arrangements for keeping cool. It is not impossible that we

> lose important protective advantages by failing to exercise these physiological mechanisms, which were developed through myriads of generations of our less favored ancestors.
>
> The man who daily takes a cold bath and works till he sweats may be keeping "fit" because he is not permitting a very valuable part of his bodily organization to become weakened and inefficient by disuse.

Consistent with this, Hutunnen *et al.* (1981) did find that Finnish lumbermen and other outdoor workers exposed to the cold had definite brown fat surrounding the cervical arteries and in the pericardial region, whereas sedentary office workers in the same region had not a trace. The identity of brown fat was established by a number of enzymatic studies. Acheson *et al.* (1980), however, could find no seasonal difference in body weight and body fat by skinfold measurements in members of an Antarctic expedition. Perhaps conditions were not sufficiently rugged. O'Hara *et al.* (1979) have studied the body composition of moderately obese middle-aged men exercising in a cold chamber 2.5 hours a day for 2 weeks in contrast to those engaging in similar exercise at a reasonable temperature. Significant differences in relative body composition were found only in those who exercised in the cold, and these were attributed to new protein synthesis, ketosis, and a small energy deficit.

Using a more definitive protocol Sheldahl in Buskirk's laboratory (1980) persuaded seven obese women to ride ergometer bicycles in 17–22°C water for 90 minutes five times a week for 8 weeks. They found little net heat loss and suggested that body heat stores were slowly repaid during metabolic heat production associated with a reduced rate of loss of body heat. They could find no evidence of cold adaptation. Perhaps cutaneous vasoconstriction plus the added insulation of fat buffered the response. Another group of women exposed to cold, Korean divers, was studied by Kang *et al.* (1970). There was a slight increase in excretion of norepinephrine and a slight increase in the response to infused norepinephrine in the divers in winter; they considered these changes too small to attribute to nonshivering thermogenesis. More recently Macdonald *et al.* (1984) demonstrated that the core temperature during cooling could be maintained after 12, but not after 48, hours of fasting. Increased forearm blood flow with decrease in hand blood flow was produced, but catecholamine measurements were inconclusive. Kinetic studies will be required to define the role of norepinephrine in these responses.

2. *Thermogenic Response to Excess Caloric Intake*

The thermogenic response of small animals to diets low in protein and the mechanisms involved have already been considered. In rats the facultative response can be evoked equally well by isocaloric diets high in fat as by control diets fed at a level 2.5 times above maintenance, but the effect is masked by the greater efficiency of triglyceride deposition from dietary fat (Rothwell *et al.*, 1985).

The critical question is whether a facultative increase in thermogenesis in normal man serves to buffer the effects of overeating and whether a decrease in such a protective mechanism may contribute to some subtypes of obesity. The experimental evidence is conflicting and is a source of much controversy. Recent reviews include that of Rothwell and Stock (1983), with a dissenting view by Hervey and Tobin (1983) and by Himms-Hagen (1984), which provoked a rebuttal (Seaton and Welle, 1985) and counterrebuttal (Himms-Hagen, 1985). It is because there has been so much disagreement between results of studies from competent laboratories that I have examined the available reports in some detail in the hope of finding sources of the discrepancies which may be taken into consideration in future studies. I believe that the bulk of the most reliable evidence favors a facultative component to diet-induced thermogenesis in normal man and that the main sources of contradictory results lie in the heterogeneity of the subjects and in certain limitations of the methods and protocols employed. In one of the earliest studies of the reaction to a diet low in protein (Stirling and Stock, 1968), emphasis was on the liver, which showed an increase in α-glycerol-phosphate dehydrogenase, leading to less efficient formation of ATP. However, later studies indicated that all but a small fraction of the facultative heat production can be accounted for by brown adipose tissue (Rothwell and Stock, 1983). T_3 is increased in all cases of cold- and diet-induced thermogenesis and is apparently needed for the necessary metabolic adaptation, but not for thermogenesis induced by BAT per se.

The concept of disposing of excess energy in the face of caloric excess is not new. In 1881 Voit advanced a theory of plethora. This was consistent with Max Rubner's later statement (1902): "We must distinguish between the period of under-nutrition, of nutritional equilibrium, and of pure weight gain, and the period of heat increase. The stream of food increases, but it does not determine the size of the consumption. Apparently the organism does."

While Rubner was writing this Neumann (1902) also in Germany was observing changes in weight and nitrogen balance in himself as he varied his intake of food over a considerable time. During one period his intake included 670 calories as beer. It was he who coined the word *Luxuskonsumption*. Gulick (1922) performed a similar long-term experiment on himself. Neuman's findings, as well as Gulick's, are often misquoted. Their weight did not remain "constant" in spite of wide variations in caloric intake, but did reach different plateaus of weight on shifting intake. The results of our Vermont Study of experimental obesity in man have been similarly misquoted in the lay press. Forbes (1984) has done a service in pointing out that Neuman and Gulick's weights were far from constant. He showed a linear relationship between caloric intake and change in body weight in the two experiments. The slopes are indeed steep, but as he pointed out the changes are small. The scale on the abscissa is multiples of 1000 kcal intake independent of duration of overfeeding while that on the ordinate is in multiples of 100 g. The still-unresolved question is whether compensatory mechanisms were operative over and above the effect of change in lean body mass, in the effort needed to move the increased weight, and in the obligatory costs of metabolizing the various substrates derived from the food.

The studies of Miller and Mumford (1967a,b) of the effects of overfeeding in man on body weight and the cost in energy of exercise, as well as our Vermont Study, served to rekindle interest in this area (Sims *et al.*, 1968, 1975, 1976; Goldman *et al.*, 1975). In an incisive paper Garrow (1978) summarized the 16 studies of overfeeding through 1977. His scoreboard indicated that 11 of the 16 investigators concluded that energy expenditure was increased. Five considered that there was unexplained loss of energy, six considered that they could balance the energy books, three were uncertain, and two abstained. Garrow suggested that it was not until an intake of approximately 20 Mcal (82 MJ) was exceeded did a measurable degree of facultative thermogenesis become apparent.

Studies of normal, preferably free-living subjects which include complete balance of intake and output of energy and change in body composition are difficult. Durnin, who has done much to keep investigators in this field honest, has outlined some of the problems and also criteria for adequate studies (Durnin and Ferro-Luzzi, 1982; Durnin, 1982, 1983), and Jequier (1984) has discussed newer approaches. Advances in technology, including the availability of chambers for indirect or direct calorimetry, have improved the situation, but still have not solved all the problems. These include all the variables considered in Section II. I have summarized in Table I the studies in normals since Garrow's review, with apologies to any relevant studies I may have missed. Only three of the overfeeding studies are 3 weeks or longer in duration and exceed Garrow's possible threshold figure for intake of 20 Mcal. The resources of the chambers for calorimetry have been variously exploited in three studies of shorter duration. Review of these and other studies of thermogenesis reveal many of the variables contributing to the conflicting results. These are deferred to Section V,B,20, which describes the thermogenic response of the obese to overfeeding, since many points apply equally well to lean and obese.

A study by Olefsky *et al.* (1975), not included in the table, was designed to test whether endocrine and lipid changes develop before significant weight gain during overfeeding and not to test the theory of luxuskonsumption. There was increase in plasma insulin and in triglycerides, but no measured change in insulin resistance. The estimation of energy balance is simplistic, in that predicted gain is based on the intake divided by the 3500 kcal per pound of adipose tissue. The mean active gain was 4.4 kg. The finding of most interest was that even within age groups there was marked variation in the actual weight gain independent of the degree of fatness, and also that two subjects with a family history of diabetes in a parent stood out, perhaps only by coincidence, in their ease of gaining (6.0 and 6.6; mean for the group 4.4 kg). As in Mann's study (1955) and others, the rate of gain was reduced in the third week.

Norgen and Durnin (1980) have extended their overfeeding study of 1969. Food intake was calculated from tables, with an unspecified number of checks by bomb calorimetry of food, feces, and urine. The six subjects were generously overfed for 42 days with a total of 62 Mcal. The increase was mainly as fat, and the actual composition of the daily diet varied from subject to subject. The metabolic rates for standard tasks were increased 10% after overfeeding, but were not increased in relation to total body weight. There was a discrepancy between the weight gained and the caloric intake, which Norgan and Durnin attributed to probable error in calculation based on the variables involved. Degree of physical activity was not assessed. There was no correlation between ease of weight gain and degree of fatness. Again, they pointed out that there was considerable individual variation in ease of gaining and that the "causes for the individual differences are obscure."

The study by Welle and Campbell (1983), discussed in the subsection below on catecholamine effects, also involved an estimate of the effect of long-term overfeeding on diet-induced thermogenesis and the cost of exercise.

The most complete study of dietary thermogenesis employing an open-circuit chamber for indirect calorimetry is that of Ravussin *et al.* (1985a) in Jequier's laboratory in Lausanne. The chamber was equipped to record periods of physical activity by the Doppler principle with radar (Schutz *et al.*, 1982b). Although the radar does not directly

TABLE I

RECENT STUDIES OF THE EFFECT OF EXCESS CALORIC INTAKE ON THERMOGENESIS IN NORMAL SUBJECTS[a]

Investigators	Subjects	Study type	Overfeeding: Days form	Overfeeding: Excess kcal P-F-C (%)	Test MR duration	Facult. DIT	NE	NE infusion	Beta block	Serum T_3	Exercise cost	Conclusions regarding facultative thermogenesis
Studies not supporting a facultative component												
Norgan and Durnin (1980)	6	Effect of overfeeding of F on total balance	42 M	1483 16-47-37	2–4 hours	—	—	—	—	—	No change per kg	Gain less than intake attributed to errors. Much individual variation
Welle and Campbell (1983)	7	Overfeeding of C	20 M	1810 9-11-80	120 minutes	No	—	Effect on VO_2 same	No effect on VO_2	Increased	—	Thermic effect unaffected by beta block. No increased sensitivity to NE infusion
Ravussin *et al.* (1985)	5	Chamber studies of effect of mixed overfeeding on balance and body composition	9 M	60% increase 15-40-45	Chamber, 24 hours	—	—	—	—	No change	—	Possible to account for all ingested energy in excess of maintenance. Activity monitored
Katzeff *et al.* (1985)	6	Effect of overfeeding on stepwise NE infusions and cost of exercise	18 M	1000 15-35-50	1 hour	—	Clearance increased	(Stepwise)	—	Increased	No change	No increase in thermogenic response to NE
Forbes *et al.* (1982)	6	Overfeeding, mainly of C (Polycose); body composition determined by total body potassium	17–19	1200–1800 8-22-70	BMR only	—	—	—	—	—	—	No evidence of facultative response; checked only in subjects who gained over 4 kg

					Studies supporting a facultative component							
Dauncey (1980)	8	Overfeeding 1 day only; chamber study	1 M	1300 26-34-50	Chamber, 24 hours	—	—	—	—	—	—	Effects similar to longer studies. Individual variation. Increased RMR 14 hours after last meal
O'Dea *et al.* (1982)	6	Low, maintenance, and high intake; constant-proportion mixed diet	10 × 3 M	1700 15-40-45	—	—	Turnover increased	—	—	Increased	—	NE turnover and thyroid hormones increased with no change in plasma NE. Included smokers and coffee drinkers
Webb and Annis (1982)	9 (12×)	Overfeeding of high P and F, or high C; "space suit" calorimetry	30 M	1000 Variable	"Space suit"	Variable	—	—	—	—	—	Caloric intake of excess protein and fat not accounted for
Dallasso and James (1984)	8	Chamber study, effect of overfeeding on thermogenesis and cost of exercise	7 M	50% increase as F	Chamber, 36 hours	Yes	—	—	—	—	Increased	Thermic effect of meal (TEM) increased but no interaction between TEM and exercise
Schutz *et al.* (1985)	3	10-day chamber study; stepwise increase in C intake	7 M	1550 high C	24 hours	Yes	Urine catecholamines	—	—	—	—	Marked increase in thermogenesis, attributed to increase SNS stimulation and lipogenesis

[a] P, Protein; F, fat; C, carbohydrate; BMR, basal metabolic rate; Beta block, propranolol block; Facult. DIT, facultative component of diet-induced thermogenesis; M, full meal; NE, norepinephrine; RMR, resting metabolic rate; SNS, sympathetic nervous system; T_3, triiodothyronine; —, not tested.

give a quantitative estimate of the work done, extrapolation to zero of the plot of activity versus oxygen consumption can permit an estimate of the cost of activity above the resting metabolic rate. The subjects also wore pedometers and accelerometers on the nondominant wrist during the 3 weeks of the study. There were no smokers among the young subjects and they had been at constant weight for over 2 years. Caffeine was avoided. Change in body composition was estimated by underwater weighing and by nitrogen balance during two 3-day periods. Intake of food was estimated from standard tables, without bomb calorimetry. After a 13-day period of dietary equilibration the subjects increased their caloric intake by 60%, while maintaining the same proportions of 15% protein, 40% fat, and 45% carbohydrate in a mixed diet. This amounted to an excess of about 18 Mcal.

The dietary excess was sufficient to cause a modest increase in plasma insulin, but no increases in thyroid hormones or catecholamines, i.e., the changes that occur with more prolonged or vigorous overfeeding. Energy expenditure was measured at the end of the baseline period and on the second and nineth day of overfeeding. Weight increased by 3.2 kg, of which underwater weighing indicated 56% to be fat, while computation from nitrogen and energy balance indicated 40% was fat. It was estimated that 24-hour energy expenditure increased by approximately 490 kcal, of which a third could be explained by increase in the basal metabolic rate. Ravussin *et al.* considered that the remainder could be attributed to the obligatory thermic effect of the food, which increased in proportion to the excess energy intake and to the extra cost of the physical activity related to increase in body weight. Seventy-five percent of the energy was stored in the body. Thus they believed that all the energy could be accounted for without calling on a facultative or adaptive component. The study was meticulously carried out, but there still must remain some uncertainty regarding the caloric intake derived from tables and particularly regarding deriving the composition of weight gain from body density when relatively small quantities are involved. It is reassuring to see that the figures for body composition derived by the body density and the balance techniques were in fair agreement.

Forbes *et al.* (1982) measured the thermogenic effect of overfeeding six subjects for 17–19 days with an excess of 1200–1800 kcal as meals, 70% of which was carbohydrate. They elected to consider only the four subjects who gained 4 kg or more, in whom they considered body composition could be more accurately measured. They could find no evidence of any facultative energy expenditure in the selected subjects who gained more readily.

The first study employing a chamber was that of Dauncey *et al.* (1980) at Cambridge, England, using a whole-body calorimeter to study the effect of a single day of overfeeding. They found a reproducibility of 1.2 ± 0.14% between two measures of 24-hour expenditure. Two subjects were outliers. Again, the individual subjects had very wide variation in response. Mean expenditure for the group of eight subjects increased 10% on overfeeding 1300 kcal and decreased 6% on underfeeding by 1100 kcal with a mixed diet. The increase on overfeeding was relatively greatest at night, and the resting metabolic rate remained elevated 12% for 14 hours. The heat loss was partitioned. They concluded that the effects of just 1 day of overfeeding did not differ appreciably from those estimated by other workers after several weeks of overfeeding.

Webb and Annis (1982) reported on 12 unique overfeeding studies of nine middle-aged subjects. The excess intake, 30 Mcal taken over 30 days after a 30-day control period, exceeded Garrow's threshold value for induction of facilitative thermogenesis. Bomb calorimetry of food and body waste was used to estimate net food intake. Change in fuel stores was estimated by change in body composition derived from density measurements. Daily energy expenditure was estimated from the net intake during the control period. Webb's water-cooled "space suit" was used for both direct and indirect calorimetry for 36 hours while the subjects were living quietly in a research center during the last week of the control period and at the end of the overfeeding period. Three different diets were used for overfeeding, one an average American diet, one high (60%) in carbohydrate, and one containing 70% protein and fat. Subjects' energy intake corresponded to measured losses while on the first two diets, but their energy intake exceeded losses by over 500 kcal per day while on the diet higher in protein and fat. There was no difference in response between lean and overweight subjects. Webb and Annis could find no easy explanation for the unaccounted calories of the third experiment. There was no apparent difference in level of activity, and they assumed the obligatory cost of deposition in stores would be measured by the calorimetry.

Dallosso and James (1984) used a chamber for indirect calorimetry to study the effect on 24-hour energy expenditure of overfeeding fat to eight subjects for 7 days. After a control week the subjects' intake of fat was increased 50% and calorimetry was carried out twice in each period, during which two levels of physical activity were maintained. The interactions between three meals and six periods of graded exercise were estimated in the complicated protocol. Energy expenditure during the period of fat feeding increased only 5.6% during low activity and 6.4% during increased activity. They found only a small increase in thermogenesis in excess of the obligatory cost of storage. Minimal effects on thermogenesis might have been expected during this overfeeding of fat, in view of the remarkably efficient gain in weight of the four subjects of the Vermont Study overfed with 1000 kcal fat/day (Goldman *et al.,* 1975). It was the impression of Dallasso and James that those with the lowest body fat showed the greater thermogenic response, although body composition was not directly measured, and they suggested that more prolonged studies with increased intake of carbohydrate and measurement of body composition were required.

Robbins *et al.* (1979) studied in our laboratory the response to slight overfeeding of a young girl with acquired lipoatrophy and no evidence of subcutaneous fat depots. Any intake above maintenance provoked a marked increase in metabolic rate. This was consistent with the suggestion of Dallosso and James (1984) that the capacity to store additional fat might condition any thermogenic response to overfeeding.

Our Vermont Study of experimental obesity in our cooperative group of volunteers at Windsor Prison (Sims *et al.,* 1968; Sims, 1976; Goldman *et al.,* 1975) is sometimes quoted as settling decisively the question of the existence of luxuskonsumption. In the lay press it is even sometimes stated that the men of the study could double their intake without gaining weight. Had this been true, the food would have been disposed of by routes other than the alimentary canal. We cannot say that we met all the criteria for an ideal study as indicated by Durnin (1983) and by Hervey and Tobin (1984). But we can say that all intake was provided from a special kitchen and the amounts actually eaten were recorded by special attendants. Reliance on standard tables for estimating intake has obvious limitations, accurate to perhaps +3% but estimates can have relative value. Change in body composition by body density, corrected for residual lung volume, was measured in all subjects. It is frequently stated that a prolonged study providing larger changes in body fat gives greater accuracy, but daily errors in estimating intake or other variables are also cumulative. A large area of uncertainty is the degree of variation in activity. The men were required to climb three flights of stairs five times a day within the research area in the institution. In terms of cost of moving the added weight, this should have limited the gain of those who gained most readily. Unfortunately other activity could not be monitored, except by pedometer readings in several groups.

In hindsight, the most impressive evidence suggesting some degree of facultative thermogenesis was the fact that after weight gain had reached a new plateau an average of 2700 kcal was required to maintain this weight, compared to approximately 1300 kcal required by the spontaneously obese individuals of comparable weight. It is difficult to believe that the measured increase in lean body mass and in cost of physical activity could explain this difference. It is true, however, that smoking, caffeine intake, and possibly anxiety contributed to the requirement for energy. A further analysis of the data from our fourth group, in which the most accurate figures of intake and losses are available, is currently in progress using newer techniques of data handling and analysis.

3. *The Role of Catecholamines and Thyroid Hormones in the Components of Diet-Induced Thermogenesis*

Another area of controversy in the field of energy balance concerns the role of the sympathethic nervous system (SNS) in the thermogenic reactions to food. Nineteen relevant studies are outlined in Table II, with emphasis on the features bearing on the response of the sympathetic nervous system and of thyroid hormones. Twelve of the studies found significant relations between the SNS and thermogenesis, whereas seven studies did not find a significant relationship. Essentially the same considerations apply to these studies as to the above studies of overfeeding. I believe that the more compelling evidence indicates that the facultative component of diet-induced thermogenesis is mediated by catecholamines and that increased insulin action is a contributor to the catecholamine response. The plasma concentration of catecholamines is, however, a poor index of catecholamine activity. Many of the considerations regarding selection of patients and variables affecting the protocols mentioned in the later section on dietary thermogenesis in obesity also help to explain the discrepancies in the results here (Section V,B,20).

a. Studies Using Single Feedings or Glucose Infusion. In 1981 Welle *et al.* measured the response during a 4-hour period to ingestion of 100 g of protein or glucose or an equivalent amount of fat (44 g). Protein gave a greater thermogenic response. Since plasma norepinephrine concentration increased significantly only after the carbohydrate feeding, they concluded that the sympathetic nervous system played no role in thermogenesis in this context. Zwillich *et al.* (1981) also found no reduction by β-receptor blockade with propranolol in the energy expenditure over 3 hours following ingestion of 250 g of carbohydrate. Thus, in general, it has been difficult to prove a function for the SNS with small oral feedings studied over a relatively short period of time. Results of recent studies of longer duration which employ a chamber suggest that such short periods of measurement are not adequate to

TABLE II

STUDIES OF THE ROLE OF THE SYMPATHETIC NERVOUS SYSTEM IN THE THERMOGENIC RESPONSE TO EXCESS CALORIC INTAKE[a]

Investigators	Subjects (obese/control)	Study type	Overfeeding: Days form	Overfeeding: kcal P-F-C (%)	Test MR duration	NE in plasma/urine	NE appearance and clearance (flux)	Beta block	Serum T_3	Conclusions and comments
Studies supporting a facultative component										
Jung (1979)	6/7 (familial)	Response to NE infusions (45 minutes)	—	—	1.5 hours (hood)	—	—	—	—	Lesser response in obese to NE
Rowe *et al.* (1980)		Euglycemic clamp with graded insulin infusion	— —	— —	Clamp	Increased	Clearance same	—	—	Dose response increases in plasma NE with insulin infusion and no change in blood glucose
Schwartz *et al.* (1982)	7/6	Response of NE and TG to mixed meal	1 L	800 15-0-85	2 hours	Plasma	—	—	—	NE increased after single, large C feeding, but no correlation with TG
O'Dea *et al.* (1982)	0/6	NE turnover during low, normal, and high intake	10 × 3 M	1700 15-40-45	—	No	Increased in 4 of 6 subjects	—	Rose with higher intake	No significant change in flux with over- and underfeeding in obese. No change in glucose utilization
Acheson *et al.* (1983)	0/9	Hyperglycemic–hyperinsulinemic clamp and beta blockade	— —	— —	7 hours	Increased	—	Propranolol	—	Propranolol lowers TG and blocks increase in glucose disposal
Acheson *et al.* (1984c)	0/9	Euglycemic clamp, increased insulin and beta blockade	2 —	— —	4 hours	Slightly increased	—	Propranolol	—	Insulin stimulates and propranolol blocks TG, SNS responsible for entire increase in TG
Schutz *et al.* (1984)	20/8	Comparison of DIT in obese and lean in chamber	— —	— —	24 hours	Lower in obese	—	—	—	Response of SNS and TG to feeding lower in obese
DeFronzo *et al.* (1984)	0/12	Alpha and beta block, euglycemic clamp	— —	— —	2 hours	—	—	See comment	—	TG and glucose oxidation reduced with beta block and not with alpha. See text

Bazelmans *et al.* (1985)	6/0	Effect of over- and undereating on NE flux and euglycemic clamp	10 M	−400, 1000 15-40-45	Clamp	—	—	—	—	No significant change in flux with over- and undereating in obese. No change glucose utilization
Schwartz (1986)	0/13	NE flux following a meal	1 M	800 kcal C 200 g C	2 hours	Increased	Appearance increased; clearance same	—	—	Changes in RMR correlated with appearance of NE only
Vernet *et al.* (1986)	9/8	TG during infusion of mixed nutrient ± beta blockade	— —	— —	4 hours	—	—	Yes for lean, no for obese subjects	—	SNS modulates TG response to mixed meal in lean but not in obese
Thorin *et al.* (1986)	0/8	Euglycemic clamp with beta-1 blockade	— —	— —	Clamp	—	—	MetaProlol (beta-1 block)	—	TG inhibited by beta-1 blockade but glucose total uptake (oxidative and nonoxidative) not affected
					Studies not supporting a facultative component					
Welle *et al.* (1981)	0/7	Response of NE and TG to P, F, or C	— L	100 g P or C or 44 g F	4 hours	Increased with C only	—	—	—	Protein gave greater thermogenesis. No apparent role of SNS
Zwillich *et al.* (1981)	0/6	Response to C feeding with beta blockade	— L	250 g C	3 hours	Increased	—	Propranolol	—	No effect of beta blockade on thermogenesis from oral C on cardiovascular response
Welle and Campbell (1983)	13/11	Response of NE and TG to oral glucose	— L	100 g C	3 hours	Increased in both groups	—	—	—	NE response same in controls and obese; no correlation between plasma NE and TG
Welle and Campbell (1983)	0/7	Response of TG and NE to high or low C intake and beta blockade	20 M	1810 8-22-70	2 hours	—	—	Propranolol	32% increased	Increased TG not blocked by propranolol. No increased sensitivity to iv NE

(*continued*)

TABLE II (*Continued*)

Investigators	Subjects (obese/ control)	Study type	Overfeeding		Test MR duration	NE in plasma/ urine	NE appearance and clearance (flux)	Beta block	Serum T_3	Conclusions and comments
			Days form	kcal P-F-C (%)						
Seaton *et al.* (1984)	0/6	Effect alpha and beta blockade on TG, NE, and insulin	— L	100 g C	3 hours	Increased	—	Propranolol	—	TG, basal glucose, and insulin not affected by beta and/or alpha blockade after oral glucose
Katzeff *et al.* (1986)	6/6	TG response to iv NE before and after overfeeding	2 M	1000 and 500	30 minutes in AM	Plasma slightly increased in lean; obese same	Clearance same in obese and lean	—	Increased in lean	No difference response to NE after overfeeding in lean or obese
Kush *et al.* (1986)	5/5 (Pimas, family history of DM)	TG response to NE and exercise after overfeeding and underfeeding	21 M	1000 kcal 20-35-45	3.5 hours total (800 kcal)	Plasma NE variable	—	—	No increase	No increase in TG response to meal or exercise in lean or obese. TG and glycemic response to NE fell more in obese Pimas

[a] L, Liquid meal; SNS, sympathetic nervous system; TG, thermogenesis; DM, diabetes mellitus. Other abbreviations in Table I.

determine the full thermic response. It is also possible that the catecholamine effect on facultative thermogenesis develops earlier after intake of substrate than does the obligatory thermogenesis and that the timing may vary with differing stimuli.

b. Studies Employing a Calorimetry Chamber. Only the study by Schutz *et al.* (1984a) has involved use of a calorimetric chamber for 24-hour studies. In this the thermogenic response to three meals was found to be less in obese subjects, and consistent with this was a reduction in the diurnal variation and urinary excretion of norepinephrine. Each subject was given an average of 41.2 kcal of energy per kilogram of fat-free mass, so that a reduction was found even though the obese actually received more food energy than the nonobese controls.

c. Thermogenesis in Response to Infusion of Glucose and Insulin during the Clamp Procedure. Acheson *et al.* (1983, 1984) reported a significant reduction in the thermic response to infused glucose during the clamp procedure when propranolol was also infused. E. Danforth *et al.* (personal communication) found an extremely close correlation ($r = 0.95$, $p < 0.001$) between the plasma appearance and clearance rates of norepinephrine and the metabolic rates and the glucose disposal rate during the euglycemic–hyperinsulinemic clamp procedure. The appearance and clearance rate also correlated well with the degree of stimulation of glucose uptake when the concentrations of insulin were varied. Norepinephrine in the plasma increased during the infusion, but the correlation with plasma concentration alone was less direct. Since the clearance of NE also increases under these conditions, the plasma concentration underestimates the activation of the sympathetic nervous system, which is better reflected in the increased appearance rates. From their data the cost of nonoxidative glucose disposal was 0.4 kcal/g and not the theoretical 0.2 kcal/g, which would have been the case had the glucose been directly converted and stored as glycogen. The excess (0.4 − 0.2 = 0.2 kcal/g) or the "facultative" cost of storing the glucose directly as glycogen varied with the increase in norepinephrine appearance. This adds further support to evidence acquired using propranolol blockade that the excess or "facultative" costs of an insulin and glucose infusion are related to activation of the sympathetic nervous system.

d. The Role of Catecholamines in Long-Term Overfeeding. In animals that are overfed, plasma norepinephrine is increased, and the response to infused NE is enhanced, consistent with hypertrophy of brown adipose tissue. In a further study Weele and Campbell (1983; Welle, 1985) overfed seven normal subjects with 36 Mcal over 20 days. Basal oxygen consumption was increased by 7.4%. Overfeeding did not affect the thermic effect of a standard meal, which was measured, however, only over a 2-hour period, nor did it affect the response to infusion of norepinephrine. Catecholamines were not increased in plasma or urine, and propranolol, given to block β-adrenergic stimulation, produced the same effect on oxygen uptake after as before the overfeeding. Neither was there an increase in thermic effect of a standard meal after overfeeding.

These findings were consistent with those of Katzeff *et al.* (1985) in Danforth's laboratory, who studied the role of the sympathetic nervous system after overfeeding (18 Mcal) six normal subjects over 18 days. They did find a similar increase in resting oxygen consumption of 6.6% and a logarithmic relationship between NE concentrations in plasma and oxygen uptake after graded infusions. The response to graded infusions of norepinephrine was unaffected by overfeeding. Overfeeding caused a minimal increase in plasma concentrations of norepinephrine. Finally, the thermic response to graded bicycle exercise was unaltered by over- or underfeeding.

In an important study, O'Dea *et al.* (1982) applied kinetic studies of norepinephrine to man. They measured both appearance and clearance of norepinephrine by infusion of tritiated norepinephrine in six subjects given low-caloric, weight-maintaining, or high-caloric mixed diets for 10-day periods. Both appearance and clearance, i.e., turnover (flux or spillover), of norepinephrine were increased in four of the six subjects and the mean was significantly increased. The plasma concentration, previously used as an index of sympathetic stimulation, was not significantly changed. Thus the kinetic measure is apparently a more reliable indicator of such stimulation than the plasma concentration alone, and it may also be that this measure will turn out to be a valuable indicator of facultative or adaptive thermogenesis (Esler, 1982). In a related study, Mancia *et al.* (1983) found in subjects with essential hypertension a poor correlation between plasma concentrations of NE and blood pressure.

Acheson *et al.* (1981) have shown by selective blockade that the facultative component of the thermic effect of intravenous glucose and insulin is dependent upon β-adrenergic stimulation, while DeFronzo *et al.* (1984) found that α-blockade was without effect. Thorin *et al.* (1986) have further shown that the stimulation is specifically mediated by the β-1 receptors. Macdonald *et al.* (1985) reviewed the evidence that relatively small increases in plasma catecholamines can produce substantial effects. On the other hand during 20-day overfeeding of approximately 1200 kcal to normal subjects, Seaton *et al.* (1984) and Welle (1985) could find no evidence whatever of increased sympathetic activity in association with the increased thermogenesis. This negative finding may be in part due to selection of subjects or to the fact that the concentration of plasma catecholamines is an imperfect index of sympathetic activity.

e. The Synergistic Role of Thyroid Hormones. Smith and Edelman (1979) have reviewed the evidence that the major thermogenic action of thyroid hormone is effected through stimulation of Na^+,K^+-ATPase, the enzyme critical in maintaining the intra- and extracellular gradient of sodium, a process responsible for much of the resting metabolic rate. This enzyme is also a target for catecholamines through stimulation of β-noradrenergic receptors (Swann, 1984). Larsen *et al.* (1981) recently reviewed the intracellular action of thyroid hormones, and Danforth and Sims (1983) reviewed the deiodination of thyroxine to its active and inactive metabolites in relation to nutrition.

O'Dea and associates (1982) found a significant decrease in serum T_3 and an increase in reverse T_3 on overfeeding normal subjects. This is consistent with the changes with overfeeding reported by Danforth *et al.* (1979). Acheson *et al.* (1984b) have also dissociated the effect of T_3 on the resting metabolic rate, versus any possible effect on the efficiency of exercise or utilization of food. They blocked endogenous thyroid hormone production with T_4 and gave T_3 in amounts sufficient to reproduce the serum concentrations previously produced by a degree of overfeeding carbohydrate that had apparently given a facultative increase in thermogenesis. They found that the increase in plasma T_3 concentration could explain corresponding increases in metabolic rate, but not the changes in efficiency. This does not rule out a synergistic action of the T_3 in the effect of norepinephrine. Possible changes in NE turnover were not measured in this study. Jung *et al.* (1980) have found that propranolol blocks a portion of the RMR in overweight subjects taking a maintenance diet, but that it is without effect during caloric restriction. Since the fall in serum T_3 and increase in reverse T_3 from propranolol was the same with both diets, the catecholamine effect is presumably the greater.

4. *Summary and Conclusions Regarding the Components of Diet-Induced Thermogenesis*

Application of the newer techniques to the question of facultative thermogenesis has not yet given clear-cut answers. The many variables affecting thermogenesis considered in this section (and considered again in Section V,A) make the perfect study difficult to attain. The availability of chambers for direct or indirect calorimetry has solved problems of too-brief calorimetry, but others remain. Chamber studies to date have been limited to the short term, and confinement in the chamber interferes with an individual's spontaneous physical activity.

Competent investigators in different laboratories, many employing state-of-the-art techniques, have carried out 26 studies by the time of writing and have obtained contradictory results. Some of the contradictory results of the many studies perhaps again reflect heterogeneity of the subjects studied. We were certainly surprised and impressed by the degree of variation in ability to gain of the volunteers in the Vermont Study. Some have attributed variation in data to technical error. I recall my former mentor, John P. Peters, saying that the truth may often be found in the response of the outliers as well as of those whose data appear reasonable. Other contradictory results again probably can be explained by limitations of the protocols employed.

Individuals may differ in spontaneous activity and also apparently in the ratio of resting metabolic rate to their fat-free mass. In 1961 Rose and Williams at Johns Hopkins University studied students who were large or small eaters. In six such pairs the most discriminatory finding out of a battery of tests was the rate at which the subjects walked in carrying out assigned tasks. Jayarajan *et al.* (1986) in Shetty's laboratory in India studied the cardiovascular and β-adrenoreceptor responsiveness of lean versus normal-weight subjects of the same social class apparently with similar intakes of energy. The increase in heart rate and fall in blood pressure in response to isoproterenol were greater in the lean subjects, suggesting a generalized increase in adrenergic responsiveness. Other studies have shown that at least some of the obese may be more economical of their physical effort than lean persons (Mayer, 1965b). The study of Poehlman *et al.* (1985) of identical twins in Bouchard's laboratory showed concordance in their capacity for diet-induced thermogenesis. The ratio of RMR to FFM apparently differed genetically, although one cannot entirely rule out environmental factors. The possibility that the genetic difference may be found in part in mitochondrial DNA is an intriguing possibility. See also Section V,B,20.

Further progress in this area should be made not only through further application of direct and indirect calorimetry, but also by exploiting new techniques (Schoeller, 1983; Ravussin *et al.*, 1985d). The use of doubly labeled water may permit estimating long-term energy expenditure over long periods in free-living subjects. The measurement of the turnover rate of norepinephrine, rather than plasma concentrations alone, should be helpful in unraveling the question of facultative thermogenesis and perhaps in identifying those who may be deficient.

It is certainly important to know whether man as well as animals shares in this adaptive mechanism before considering whether some obese persons may partly lack this ability.

Another long-term overfeeding study, at least longer than 3 weeks, with attention to hard and easy gainers could give useful information through the techniques now available. It does seem a pity that past abuses make prison populations inaccessible for such studies. In our experience such a study can be successful from a humane point of view. The men in our studies profited from working with a group, from the gourmet diet, and from companionship with the staff of our Vermont Study. Unfortunately, it is difficult to guard in such situations against possible coercion, though in one area prisoners have petitioned for the right to take part in research studies like other people.

On reviewing the evidence to date my personal bias is that a facultative component of dietary thermogenesis is operative in normal persons who are overfed, particularly with carbohydrates. A logical sequence might be increase in insulin effect, stimulation of critical hypothalamic centers, increased turnover of norepinephrine, and stimulation of metabolic pathways and processes involving lower efficiency. These may involve brown fat that is residual in the adult, but are not dependent upon it.

B. Increased Thermogenesis in Pathological States

1. *Thermogenesis of Trauma and Fever*

This important topic, beyond the scope of the present review, has been considered recently by Aulick and Wilmore (1984) and by Eiger and Kluger (1984).

2. *Hypermetabolism of Mental Stress and Anxiety*

Over 30 years ago Friedman (1950) reviewed the evidence for "psychogenic" or "neurogenic" fever. To a large extent this was a diagnosis of exclusion using the techniques available at the time. He described 30 patients whom he considers fall into the category of neurogenic hyperthermia and pointed out that the fever invariably subsides during sleep and that fever can be elicited more readily by the usual fever-provoking stimuli. Quite possibly such patients warrant investigation by modern methods.

It does seem likely that anxiety can increase the resting metabolic rate and may increase sensitivity to catecholamines. Under the moderately stressful conditions of laboratory studies in the field of energy balance, such as the glucose clamp, this may be a confounding factor.

3. *The Hypermetabolism of Hyperthyroidism*

Gelfand *et al.* (1985) studying the effect of T_3 in normal subjects, stated in a preliminary report that T_3 increases the sensitivity to the calorigenic action of epinephrine and increases leucine flux and oxidation. Beta blockade, however, did not affect basal metabolic rate or amino acid flux. They concluded that in thyrotoxicosis there is inhibitable hyperresponsiveness to the catecholamine, but that the hypermetabolism and increased protein breakdown are not adrenergically mediated.

4. *Luft's Syndrome*

Two cases of extraordinarily severe hypermetabolism in young girls have been reported (Luft *et al.,* 1979; Haydar *et al.,* 1971). The unfortunate girl reported by Haydar was required to stay constantly in the draft of two fans and to lie in a cool bathtub in warm weather. Both displayed overgrowth of anatomically abnormal mitochondria with uncoupled phosphorylation.

5. *Congenital Lipoatrophy*

The composition of the diet as well as the metabolic route taken by the various substrates influence the thermogenic response to food. Robbins *et al.* in our laboratory (1982) studied a young girl with lipoatrophy with no fat depot other than intraabdominal. A modest increase in caloric intake above maintenance produced a marked hypermetabolic state as noted. This is consistent with the suggestion of Dallosso and James (1984) that the size of the depot available for fat storage may be another factor modifying the thermogenic response.

6. *Smoking as a Possible Cause of Increased Thermogenesis*

Fear of gaining weight is frequently strongly advanced as a reason for not giving up smoking (Wack and Rodin, 1982). In 1970 Glauser *et al.* reported that gain in weight during the month after stopping smoking was associated with a decrease in metabolic rate and in serum protein-bound iodine. We have studied a limited number of moderate young smokers (only four to date) during 2-week periods before stopping smoking, during abstinence, and on resuming smoking. Dietary intake was kept entirely constant by controlled use of TV dinners. In collaboration with Burse of the United States Army Research Institute of Environmental Medicine at Natick, Massachusetts, measurements of resting, postprandial, and exercise metabolic rates were carried out with the aid of an environmental chamber. There was a central stimulation of the hypothalamus which persisted for at least 12 hours after the last cigarette, in that the response of TSH to TRH, but not of prolactin, was significantly increased during the two periods of smoking. Appetite, estimated by rating scales, was significantly increased while not smoking. This may apparently be a major factor promoting weight gain. Changes in body weight and body composition and in the parameters of thyroid function (serum TSH, T_3) and in metabolic rate were all in a direction consistent with an increase in thyroid-stimulated increase in thermogenesis, but with the small number of subjects none of the changes by themselves were statistically significant. In order to help people to stop smoking, we need to learn more about the effects of smoking on appetite and its thermogenic effects.

7. *Caloric Excess, Obesity, and Hypertension*

A close association between obesity and hypertension has long been recognized. Not all obese are hypertensive, but the incidence is higher in those with central distribution of body fat (Sims, 1985). The first international meeting to probe the possible mechanisms relating obesity and hypertension was held in Florence in 1980 as a satellite of the International Congress on Obesity (Berchtold *et al.*, 1981). A relationship was brought out between hyperinsulinemia, increased plasma norepinephrine, and sodium retention, which may contribute to hypertension in those genetically susceptible. These interrelationships were further explored at the symposium held in Princeton in 1982 (McCarron *et al.*, 1982; Sims, 1982). It has since become apparent from the work of Rowe *et al.* (1981) that physiological concentrations of insulin can directly stimulate catecholamine turnover. These relationships are potentially important, since the insulin resistance and hypertension of the overweight and those suffering from non-insulin-dependent diabetes can be greatly reduced by change in the composition of the diet, the caloric intake, and the level of physical activity (Sims, 1982, 1986). Such an initial approach to management of mild to moderate hypertension is preferable in the long run to the use of drugs as a first step in treatment, particularly since the pharmacological approach carries the risk of exaggerating other risk factors (Dustan, 1984).

8. *Caffeine*

It has been known for many years that caffeine causes an increase in the metabolic rate. Acheson *et al.* (1980) found that a large dose (equivalent to five to six cups of coffee) caused an increase in the metabolic rate in normal subjects with a doubling of free fatty acids in the plasma and an increased oxidation of fat. An amount equivalent to three cups of coffee in normal subjects similarly mobilized free fatty acids and increased fatty acid oxidation and energy expenditure, but in obese subjects only the increase in thermogenesis was noted. Coffee taken with a large meal increased its thermic effect. Jung *et al.* (1981) investigated the role of catecholamines in the thermic effect. They found a similar thermic effect of caffeine in lean and obese subjects, which was thus independent of other subnormal thermic responses of the obese. The response was not affected by β-adrenergic blockade, and the degree of thermic effect correlated with the rise in free fatty acids. Previously obese women showed a diminished response to caffeine. Currently Poehlman *et al.* (1986) report that caffeine produces less thermic effect in trained athletes than in sedentary subjects.

IV. Situations in Which Thermogenesis May Be Reduced in Normal-Weight Individuals

Physiological and Environmental

1. *Age*

The changes in thermogenesis in the various stages of life have been considered in Sections II,C.

2. *Acute and Subacute Caloric Deprivation*

At least since Benedict's classic study (1919) of starvation in the Maltese lawyer, Mr. Levanzin, it has been known that the metabolic rate declines in the face of caloric deprivation. The metabolic adaptations have been summarized in Cahill's classic paper on starvation in man (1970). Such reactions are clearly of survival value. The outstanding question has been whether the reduced caloric needs simply reflect a reduced respiring mass and perhaps reduced activity, or whether there is a facultative reduction in thermogenesis as well.

a. The Role of Thyroid Hormones. The thyroid has long been suspected of mediating such a response, and the decrease in the active form of thyroid hormone, T_3, and increase in the inactive form, reverse T_3, is well known. This is seen not only during caloric deprivation, but also with a variety of illnesses involving malnutrition in what has been called the "euthyroid sick." Recent *in vitro* studies of rat liver homogenates by Chopra *et al.* (1985) suggest that there may be an inhibitor of nonthyroidal conversion of thyroxine to T_3 operative in such nonthyroidal illnesses.

b. The Role of Catecholamines and of a Possible Facultative Component. The pioneer work of Landsberg and Young (1978) showed in rats that the tissue turnover rate of norepinephrine is decreased by undernutrition, and studies of norepinephrine flux in man by O'Dea *et al.* (1982) provided similar evidence. It is not yet clear what energy-consuming processes are affected. Garrow (1978) stated that his favorite candidate is the rate of protein turnover. Substrate cycling or electrolyte pumping are other candidates (see Section II,E,1–3).

Since Keys (1950) classic war-time study of semistarvation in volunteers there have been few studies of the mechanism of the reduced metabolic rate in normal fasting subjects to learn whether man responds to caloric deprivation as do smaller animals. Bray (1969) found a reduction in adipose tissue of patients undergoing weight reduction of the two α-glycerol-phosphate dehydrogenases which could account for less efficient generation of ATP in mitochondria from oxidation of substrate. Other investigators have looked for consistent changes in catecholamines and in thyroid hormones to explain the changes in undernutrition, with inconsistent results. In an important study by O'Dea *et al.* (1982) in Esler's laboratory, it was shown that during modified fasting there is a change in the turnover or spillover rate of norepinephrine, which is strong evidence for a facultative control (see Table IV). This response would be expected, since insulin concentrations are modulated by caloric excess and deprivation, and in turn this hormone within physiological range can affect the concentration of norepinephrine. Other studies investigating possible facultative changes in thermogenesis in response to fasting have involved both normal and obese subjects and are considered in the next section (Section V,B,21).

3. *Chronic Caloric Deprivation*

In 1973 four English investigators (Durnin *et al.*) raised the question of whether the caloric needs of man may not be overestimated. The metabolic rate in relation to lean body mass under a variety of conditions is held to be quite constant and not altered by brief caloric deprivation (see Section II,B). There have, however, been reports of workers in various parts of the world carrying out physical work with surprisingly small rations (James and Shetty, 1982). Narasinga Rao (1985) recently reviewed the metabolic adaptation and placed emphasis on growth retardation in childhood, a lower basal metabolic rate, and reduced work capacity in adults. Reduced protein turnover and reduced activity of enzymes involved in substrate catabolism may be contributory. However, it is not clear whether there is an adaptive reduction in metabolic rate related to the fat-free or respiring mass.

On his return to India from work in the Dunn Laboratories in Cambridge, Shetty (1984) studied 14 undernourished, unskilled laborers and compared them with more privileged controls of their same age. The protein intake of the workers was only 35 g per day, and their body fat was 6.1%. Body composition was estimated from skinfold thickness with standards related to the Indian population. This was presumably a reasonably accurate index of body fat within the low range involved. The RMR of the workers was 111.6 ± 1.89 kJ/kg FFM/day versus 129.5 for the controls. The workers were judged to be physically fit with normal cardiovascular function on the basis of standard tests and showed significantly lower serum cholesterols and free fatty acids. The lower caloric needs of the laborers could be explained in large part by reduced lean body mass (42 versus 53 kg) and by lowered requirement for movement, but it appears that their metabolic efficiency may have also been increased. Unfortunately there are limitations to the estimation of lean body mass by any method. Laborers doing hard physical work, for instance, could be expected to have more dense bones, which would increase the apparent efficiency. Clearly, however, there is much to learn regarding the optimal caloric intake of man. Measurements of such a population using a battery of the most refined methods for body composition would be useful.

V. Factors Promoting Weight Gain and Persistence of Obesity

The various syndromes of obesity are certainly some of the major problems of preventive medicine both in the United States and abroad in their relation to the ubiquitous type II diabetes, hypertension, hyperlipidemia, and human misery in general (Bray, 1979; Hirsch *et al.*, 1985). Helping the overweight to combat these problems can be an exercise in frustration. The 1959 reference of Stunkard is all too frequently cited as evidence that little can be done, though some progress has been made since that time (Garrow, 1981).

We should be more successful in helping the overweight if we can gain more understanding of their individual problems. A wide assortment of derangements have been pinpointed in animal species subject to obesity, and it seems likely that there are as many potential derangements in man (Bray and York, 1971; James, 1979). The goal of this section is to outline possible derangements as a basis for planning realistic strategy and reasonable goals for a given individual and as a basis for evolving a useful data base to aid in planning and interpreting clinical investigation in this area. First we should consider the population concerned.

A. Who Are the Sufferers from Plenitude?

Putatatively prestigious tables and various indices for normal weight are used to estimate the degree of obesity and the risks engendered. These guidelines, recently reviewed at a National Institutes of Health Consensus Meeting in Washington (1985), are useful to a degree, but are not adequate for clinical investigation or for clinical care of individuals, and they do not discriminate between those with normal or abnormal distribution of body fat. Ruderman *et al.* (1981) described subjects who are normal in weight by the usual criteria, but who display the metabolic and endocrine changes of the obese. Such individuals are presumably inactive and have a reduced muscle mass and a proportionate increase in body fat. There are also the successfully reduced obese, who include the restrained eaters (Herman and Polivy, 1980). They share with obese patients who have acutely lost weight the continual tendency to return to their habitual weight, particularly if they have hyperplasia of adipocytes. Such successful persons tend to be overlooked, while those who fail to maintain a reduced weight are more apt to find their way into the medical literature. A final group is the familial "obese" who in reality are active, have adipocytes of a reasonable size in a normal distribution, have normal metabolic responses, and may be at no increased risk of cardiovascular or other diseases. They should not carry a burden of guilt because they exceed some statistical cutoff value of normal risk.

B. Potential Problems of the Frankly Obese and Some Implications for Management

1. *The Attitude of Physicians and Others toward the Obese*

No matter how much we may learn about the ingrained metabolic problems of the obese I must confess that one still tends unconsciously to blame severely overweight persons for what we have been conditioned to regard as simple lack of care and control; but they truly have demons with which to contend (Astwood, 1962; Sims, 1984).

2. *Problems of Inheritance*

Obesity nowadays is a source of discrimination (Mayer 1965), but it once had survival value (Neel, 1962). The genetic component is apparent, but difficult to dissociate from environmental factors. Early studies have been reviewed by Mayer (1965) and more recent studies by Mueller (1983). Withers (1964) was one of the first to try to dissociate the genetic factor in his study of adopted twins. He did find a closer correlation of obesity with true as opposed to foster parents, but adoptions were not made until an average of 14.5 months, with a range of 10 days to 8 years (R. F. J. Withers, and personal communication). Bouchard *et al.* (1985) extensively studied both adopted and biological siblings. Correlations of body composition increased with increasing degree of relatedness and included the ratio of trunk to peripheral fat. Poehlman *et al.* (1985a,b) studied the increase in thermogenic response to meals after a period of overfeeding in identical twins and found a close correlation. In another recent twin study DeLuise and associates (1985) found that the Na–K pump density in erythrocytes and lymphocytes may be genetically determined. In an earlier study DeLuise (1983) had found that the pump density was unaffected by short- or medium-term variations in nutrition. Unfortunately, even among identical twins environmental factors can be confounding, except with twins who have lived apart from birth.

Type II non-insulin-dependent diabetes is well known to be strongly inherited, and obesity in the type IIB subtype may precede overt diabetes by many years. It is often argued that the obesity causes the diabetes, and at times the Vermont Study is cited as evidence, since overeating and weight gain increased insulin resistance and glucose tolerance. This, however, only indicates that these factors may contribute to insulin resistance and could accentuate a latent genetic tendency.

Although several of the obesity syndromes are known to be genetic in origin, the evidence is less clear for familial obesity. In one study (Fumeron and Apfelbaum, 1981) an association with HLA B-18 was shown, but patients with subclinical diabetes were not excluded. Digby *et al.* (1985) could not confirm this, but found an association with Bw35 and Cw4. Subjects with abnormal glucose tolerance were excluded, but curiously data for family history of diabetes were not noted.

3. *Intrauterine Effects*

The thoroughly documented longitudinal studies of the Pima Indians at Sakaton in Arizona has made it possible to evaluate the effect of maternal diabetes on later development of obesity. Pettitt *et al.* (1983) found that overt diabetes in Pima mothers at the time of pregnancy constitutes a greater risk for obesity in the offspring in later years. The risk is greater than for offspring with one or two grandparents or parents with diabetes. On the other hand, mothers with strong genetic traits for diabetes would be expected to develop diabetes in an early pregnancy and to pass on the genetic trait, even though diabetes in the pregnancy did not influence the outcome. We do know from Naeye's work that maternal hyperglycemia can lead to hypercellularity of the islets of Langerhans of the pancreas (Naeye and Roode, 1970). Results of a Dutch study of 300,000 draftees whose mothers had been exposed to famine during the latter half of pregnancy were consistent with a reverse effect as a result of malnutrition (Ravelle *et al.,* 1976). However, famine in the first half of the pregnancy was associated with an increased incidence of obesity, which Ravelle *et al.* attributed to possible damage to hypothalamic centers. This gives an added importance to close monitoring of pregnancy for gestational diabetes in those with a strong family history of diabetes or obesity.

4. *The Legacy of Pregnancy and Lactation*

Weight gain, associated with successive pregnancies is normally quite small, in relation to that expected for age, and averages 1.9 kg between first and fourth pregnancies (Billewicz and Thompson, 1970). Those who are overweight to start with, however, triple the net gain of those initially underweight, and weight gain between pregnancies is associated with further net gain from pregnancies. Beasley and Swinhoe (1979) found in another series of studies that return to a weight below that at 20 weeks is less likely after the third pregnancy. Thus it is important to identify those at risk. Hilton and Treharne (1985) have emphasized that after an obese woman delivers, caloric restriction does not inhibit lactation, and breast feeding favors return to more normal weight.

5. *Increase in Opioid Peptides: β-Endorphin and β-Lipotrophin*

There is considerable evidence that early in the development of obesity in animals pituitary levels of β-endorphin are increased, and injection of the opioid peptide into the ventricles of rats and sheep increases food intake. In obese human beings these peptides may be markedly elevated (Given *et al.,* 1980; Genazzini *et al.,* 1986). The opioid inhibitor naloxone reduces hyperphagia in patients with Prader–Willi syndrome. Genazzi *et al.* (1986) recently reported on six prepubertal and six adolescent children more than 40% above ideal weight who showed concentrations of each peptide more than twice normal in plasma. In the prepubertal children circadian rhythms, including that for cortisol, were preserved. In the pubertal children β-endorphin tended to remain constant throughout the day, as has been reported in adults, raising the possibility of an extrahypophyseal origin. These important observations raise the possibility that there may be a subtype among severely obese persons in which a disturbance of the opioid peptides is primary and for which specific treatment may be developed. There remains the possibility that the changes in opioid secretion might be secondary to the obesity of hyperphagia. Somewhat against this is the finding that in the modestly obese subjects of our Vermont Study, the normal circadian rhythm of cortisol secretion was not abolished by experimental obesity.

6. *The Distribution and Character of Body Fat*

Ascertaining the distribution of body fat and the degree of hypercellularity can aid in predicting success with weight reduction programs. In general, hyperplastic obesity is associated with poor success either through exercise or dietary measures (Björntorp, 1980, 1985). The hypertrophy of adipocytes is less resistant to streamlining. On the other hand, central obesity with truncal and intraabdominal deposits of fat, as already discussed, is associated with increased insulin resistance, which in turn places a limitation on the thermogenic response to food.

7. *Possible Inhibition of Glucose Metabolism by Increased Lipolysis (the Hales–Randle Effect)*

In 1966 Hales and Randle at Cambridge, England, suggested that increase in the fatty acid cycle of esterification and lipolysis reduced insulin sensitivity and glucose metabolism. This concept has been reviewed and further tested recently by Ferrannini *et al.* (1983). In the course of hyperinsulinemic–euglycemic clamp studies in Pima Indian women, Lillioja *et al.* (1985) found a reciprocal relation between lipid and glucose oxidation, which was consistent with the interaction proposed by Randle. In contrast, there was no correlation in this obese subgroup between percentage body fat and basal fatty acid concentration, free fatty acid turnover, or basal or "clamp" lipid oxidation. Thus changes in lipid availability did not appear to be critical in the relation between obesity and *in vivo* insulin resistance.

8. *Increased Thermal Insulation by Body Fat*

An increased layer of subcutaneous fat can be an asset in improving tolerance to exercise in the cold. Jequier and associates (1974) have studied by direct calorimetry heat loss in the obese during moderate cold exposure and estimated that a conservation of heat is accomplished both by increased insulation and by vasoconstriction of subcutaneous vessels. The increased insulation can also be a handicap in our present society in two ways. Although vasodilatation can compensate in part by bypassing the insulating layer of adipose tissue, body heat loss is reduced, and discomfort and excess sweating can inhibit needed exercise. The increased ability to maintain body heat can also reduce caloric needs. Quaade (1963) carried out standardized tests of exposure to a 4°C cold blanket and found in a majority of obese subjects a slight decrease (2.5%) in the thermic response over that of normal-weight subjects and 13% over that of lean subjects. A quarter of the obese subjects, however, displayed a striking increase in thermogenic response for unexplained reasons, which quite probably reflected the catecholamine response.

If, as indicated by the Finnish studies of Huttunen *et al.* (1981) already cited, chronic exposure to cold can maintain brown fat throughout the adult years, it seems quite possible that the insulation of increased fat may make it even more unlikely that a capacity to adapt to caloric excess with an increase in thermogeneis might be preserved. The hothouse environment from central heating and closed bedroom windows at night thus may all contribute to the tendency of the overweight person to become more so. Quite seriously, might it not be desirable to rear children with a genetic background of obesity in cooler surroundings?

9. *Preferential Diversion of Substrates into Body Fat Stores*

The role of the adipocyte in obesity was the subject of a conference a few years ago at the University of Toronto (Angel *et al.*, 1983); a number of mechanisms which may make adipocytes tend to trap triglycerides were discussed.

a. Effect of Steroid Hormones. The effect of steroid hormones and their potential effects on energy balance and fat distribution were discussed in Section II,F,2,e. The obese may harbor endocrine derangements more subtle than overt endocrinopathies, which nonetheless may be important. Using a continuous sampling procedure to obtain hormonal profiles throughout an entire day Copinschi *et al.* (1978) found that, while there were no differences between obese and normals with respect to integrated concentrations of cortisol, there was a suggestion of a reduction in the diurnal pattern of plasma growth hormone and prolactin which returned to normal after fasting. The study was limited, however, by the wide age range and the heterogeneity of the subjects.

Obesity is a common accompaniment of the syndromes involving polycystic ovaries (Yen, 1980) for reasons not clear. It may also be associated with acanthosis nigricans, anti-receptor antibodies, or post-receptor defect in insulin action. Pasquali *et al.* (1982) studied the insulin response to oral glucose in 16 patients with polycystic ovaries and 16 controls carefully matched for age, relative weight (but not body composition), basal glucose concentrations, and total increment with oral glucose. Those with polycystic ovaries had a much greater response to both insulin and C-peptide. The ratio sum of insulin to sum of glucose was the most discriminatory. Burghen *et al.* (1980) found in similar patients a correlation between the increase in plasma insulin and the increase in androgenic steroids. This is of particular interest, since it has been reported that women with central distribution of body fat, who are now known to be particularly susceptible to diabetes and hypertension, have increased serum androgenic steroids (Evans *et al.*, 1983). The two disorders thus may be distant cousins, with a common denominator of disturbed steroid metabolism and central obesity.

b. Altered Response of Adipocytes in Obesity. There is conflicting evidence as to whether in massively obese subjects adipocytes of some depots or all show inherent tendencies toward replication. Roncari *et al.* (1981, 1983, 1985) found that differentiated omental adipocytes from such subjects regain the ability to replicate in culture and do so at higher rates than cells from normal subjects. Fried *et al.* (1985) reported similar findings of intraabdominal fat cells, together with increased lipolysis. This could produce greater delivery of free fatty acids to the liver, which in turn could contribute to inhibition of carbohydrate metabolism by the Hales–Randle effect. A more recent study by Pettersson *et al.* (1985) yielded contradictory findings. Adipocyte precursors from the stromal–vascular fraction of adipose tissue from hyperplastic obese and nonobese subjects were tested in an enriched medium to optimize conversion to adipocytes. There was no difference in replication rate between cells from obese or nonobese donors or among cells taken from various depots. Pettersson suggested that environment rather than genetics is the more important factor.

The enzyme glycerokinase promotes the reuse of glycerol released by lipolysis for synthesis of triglyceride. Chakrabarty *et al.* (1984) employed a sensitive radioassay to measure this enzyme in a heterogeneous group of normal-weight and obese patients undergoing elective surgery. They found that tissue from a small subsection of obese patients had a high potential for glycerol phosphorylation, and they proposed that this made weight loss more difficult in these subjects. The study certainly warrants repeating with a more controlled group of subjects.

Leibel and Hirsch (1986) studied the rate of lipolysis in adiopocytes from normal, fasted normals, morbidly obese, and reduced obese and pointed out that the reduced obese person in many ways resembles a normal person undergoing fasting. The obese may have the same symptoms of dysphoria, depression, cold intolerance, hunger, and amenorrhea. By use of a radioisotopic technique to measure molar ratio of fatty acid to glycerol leaving the adipocyte and thus the rate of endogenous fatty acid reesterification, Leibel and Hirsch found in normals that this rate falls from 50% in the fed state to 10% in the fasted state. Obese subjects stable in weight do not differ in this respect from normal, but weight-stable, formerly obese subjects with nearly normal-sized adipocytes have a higher molar ratio of FFA to glycerol resembling that of fasting. This raises the possibility that they are sending a stronger systemic signal which may affect appetite. Such reduced morbidly obese people thus truly have a "demon within" that makes maintenance of a weight which we may consider ideal for them difficult, if not actually counterproductive. The question whether this applies to patients with other subtypes of obesity must await further research. The mean energy requirements of such persons undergoing reduction in weight are discussed in Sections IV,A,2 and V,A,17.

It is a source of frustration to many patients, particularly women, that with serious attempts at weight loss, certain depots are particularly resistant to reduction. The characteristically feminine gluteal–femoral fat depot contains larger cells and is more richly supplied with lipoprotein lipase (Rebuffe-Schrieve *et al.,* 1985). There is also increased sensitivity of these cells to estrogens, as can be seen in the response of adipocytes of men treated with estrogens for malignancies (Krotkiewski *et al.,* 1981).

c. Increase in Lipoprotein Lipase. Most of the triglyceride stored in adipose tissue is derived from triglyceride transported in very-low-density lipoproteins in plasma. The enzyme lipoprotein lipase is secreted by parenchymal cells and attached to endothelial linings and is rate limiting for incorporation of triglyceride into cells. In view of this key role, it has been extensively investigated in obese animals (Greenwood, 1985) and in human beings (Pykalisto *et al.,* 1975). Schwartz and Brunzell (1981) have shown that this enzyme is elevated in adipose tissue from obese subjects and that it increases further after weight reduction when a new equilibrium has been maintained. When weight is regained it drops to the initial level, indicating feedback control. This represents a powerful mechanism for maintaining fat stores at a level appropriate to a given individual's complement of adipocytes. Lewis Thomas, writing of our symbiotic relationship to the mitochondria that invaded our cells sometime in the past, stated that he was never quite sure when he went for a walk whether he was taking his mitochondrial for a walk or they were taking him for a walk. In much the same manner a severely obese person may be eating to answer the demands of his avaricious adipocytes rather than to satisfy his own appetite. There is evidence that insulin stimulates activity of lipoprotein lipase in rats (Ashby and Robinson, 1980). Lipoprotein lipase activity is also increased in adipose tissue of young patients with the severe progressive obesity of the Prader–Labhart–Willi syndrome (Dunn, 1968), and it is not reduced by fasting (Schwartz *et al.,* 1979). However, on the basis of detailed functional studies of six of these unusual patients, Bier and associates (1977) could find no evidence of abnormal regulation of fat mobilization or of lipogenesis.

Hyperinsulinemia is associated with experimental obesity in man (Sims *et al.,* 1973), but this does not require that hyperinsulinemia in the spontaneously obese is secondary to simple weight gain from overeating. The insulin resistance of the obese and of the obese diabetic may lead to a vicious cycle in which hyperinsulinemia leads to increased fat stores, which in turn lead to greater insulin resistance. Unfortunately, the insulin resistance of the obese does not protect them from the antilipolytic action of insulin, as Howard *et al.* have shown (1979). Even in obese, highly insulin-resistant subjects, physiological amounts of infused insulin produce a prompt decrease in serum triglycerides and glycerol.

d. Effects of Weight Cycling, Nibbling, and Gorging. Twenty years ago Leveille found that rats trained to eat a day's supply of food within a short period lay down more body fat than those taking the same amount by nibbling throughout the entire night (Leveille and Hanson, 1966). This was particularly true if the diet was high in carbohydrate. Glucose-6-phosphate dehydrogenase and NADP-malic dehydrogenase in adipose tissue were increased by gorging. Soon after this, Bray (1972) found an increase in the enzymes favoring deposition of fat in adipose tissue from women taking a single large meal per day. Many overweight people and those with early non-insulin-dependent diabetes habitually take no breakfast, a small lunch, and a heavy evening meal, which according to the best evidence should promote weight gain. It is not clear whether such a shift in pattern of eating is secondary to a metabolic change within the person, perhaps a change in circadian rhythms, or whether a change in eating pattern itself imposes a change in endocrine response.

A study led by Graeber of the United States Army Research and Development Command at Natick, Massachusetts, was directed toward the latter question (Graeber *et al.*, 1978). The response of subjects eating only a breakfast averaging 1713 kcal for 3-week periods was compared with that of subjects switched to a dinner averaging 2139 kcal. The former lost more weight, but interpretation of the results is difficult since some degree of free choice was allowed. Mood and the rhythms of skilled performance were unaffected. It was apparent, however, that mealtimes were an important moderator of circadian rhythms. Of most interest were the changes in endocrine circadian rhythms. Peak insulin secretion shifted as expected. The peak of cortisol concentrations was shifted from 1.5 hours after awaking with ad lib feeding or the breakfast-only regimen, to 1.5 hours later when dinner was the only meal. Controlling the timing of the major intake of food as well as the caloric content could be of importance in programs for the obese, and a study of the response to shifting the time of day of the main meal in overweight subjects who have gravitated toward evening feeding could be of value.

10. *The Possibility of a Lowered Resting Metabolic Rate in Relation to Fat-Free Mass*

The recent evidence that the resting metabolic rate does not necessarily bear a fixed relationship to the fat-free mass has been considered in Section II,B. We now must admit that there may be truth in the statement of some overweight patients that they "have a low metabolism," at least lower than others. Those with a higher ratio of RMR to fat-free mass may include those who "fidget" more as described by Ravussin and Bogardus (1985; see Section V,A,13).

11. *Hypothalamic Disturbance with Somnolence and Weight Gain*

There are many examples in the animal kingdom of seasonal variation in energy balance, from the premigratory fattening of the hummingbird to the prehibernation gain in weight of the woodchuck (Young, 1976, 1982). When the latter is sufficiently fortified with fat in the fall, it progressively drops its body temperature each day during sleep until it slips into the hypothermia of true hibernation. Mrosovsky (1985) recently reviewed the mechanisms of hibernation, which are relevant to some of the more rare disorders in man. Some of the earliest descriptions of cases with abnormal somnolence are reported by Harvey Cushing and Goetsch (1915). Bray (1975, 1984a) has summarized the reported cases of severe obesity that are associated with hypothalamic injury or disturbance.

One type, Kleine–Levin syndrome, a bizarre and fortunately rare disorder of unknown etiology, is characterized by bouts of somnolence and uncontrollable overeating (Yitzhak *et al.,* 1974). But again, as in the case of overt endocrine disorders associated with obesity, we must ask whether milder forms or hypothalamic disorders may not exist among those who become characterized as lazy and gluttonous.

12. *Exaggerated Insulin Response*

The effects of insulin on the central nervous system in relation to feeding have already been discussed (Section II,C,1). There is now considerable evidence that the obese secrete more insulin just on sight of food. In 1966 Pernick *et al.* (1966) found that the mere sight of food could induce a fall in serum free fatty acids, and Parra-Covarrubias *et al.* in 1971 found a 20% increase in insulin above baseline in adolescent obese children. As noted, Sjöstrom *et al.* (1980) found that the cephalic response to food-related stimuli was significantly higher in obese women than in normal subjects. Also as noted, the Yale group (Rodin *et al.,* 1985) has shown a specific relationship between hyperinsulinemia and perceived sweetness of sucrose in normals, but obese subjects have not yet been studied. It will be valuable to learn whether subtypes of the obese differ in responsiveness.

13. *A Possible Adverse Effect of Sugar Substitutes*

Sweeteners are consumed in formidable amounts by persons concerned with gaining weight. It seems probable that a conditioned cephalic insulin response could develop from drinking a no-calorie soft drink instead of tap water. In this event hunger and appetite for a meal several hours later could increase. It does seem important to establish whether such drinks should be labeled by the Surgeon General as dangerous to health in the overweight.

14. *Increased Responsiveness to External Stimuli*

Twenty years ago Schachter (1968) carried out studies on spontaneous eating habits of Columbia undergraduates under various conditions of caloric preload, manipulated clock time, and availability of food. He concluded that obese subjects responded excessively to external cues and stimuli. This was put to further test in a hospital cafeteria by Meyers and Stunkard (1980). Over 6 days the accessibility of low- and high-caloric foods was manipulated. No difference in range of selections of normal, overweight, or obese persons could be detected. Rodin (1976) reviewed the current evidence and concluded that both genetic factors and early experience appear to influence responsiveness to external cues and can lead to overeating when food is freely available. This is consistent with Garn's emphasis (1984) on the importance of influences within the family in determining what might be interpreted as genetic in origin. Drewnowski and Greenwood (1983) have used a novel three-dimensional method of analyzing the overall pleasantness and appeal ("hedonic ratings" to the trade) of various foods containing fat and carbohydrate. They concluded that the content of fat is an important component. In view of this, the increasing content of fat in the American diet is a matter of concern. Again, this is an area in which it is difficult to generalize, and characterization of individuals is important for providing optimal help.

15. *Decreased Physical Activity*

The role of physical activity in obesity was the subject of a major section of the Third International Congress on Obesity (Björntorp *et al.*, 1981) to which the reader is referred for more detailed review.

Long-term physical training of obese persons yields the same benefits as in the lean, with added advantages (Mayer, 1965b). Reduced physical activity and excessive weight seem to go together. For survival this may make sense; accumulated fuel stores can be conserved in anticipation of a later famine. It was our impression that as the volunteers of our Vermont Study approached peak weight they lost initiative for independent projects, and the supervisors of their work assignments reported the same. Even when engaging in group activity, overweight young persons move less. In a famous study with Mayer, Bullen *et al.* in 1964 documented the reduced spontaneous activity of obese adolescent girls. Analysis of moving picture films of those taking part in activities such as swimming indicated that in spite of the greater energy required to move their bodies, they were remarkably economical of effort. Rose and Williams (1962) study on students indicated that the characteristic correlating best with normal weight maintenance whether a large or small eater was the speed of spontaneous walking.

Ravussin and Bogardus (1985) have made a preliminary report of an important component of daily activity, namely, "fidgeting." They studied 60 subjects with body fat ranging from 7 to 52% in the new human respiratory chamber in the National Institutes of Health Research Center at Phoenix and recorded fidgeting motions by means of radar and a wrist sensor. They calculated that while the thermic effect of food ranged from 55 to 363 kcal per day, the activity factor, even within the confines of the chamber, could account for 75–790 kcal per day. Thus the level of spontaneous activity or its lack can make a considerable difference. As part of a rehabilitation plan for the obese some conscious activity has to be fitted into the life pattern.

Reduction of energy expenditure can be important in two ways for the person wrestling with the problem of obesity. Reduction of caloric intake in normals may be accompanied by a reduction in discretionary or obligatory physical activity (*Nutrition Reviews,* 1984). Reduced physical activity could also be a primary factor in the production and maintenance of obesity. Once again, the problem may be the heterogeneity of obesity; some may and others may not reduce activity. In some, inactivity may precede the development of obesity, as in the *ob/ob* mouse, and in others it may be a consequence of obesity. There may be multiple factors tending to reduce physical activity. Mayer's review (1965b) could as well have been entitled "Obesity as a major factor in physical activity." Not all children react the same way to environmental factors. Those with the genetic background for becoming MODY (maturity-onset diabetes of youth) or adult type II diabetics may be less inclined to sports than their peers. As Mayer pointed out, once obesity is established the heavy burden of self-blame and inferiority sets up a vicious cycle in which activity may be further reduced and obesity ultimately increases.

There is evidence that at least some obese persons differ in response to exercise. Short periods of exercise by normal persons increase resting metabolic rate and the thermic response to meals or infused glucose and insulin for as long as 18 hours (see Section II,E,4). Conversely, Segal and Gutin (1983) found that the striking increase in thermogenic response to exercise taken after a meal was reduced in obese persons. Dallasso and James (1984a) did not find the converse, however. In studies employing a calorimetry chamber there was no apparent interaction between exercise and the thermic effect of a meal in normal or overfed subjects.

Devlin and Horton (1985) studied the effect of exercise to exhaustion 12–14 hours previously in six obese subjects (30.4% fat) and six normal subjects (14.5% fat) on the response to a euglycemic–hyperglycemic insulin clamp procedure. Splanchnic glucose production was estimated by means of D-[3-^{3}H]glucose. The exercise consisted of cycle riding at 85% of VO_2 max in short bouts until exhaustion of the quadriceps. Serum insulin concentrations were raised to 95–150 and to 3300–5000 μU/ml with serum glucose maintained near 90 mg/dl. The initial disposal rates were not significantly different either before or after exercise. During the low- and high-insulin infusions the lean showed an increase of 2.7 and 16% in total glucose disposal after the exercise, respectively, and the obese 35 and 25%. Only the latter was significant. In the obese subjects, insulin-stimulated glucose disposal was increased significantly by the prior exercise, but not entirely to normal.

In both groups there was a comparable increase in nonoxidative glucose disposal, with reduced glucose and increased lipid oxidation. Thus the major effect was to alter the pathways of glucose disposal in favor of the nonoxidative. It is difficult to draw conclusions regarding possible differences between the response of the lean and obese, because of variation within the latter group. The obese group displayed extremely wide ranges for serum insulin (mean 34 μU/ml; standard deviation 32) and three of the group showed impaired tolerance to a 75-g glucose test. Standard deviation of the percentage body fat was 5.4 with a mean of 30.4. Thus among the obese there may well have been representatives of subgroups with quite different responses.

Exercise yields additional dividends for the obese in a program of dietary therapy. Bogardus *et al.* (1984), when in our laboratory, studied the effect of 3-day-a-week aerobic training added to dietary restriction in a group of patients with obesity and mild non-insulin-dependent diabetes. Those with added exercise had a 30% increase in glucose disposal during a euglycemic–hyperinsulinemic clamp study. Both groups showed improved glucose disposal, but only the physically trained developed an increase in nonoxidative glucose disposal, presumably reflecting an increased conversion of glucose to glycogen. There was considerable heterogeneity among subjects, particularly with respect to their results for fasting plasma insulin concentrations (163 ± 96 and 143 ± 76 pmol/liter in the two groups) and the range of response to stimuli was also large. Thus one cannot know how subjects at various stages of the disorder might respond to the two regimens. The overall follow-up of this study, however, was discouraging. The subjects, mean age 45 years (± 10) and varied in duration of diabetes, took part in an intensive and supportive program, in which investigators actively shared in the training sessions. The follow-up at 1 year in regard to sustained weight loss and continued exercise was moderately encouraging, but at 2 years it was thoroughly disheartening. Only 2 of 18 subjects returned questionnaires, and they reported no progress. This illustrates the main limitation, with this age group and duration of diabetes, of this approach to insulin resistance in obesity and in obesity with diabetes.

In Woo's studies on increased physical activity and food intake, overweight, exercising subjects failed to eat enough to maintain body weight (Woo *et al.,* 1982). This was in contrast to the response of lean subjects (Woo *et al.,* 1985). It is uncertain whether this difference applies to the free-living person. One possible limitation of inpatient studies is that institutionalized obese subjects almost uniformally fail to maintain weight even during the baseline period. This is strikingly illustrated by the studies of Hashim *et al.* (1965) employing a syringe feeding device, and those of Pi-Sunyer *et al.* (1984) using covertly monitored meals. This limitation may also explain why Schutz *et al.* (1982b) were unable to detect a difference in spontaneous activity between lean and obese subjects confined to a respiratory chamber to monitor physical activity.

16. *Possible Decreased Na^+,K^+-ATPase and Sodium Pump Activity*

A large part of our resting energy expenditure, variously estimated as 20–50%, is devoted to pumping the primordial seawater, acquired during the early stage of our evolution, out of our cells. In some small animals with genetic obesity there is a reduction in muscle and liver of the Na^+,K^+-ATPase required for pumping sodium to the extracellular fluid. Contradictory findings have been reported in human beings. DeLuise *et al.* (1983) described a subset of obese subjects with a reduced number of sodium pumps, as have Klimes and associates in obese Pima Indians (1982), though others reported an increase. In a recent study by Hawkins *et al.* (1984) of an assorted collection of 25 obese persons no relationship was found. Similarly Pasquali *et al.* found no abnormality of ^{86}Rb uptake of digoxin binding to erythrocytes in 34 obese patients in comparison with controls, and there was no relation between ATPase activity and serum concentrations of thyroid hormones in the obese. There were no alterations with dietary restriction. Again the subjects were minimally characterized. This is another area in which study of more fully characterized subjects is indicated.

17. *Giving Up Smoking as a Contributor to Obesity*

The possible mechanisms whereby cigarette smoking may reduce body weight in normal persons were reviewed in Section III,B. The converse is well established, namely, that it is common experience to gain weight on stopping smoking, and some with a tendency toward obesity continue smoking for this reason (*Nutrition Reviews,* 1984). This is unfortunate, for it may mean exchanging one set of risk factors for another. There is a need for more basic studies to determine how long the increased appetite and possibly decreased activity of the thyroid and metabolic rate persist and how they can best be countered.

18. *The Effect of Pharmacological Agents*

Weight gain at the times associated with hypertension has been attributed to use of oral contraceptive agents, perhaps as a result of mimicking some of the endocrine effects of pregnancy. This has been less of a problem since more effective schedules with lower dosage of diabetogenic hormones have been developed.

Experimental animals can be fattened by giving excess insulin chronically. Similarly, excess insulin in management of type I diabetes can make a patient eat in excess to counter its effect. In type II diabetes there is the hazard that weight gain during treatment with either oral agents or insulin may initiate a vicious cycle of increased insulin resistance and increased dosage. Diets acutely restricted in caloric content and in percentage of carbohydrate under appropriate supervision may be useful in interrupting such cycles.

19. *The Possibility That Some Older Obese Persons Are Limited in Cognitive Skills*

Perlmuter *et al.* (1984) released a study with sobering results of 140 patients with non-insulin-dependent diabetes. In comparison to control subjects well matched for age and past experience, the patient group was impaired in cognitive ability to a degree that could interfere with adherence to medical programs. The degree of overweight was not indicated. A third of the patients were treated by diet alone, and it is not clear how they compared with the group as a whole. There was a direct relationship between the degree of cognitive impairment and increase in glycosylation of hemoglobin, an index of the adequacy of control. These findings place a premium upon early and aggressive treatment of this common disorder. In view of the association of obesity and impaired glucose tolerance, further studies, particularly on obese subjects with milder glucose intolerance, would be of value.

20. *The Possibility in the Obese of Reduced Facultative Thermogenesis in Response to Caloric Excess and Difficulties in Its Evaluation*

I have left the two major questions to the end of this section. First, there is conflicting evidence and much controversy whether the obese gain more efficiently than normal subjects when taking calories in excess of maintenance requirements. Second, do the obese retain fat stores more avidly at their weight than do normal subjects at their weight when caloric intake is reduced?

James *et al.* (1978) and others have shown that in the obese increased lean body mass leads to increased energy expenditure (James *et al.*, 1978). Ravussin *et al.* (1983, 1985e) showed in our laboratory that the resting metabolic rate related to fat-free mass of obese patients with non-insulin-dependent diabetes was significantly greater than that of obese subjects with normal glucose tolerance and a comparable lean body mass. One might then ask, if this is so, why should a possible reduction in a process that might at most account for perhaps 10% of total energy expenditure be of any importance? But both the adult lean and the obese are essentially at equilibrium most of the time and the latter unfortunately usually are slowly gaining. If both attend a banquet and take on a given excess of calories, it is a matter of importance if the overweight and insulin-resistant person retains more energy. On the other hand, the apparent increased metabolic "efficiency" of the obese when attempting weight reduction appears to be a response shared with the lean upon caloric restriction. They differ in the range of weight at which the adaptation is called into play. Perhaps efficiency is not the right word, since housekeeping tasks such as repair of body protein are retarded during such weight loss in the interests of survival.

A decreased faculative thermogenesis can be only one of the many potential problems of the obese. A seer once remarked, "There is a simple answer to any problem, and it is most often wrong." There is no simple answer to the multiple problems that may be brought out by plenitude.

We reviewed in Section III,A,2 and Table I recent evidence for and against the existence of facultative or adaptive increases in thermogenesis in normal persons in response to caloric excess similar to that in smaller animals. Realizing that one cannot do justice to careful and perhaps intricate protocols in this way, I have outlined in Table III 26 studies carried out within the past 10 years which bear on the problem. In only approximately two-thirds of the studies is it concluded that there is defective thermogenesis with overfeeding in the obese. Certain sources of bias have been partially avoided in some of the later studies, and thus I believe that the weight of evidence favors the existence of a defect in a facultative response to caloric excess in the obese.

It may be useful to those reviewing past studies or planning future ones to review the many variables outlined in Section II,E that can affect the thermogenic response. It is apparent that many of these variables can bias the results. Clinical investigation is admittedly difficult, however, and some compromises must be accepted. A detailed consideration follows in the sections below.

a. The Characteristics of the Test Meal. Le Blanc *et al.* (1985) have shown that the thermogenic response to reasonably appetizing meal is greater than to the same ingredients ground and made into unappetizing wafers. In many of the studies in the obese unappetizing, and perhaps nauseating, liquid test drinks were used. There were too few meal tests to say whether this affected the results.

b. The Size of the Challenge. Of the studies in Table III there were three times as many positive results using a test feeding containing 400 or more kcal. The results in the two studies in which less was given were divided. In some studies the size of the test feeding was matched to the size of the patient, but, as Hill *et al.* (1984) have shown, the size of the thermogenic response bears a direct relationship to the size of the challenge. Garrow putatively stated, "A log of a given size gives off the same amount of heat in a small or large stove," but the degree of sympathetic response can vary.

c. Heterogeneity of Experimental Subjects. In nine of the studies no useful details were provided to characterize the obese as to age of onset, family history of diabetes or hyperlipidemia, evidence for insulin resistance, or differences in distribution of body fat (though a number of investigators had taken skinfold measurements). In five studies childhood onset was mentioned, and diminished thermogenic responses were reported in three of these. The central type of obesity in adults is now well known to be more strongly associated with metabolic disease. In one study in which the subjects were stated to have obesity of central distribution, Schwartz *et al.* (1985) reported that there was definite evidence of reduced thermogenesis. The A/H ratio (abdominal/hip circumference) should now be part of the data base for subjects in this field. The need for this was further emphasized at the recent meeting in Marseille (Vague *et al.*, 1985).

d. Degree of Hyperinsulinemia and Insulin Resistance. The concentration of insulin in the plasma may also be useful in characterizing experimental subjects and in the selection of suitable controls. It is not surprising that plasma insulin should appear to be a predictor of the thermogenic response. Cunningham *et al.* (1983) found that rats with a reduced glucose tolerance gained most readily when given a cafeteria diet. Schwartz *et al.* (1983b) found that patients with increased insulin resistance tended to show diminished thermogenic reactions, and Golay *et al.* (1983) and Schutz *et al.* (1984b) reported that the same was true for obese patients with frank diabetes. The difference noted by Golay *et al.* was significant relative to young or age-matched controls. While working in our laboratory Ravussin and Bogardus (1985a) showed by means of the euglycemic–hyperinsulinemic clamp technique with simultaneous calorimetry that the thermogenic response varied inversely with degree of insulin resistance and rate of glucose disposal. In an ingenious experiment in the Lausanne laboratory, using a reverse clamp procedure and indirect calorimetry, Ravussin, Danforth, and others studied the relation between rate of glucose disposal and increase in thermogenesis (Ravussin *et al.*, 1983). A given rate of glucose disposal ("M" value) was associated with the same thermogenic response in lean as in obese subjects. The study was accomplished by varying the amount of infused insulin rather than of glu-

TABLE III

STUDIES OF THE EFFECT OF EXCESS CALORIC INTAKE ON THERMOGENESIS IN OBESE SUBJECTS[a]

Investigators	Subtype subjects (obese/control)	Study type	Overfeeding		Test MR duration	Facult. DIT	NE in plasma/urine	NE appearance and clearance	Serum T_3	Exercise cost	Fasting insulin ratio of insulin to glucose	Conclusions and comments
			Days form	kcal P-F-C (%)								
Studies supporting a facultative component												
Kaplan and Leveille (1976)	Childhood 4/4	TG after meal; indirect calorimetry	— L	832 82-2-16	5 hours	Less	—	—	—	—	Increased 50% 0.17	TG reduced in obese per weight and per fat-free mass
Pittet *et al.* (1976)	No details 11/10	TG from C; direct and indirect calorimetry	— L	50 g C (2–4 hours)	2.5 hours	Less	—	—	—	—	? ?	Obese have greater lipid oxidation. Thermic effect less in obese
Zahorska-Markiewicz (1980)	— 14/10	RMR measured after meal and exercise; indirect calorimetry	— M	Mixed meal	1.5 hours + exercise time	Less	—	—	—	Decreased in control only	—	TG increased in both obese and control groups after meal. Exercise increased TG further only in control group
Shetty *et al.* (1981)	Healthy, euthyroid 5/5	TG from mixed diet; indirect calorimetry	— L	580 21-47-32	2 hours	Less	Increased in obese	—	Same	—	Increased 28% 0.14	Familial and reduced obese showed half the TG response
Golay *et al.* (1982)	Normal glucose tolerance	TG from C; indirect calorimetry	— L	100 g C	3 hours	Less	—	—	—	—	Increased 36% (85%+ in DM)	TG less in obese and in obese non-insulin-dependent DM versus own controls
Sharief (1982)	— 5/6	TG from sucrose or glucose	— L	5 g/kg ideal body weight	3 hours	Less	—	—	—	—	—	TG greater in controls after sucrose than glucose but not significantly different in obese
Segal and Gutin (1983)	Few details 10/10	TG during exercise after meal	— M	910 kcal 14-40-46	4 hours	Same	—	—	—	Decreased	—	TG less in exercise postmeal in obese

Ravussin *et al.* (1983)	Age 29–33 7/10	TG during euglycemic clamp	— —	iv C (clamp)	4 hours	—	—	—	—	—	Increased 175% 0.11	TG decreased in obese
Schwartz *et al.* (1983a)	Adult 6/7	TG from C; indirect calorimetry	— L	800 15-0-85	2 hours	Less	Same	—	?	—	— —	TG less in adult-onset centripetally obese. Much individual variation
Bessard *et al.* (1983)	Childhood onset 6/6	TG after mixed meal; indirect, 24 hours	— L	60% basal 17-29-54	Increased with 24 hours	— Less	— —	— —	—	—	Increased 120% 0.28	TG less in obese and reduced obese. Total RMR greater
Schutz *et al.* (1984b)	±DM 32/30	TG from C; indirect calorimetry	— L	100 g C	3 hours	Less	—	—	—	—	Increased ?	TG reduced in all obese versus age-matched controls
Schutz *et al.* (1984a)	Young, middle-aged 20/8	TG response to 3 meals; in chamber with activity monitor	— M	3 meals 15-40-45	24 hours	Less	—	—	—	—	— —	TG corrected for activity and night NE excretion less in young obese
Bogardus (1985)	Pima/Caucasian 11–13/11–13 (matched)	Response to low or high dose of insulin; clamp			Clamp	—	—	—	—	—	—	Reduced thermic response to low insulin dose in Pimas. Same as high dose
Segal (1985)	30% body fat 8/8	TG response to food ± exercise, weight matched	3 M	750 14-32-54	3 hours	—	—	—	—	Less	Increased 100% 0.27	With same BMI, TG less in obese (total and per fat-free mass)
Vernet *et al.* (1986a)	No family history of DM 9/8	Response to iv nutrient and propranolol	— iv	Double 18-30-52	4 hours	Same (iv)	Lower	—	—	—	Slightly increased	SNS modulates RMR and iv response in lean but not in obese
Bazelmans *et al.* (1985)	Childhood onset 6	Response of NE flux to overfeeding	10 M	1000/m^2 body surface 15-40-45	None	—	Erratic	—	—	—	— —	NE flux did not change with body weight as in lean

(*continued*)

TABLE III (*Continued*)

Investigators	Subtype subjects (obese/control)	Study type	Overfeeding: Days form	Overfeeding: kcal P-F-C (%)	Test MR duration	Facult. DIT	NE in plasma/urine	NE appearance and clearance	Serum T_3	Exercise cost	Fasting insulin ratio of insulin to glucose	Conclusions and comments
Studies not supporting a facultative component												
Glick *et al.* (1977)	Childhood onset 4/4	TG after mixed meal and during exercise	5 M	2300 Mixed	3× a day	Same	—	—	—	Same	— —	No increased TG in normal or obese (25% controls had family history of diabetes)
Nair *et al.* (1983)	"Healthy" 5/5	TG from P, F, or C	— L	300 kcal (P, F, or C)	2.5 hours	Same	—	—	—	—	Increased 18–200%	TG same as in lean. Glucose oxidation same
Felig *et al.* (1983)	Childhood onset 10/10	TG from meal; indirect calorimetry	— L	800 kcal 15-40-45	3 hours	Same	Increased in obese	—	—	—	? Increased 30% 0.25	TG response same as in lean. RMR obese same per lean body mass
Welle and Campbell (1983)	No details 13/11	TG from C; indirect calorimetry	— L	100 g C	3 hours	Same	Same	—	—	—	? Increased 50% Both low	TG same as in lean. Obese slightly more hyperinsulinemic

Blaza and Garrow (1983)	Age 20–46 5/5	Effect of exercise, cold, and food	— M	4–4.4 MJ 11-44-45	Chamber (direct)	Slightly more	—	—	—	Same	— —	Same response with food or exercise as lean
Webb and Annis (1983)	Age 40–50 5/5	Effect of overfeeding; direct and indirect calorimetry	30 M	1000 Varied	24 hours "space suit"	Raised with high P and F	—	—	—	—	— —	Inefficient gain with P and F. Lean and obese same response
Katzeff *et al.* (1985)	Childhood onset 6/6	TG from NE and exercise after overfeeding	21 M	1000 15-35-50	3 hours	—	Lower	Mean rates of clearance similar	Same	Same	Same ?	No differences in lean versus obese (both same fasting insulin)
Kush *et al.* (1986)	Pima Indian 5/5	TG from food, iv NE, and exercise	21 M and L	1000 20-35-45	3.5 hours (800 kcal)	Same	Same	—	—	—	—	RMR, TG response to meal and exercise same in lean and obese. NE response same with comparable concentrations
Vernet (1986b)	Moderate 10/10	TG response, iv and intragastric	— L	— 18-30-52	6 hours	Same	Same	—	—	—	— —	Facultative TG same in lean and obese; iv and intragastric TG same
Ravussin *et al.* (1986)	Pbese 9/6	TG with same glucose disposal. Clamp	— —	— —	4 hours	—	Increased	—	—	—	—	Same TG with same rate of uptake

[a] For abbreviations see Tables I and III.

cose. In spite of their greater insulin resistance there was no difference under these conditions between the lean and the obese in "obligatory" and "facultative" components of thermogenesis. This indicates that under conditions in which the insulin resistance is overcome, the obese (and presumably also the obese type II diabetic) do not differ in thermogenic response from the normal. But this, of course, is not the natural condition, and they do differ under usual circumstances.

Values for fasting and sometimes postprandial plasma insulin concentrations are provided in 11 of the studies of thermogenesis in obesity in Table III. In eight of these there was definite relative hyperinsulinemia, and in seven there was evidence of a facultative increase in thermogenesis. In at least one study the fasting insulin concentration was increased in both experimental and control groups (Nair *et al.*, 1983). In another study (Katzeff *et al.*, 1985) fasting insulin values and their ratio to glucose were so low in both groups as to suggest that these relatively young obese volunteers, ranging in age from 20 to 29, may have been physically active with minimal insulin resistance. Insulin concentrations alone, however, are not always an adequate indication of the degree of insulin resistance. The mean fat-free mass of the two groups was similar. Thus the experimental subjects may not qualify as representative of obesity in general, as usually seen in the adult population.

e. The Age of the Subjects. The choice of age of subjects raises a number of questions which have been discussed in Section II,C. As noted, any change in resting metabolic rate may be more a reflection of change in the fat-free mass than of age per se.

f. Heterogeneity of Control Subjects. Ideally subjects should be matched on the basis of respiring mass, but in view of the changes usually associated with age, matching for age is a second best. Schultz *et al.* (1984b) appropriately provided older controls for the older obese subjects who had either impaired or abnormal glucose tolerance. The percentage increase in thermogenic response related to glucose uptake was 8.7% in young controls, compared to 5.7% in middle-aged controls. Webb and Annis (1983), in their study of thermogenesis using a calorimetric "space suit," did limit subjects or controls to the fifth decade in age. In this study, however, two subjects classified as "obese" ranged in percentage body fat from 11 to 27%. In another study (Glick *et al.*, 1977) one of the four control subjects gave a family history of obesity and of diabetes in a close relative. It is, of course, not easy to obtain ideal experimental and control subjects. In our Vermont Study we belatedly learned that one volunteer had an obese grandmother with type II diabetes. He turned out to be an easy gainer and somewhat reluctant loser.

g. The Problem of the Physiologically Obese Control Subject and the Healthy Obese Experimental Subject. As noted in Section V,A, Ruderman *et al.* (1981) have described subjects of normal weight by the usual criteria, but physiologically obese in character. There are others who are overweight by conventional standards and have increased fat mass, but are basically very healthy. They may be at the very upper end of the distribution curve for body fat and have been above conventional weight since childhood. They are the hyperplastic obese, with an increased number of evenly distributed adipocytes, and may be vigorous and active. Those with the central distribution of fat who tend to have more insulin resistance and ultimately more impaired glucose tolerance, diabetes, and hyperlipidemia have already been referred to under experimental subjects. The increase in the concentration of insulin in the plasma should help to distinguish these physiologically obese from the healthy obese.

The relation between RMR and fat-free mass, which we now know to be somewhat variable and under genetic influence, has been discussed previously (Section II,B). No reference is ideal, but it seems more logical to report physiological variables as related to this parameter. Yet in quite a few of the studies body composition has been estimated by skinfold measures alone or not at all.

h. Duration of the Measurement of the RMR. Especially in earlier studies thermogenesis after meals had been monitored barely long enough to include the peak of the response. In none of the tests with indirect calorimetry hoods has the RMR been followed to baseline, so that the total response of control and experimental subject remains uncertain. Three out of the four studies greater than 24 hours in duration utilizing chamber calorimetry have shown a diminished thermogenic response in the obese.

i. Menstrual Cycle. The stage of the menstrual cycle must be taken into consideration because the changes in RMR already described (Section II,C) may add further to variability of results.

j. Physical Activity as a Component of Energy Expenditure. The importance of the level of physical activity for energy balance of the overweight has been considered in relation to normal subjects (Section II,E,4) and was further discussed relative to the overweight (Section V,B,15). This factor must be considered in research protocols. In most protocols the activity level of subjects while confined and under study or while free living cannot be adequately accounted for. One subject may expend calories by "fidgeting," as already noted, while another may not. The marked variability among subjects is particularly important. The long-term assay of energy expenditure by the technique of Schoeller (1983) using doubly labeled water may be useful, since measurements correlate well with those of calorimetry (Klein *et al.*, 1984; Ravussin *et al.*, 1985) while subjects follow their normal daily routines. I understand that current reports from the workshop on this technique held during the Thirteenth International Congress of Nutrition Meeting in 1985 have been encouraging. Expense and need for mass spectrometry, however, are current disadvantages.

21. *Possibly Greater Reduction of Metabolic Rate during Caloric Restriction*

The response of obese subjects to the reduction of caloric intake is the second area of considerable controversy (Table IV). The discouraging results of attempted weight reduction are all too well known. When reduced below their usual weight, the obese apparently develop the same responses as those of undernourished normal-weight subjects, as described in Section IV). It is often claimed on the basis of dietary histories that some obese persons maintain their reduced weight with very low caloric intake, but there is also evidence that for psychological reasons obese people may underreport their intake of food (Sjöström, 1985). The key question is whether a person who has lost considerable weight requires the same or fewer calories to maintain his new weight than does a normal person of similar body composition who is not restricted.

The response of normal subjects to overfeeding and the evidence of O'Dea *et al.* (1982) that norepinephrine turnover is decreased in man as well as in small animals by caloric deprivation were reviewed in Section IV. The degree of disagreement between laboratories is not quite so great here as in the studies of facultative thermogenesis in response to overeating in normals and obese, but is still considerable. Of the 12 studies, eight are in favor of an increase in metabolic efficiency with caloric restriction in the obese. Most of the studies are marred by the same limitations as those already mentioned in the section on response to overfeeding.

Welle *et al.* (1984) were unable to find any evidence of unexplained decrease in RMR after short-term weight loss, in spite of a marked reduction in total T_3. Measurement of RMR was limited to morning sessions and extrapolated over 24 hours. Measurement over a 24-hour period, as in the experiment of Bessard *et al.* (1983) in the chamber at Lausanne, is advantageous. The findings of Bessard *et al.* in obese patients undergoing weight reduction were consistent with a decrease in thermogenesis beyond that expected from change in activity and body composition. Activity of subjects in the chamber was monitored by radar. Serum insulin and its ratio to glucose, urinary catecholamines, and T_3 all decreased. Resting metabolic rate related to lean body mass decreased significantly. Diet-induced thermogenesis was less than normal before weight reduction and was unchanged by weight reduction. In subjects with familial obesity Schutz *et al.* (1984b) in the same laboratory found reduced glucose-induced thermogenesis upon weight reduction which was independent of body weight. The fact that this reduction persisted after weight loss was interpreted as indicating a primary defect. It seems equally possible, however, that different and independent mechanisms may have reduced the glucose-induced thermogenesis subsequent to weight reduction.

The original findings of Esler's laboratory (O'Dea *et al.,* 1982) in normal subjects undergoing caloric excess or restriction were tested by Bazelmans *et al.* (1985) in four to six obese subjects. None of the changes between hypo- or hypercaloric and isocaloric diets were significant. This would support the concept of limited facultative thermogenesis with overfeeding, but not that of increased efficiency of the obese with underfeeding. The number of subjects was small and the spread of data was limited, so these observations require confirmation.

Leibel and Hirsch (1984) evaluated retrospectively under clinical research center conditions the caloric requirements of 26 former patients who had lost considerable weight. The patients averaged 152 kg in weight initially and were not diabetic. When restudied over 7-day periods they required 28% fewer calories per square meter of body surface area than before weight reduction, and 24% less than age- and sex-matched controls. Total energy requirement was slightly less than that of the controls even though they weighed 60% more. Actual mean caloric requirements per 24 hour per square meter of body surface area were 1432 ± 32 for the obese, 1021 ± 32 after weight loss, and 1341 ± 33 for the controls. There was no measure of body composition, so that caloric requirement per fat-free mass could not be evaluated, and the controls, from a study of arteriosclerotic vascular disease, may not have been optimal. These figures are to be contrasted with 2300 kcal required to maintain peak weight in the experimentally obese subjects of the Vermont Study (Sims *et al.,* 1968, 1973; Sims, 1976).

The Leibel and Hirsch findings are in sharp contrast to those of Dore *et al.* (1982) in Garrow's laboratory, who made a regression analysis of 140 obese women with respect to resting metabolic rate on weight and body composition derived from total body potassium. Dore *et al.* then studied the changes in RMR and body composition of 19 severely obese women and concluded that the requirement of obese patients for weight maintenance was similar to those of comparable weight who had not reduced. The means for the RMR of the reduced obese were

TABLE IV

STUDIES OF THE RESPONSE OF OBESE SUBJECTS TO REDUCTION OF CALORIC INTAKE

Investigators	Subjects (lean/obese)	Type of study	kcal deficit/days	kcal/P-F-C (%)	RMR per lean body mass	Test MR duration	NE	NE appearance and clearance (turnover)	Serum T_3	Fasting insulin ratio of insulin to glucose	Conclusions and comments
Studies not supporting a facultative component											
Dore *et al.* (1982)	0/19	RMR after 30 kg loss in severely obese	— 365	800 P 40 (milk)	See text	Hood in AM	—	—	—	—	Mean decrease in RMR same as predicted (see text)
Webb and Abrams (1983)	1/8	Energy balance with direct and indirect calorimetry	1000 42	—	12% decreased	"Space suit"	—	—	—	—	All but 362 kcal/day accounted for; possibly less free activity
Welle *et al.* (1984)	19/6	RMR and T_3 after rapid weight loss	35	472 70-0-30	Total decreased 9.4%	Hood in AM	—	—	Decreased 46%	—	Hypometabolic response cannot explain difficult weight loss
Bazelmans *et al.* (1985)	0/6	NE turnover with under-feeding in obese	— 10	400 15-40-45	—	—	n.s.[a] versus controls	n.s.[a]	—	—	No change in NE flux in obese with under- and over-feeding
Studies supporting a facultative component											
Bray (1969)	0/14	Weight loss in "grossly" obese	3050 28	450 (liquid) ?	Total 15% decreased	5 minutes 3×/day	—	—	—	—	Increased efficiency associated with decrease in α-glycerolphosphate dehydrogenase
Jung *et al.* (1979)	0/11	Weight loss normotensive, low carbohydrate	25% maintenance 18	9.2/kg (80 g P, 10 g F)	—	—	Plasma NE decreased; HMMA decreased	—	—	—	Decreased urinary and plasma catecholamines and blood pressure

O'Dea *et al.* (1982)	6/0	NE turnover with over- and underfeeding	— 10	400 15-40-45	—	—	n.s.[a] —	All decreased ($p < 0.05$)	Decreased ($p < 0.001$)	—	NE turnover varied with short-term underfeeding. Plasma NE poor index
Bessard *et al.* (1983)	0/5	DIT and TG in calorimetry chamber (24 hours)	12.1 kg loss/77 days	60% basal rate (P suppl.) 17-29-54	Decreased ($p < 0.01$)	Chamber, 24 hours	Decreased in urine	—	Decreased 35%	23 to 13 μU 0.26 to 0.14	24-hour energy expenditure due to higher BMR. DIT less before in obese and unchanged after weight loss
Leibel and Hirsch (1984)	0/26	Intake before and after weight loss	Variable 202	(33% weight loss)	—	—	—	—	—	—	Per square meter body surface caloric requirements in obese 25% less than predicted per body size
Schutz *et al.* (1984b)	30/27 (7-DM)	Glucose-induced TG after weight loss	— 28–42	550–750 (P suppl.) fast	Total decreased	3 hours	—	—	—	Increased	Reduced glucose-induced TG in familial obese independent of body weight
Ravussin *et al.* (1985a)	0/7	24-hour energy expenditure after weight loss	Variable 60–112	800–1100 (P suppl.) fast	No change	Chamber, 24 hours	—	—	Decreased 8%	27 to 19 μU/ml 0.29 to 0.24	Reduced 24-hour energy expenditure from decreased DIT and less cost activity
Warnold *et al.* (1978)	0/8	Long-term weight loss, with estimated energy balance in hyperplastic obese	1000–500 245	1100 (Mixed)	No change	Each of 4 periods	—	—	Normal	Increased	Loss less than predicted on the basis of calibrated heart rate activity, intake, and body composition

[a] n.s., Not significant.

almost identical to that predicted from the regression equation (234 and 232), but the standard deviation of the former was large and almost double that of the latter (± 26 versus ± 16). Thus I wonder whether a form of the "constancy" fallacy described by Garrow in the revision of his book (1978) may not be involved. The means are not different, but this, as he pointed out, could mean that the changes in different directions really occur in different people or that the error of the measurement is such that the changes are not real. Thus the two means cannot be taken to be the same. Since this is meticulous work and since obesity in man is so heterogeneous, I suspect the former, and that there may be a subpopulation, perhaps more like that studied by Hirsch and Leibel (1984), which does have a lower maintenance requirement.

Ravussin *et al.* (1985a) used the indirect calorimetry chamber at Lausanne to partition energy expenditure before and after weight loss in moderately to severely obese male and female patients (146–219% ideal body weight) ranging in age from 23 to 46. Energy expenditure over 24 hours related to fat-free mass (FFM) did decrease, although half of the drop in total expenditure was related to a reduction of the FFM. Most of the remaining decline in 24-hour energy expenditure could be explained by a reduction in the thermic effect of food, and the reduced cost of physical activity due to a lowering of body weight. The authors found little reason to evoke additional mechanisms. The study was meticulously carried out and as complete as any available to date. However, the standard errors of the means for the RMR and 24-hour are large, presumably due to heterogeneity of the subjects with respect to age, sex, degree of obesity, and perhaps other unspecified variables. Again one must wonder whether there may not be obscure differences due to the existence of subtypes.

We do not yet have a way directly to evaluate in man such elements of thermogenesis as substrate cycling and sodium pumping. One study, however, directed at underlying mechanisms is the enzymatic study of Bray (1969). In 1968 Stirling and Stock had found that the caloric wasting of rats subsisting on a diet low in protein was associated with an increase in the α-glycerol-phosphate dehydrogenase (α-GPDH) in liver which enhances oxidation of α-glycerol-phosphate via the dihydroacetone phosphate shuttle yielding a P : O ratio of 2 as opposed to 3. Bray then measured the soluble and mitochondrial α-GPDH (EC 1.1.1.8 and 1.1.99.5) in adipose tissue of obese patients before and after undergoing 10–15 days of a 900-kcal diet and found a reduction coincident with the reduction in resting metabolic rate. He suggested that this might contribute to metabolic efficiency. I am not aware of further studies along these lines.

Lars Sjöstrom (1986) found normal sensitivity and responsiveness to the thermogenic effect of epinephrine in obese subjects before weight reduction, but the response curves are shifted to the right during caloric restriction and early refeeding. The affinity of β-receptors was correspondingly reduced, and this reduction was more marked in the obese.

22. *Comment and Conclusions Regarding the Possibility of Reduced Facultative Thermogenesis with Overeating and Greater Efficiency during Weight Reduction in the Obese*

It is apparent that there are many factors, both genetic and environmental, which make it difficult for the overweight to conform to our present standards for body weight. Little can be done to modify some of them, and they must be respected. It may again reflect my personal bias, but on review of the many recent studies of thermogenesis, it appears that at least some subtypes of the obese are limited in their thermogenic response to excess calories and that this is conditioned by their degree of insulin resistance. It also appears that after weight reduction they suffer from increased efficiency of foodstuff utilization beyond that attributable to reduction of lean body mass and altered activity. Lean persons show similarity enhanced utilization when reduced below their weight "set points." Further controlled work will be required to establish the extent, range, and potential reversibility of these metabolic characteristics.

It is also apparent that psychological or behavioral factors are important. Any one alone might not produce the distressing problems of severe obesity, but one may reinforce the other, perhaps setting in motion a sequence of disorders each in turn amplifying the other. There are many interrelated mechanisms, some outlined above, that can contribute to unwanted storage of fat, and we are beginning to delineate subtypes of obesity.

VI. The Need for Improved Characterization of Obesity in Human Beings

It should now be clear that one of the main difficulties in resolving the important questions concerning energy balance and thermogenesis is the heterogeneity of human beings and of their disorders, all of which in various combinations can lead to development of obesity and its complications. It would be useful if we could assign specific diagnoses, but unfortunately we do not yet know enough. But gone are the days when Noorden's classification, beautiful in its simplicity, of "A. Exogenous" and "B. Endogenous" sufficed. It is all too similar to the current limited classification of the most ubiquitous form of diabetes, non-insulin-dependent diabetes, into "Type IIA Lean" and "Type IIB Obese" (National Diabetes Data Group, 1980). I suspect that it, too, must in time undergo revision and amplification.

Many attempted classifications of obesity were reviewed in the first conference on obesity at the Fogarty International Center and a recommended data base was provisionally outlined (Bray, 1975). This has been successively refined (Sims, 1984), but the diagnostic potential is limited in requiring that patients be put in one pigeon hole or another for purposes of classification. Five years ago the Nutrition Program of the then NIAMDD of the National Institutes of Health organized a planning meeting on methods of characterization of obesity. This led to a 3-day NIH workshop on the subject held in 1982 at Vassar College, the proceedings of which have recently been published (Callaway and Greenwood, 1984, 1985). A symposium on the same subject was also held in 1983 as part of the Fourth International Congress on Obesity (Hirsch and Van Itallie, 1985). Recent emphasis has been placed on characterization, since in the present state of our knowledge, attempts at rigid classification are not fruitful and may be counterproductive. The four panels of the Vassar workshop made recommendations on types of data to be collected systematically in reference to morphology, metabolic disorders, energy balance, behavioral and psychological factors, as well as risk factors associated with obesity.

It is recognized that no single data base or final classification can meet the diverse needs of clinical work, epidemiologic studies, or clinical investigation. A manual on standardized data collection and methodology is under development (Callaway and Greenwood, 1984).

Standardized data bases for the three areas of endeavor could provide many benefits. In clinical work identification of related risk factors and problems, genetic, anatomical, and metabolic, could aid in planning rational therapy and improving cost-effectiveness. As Callaway and Greenwood have emphasized (1985) fewer specific mechanisms leading to obesity would be statistically "washed out" in clinical investigation. Contradictory results from different laboratories could perhaps be reconciled if the responses of subgroups could be studied and the way pointed toward useful further studies. Epidemiological studies could be furthered by an increased ability to identify subtypes of the obese such those with incipient type II diabetes and hyperlipidemias. With organized data collection it should be possible in time to develop a meaningful classification, reducing the number of those tossed into the wastebasket of "exogenous obesity."

As I write I am looking at the screen of one of the microcomputers that have become standard equipment in most medical laboratories and clinical and home offices. The floppy disk could well hold a suitable data base, more knowledge about the potential disorders and disease states than any one person can keep in mind, and up-to-date details of the management options. For clinical work, management options can be adapted to the situation of a particular individual, and possible hazards avoided. Techniques are rapidly developing for handling data and for aiding in decision making. A promising one for this purpose is the Problem-Knowledge Coupling system developed by Weed (Sims *et al.*, 1985). I believe that development of a comprehensive system of this type should be given high priority and am pleased to share in this effort.

VII. Summary and Conclusions

In this article studies relevant to a number of important and controversial topics have been revisited in the hope of finding a consensus. A consensus remains elusive, but a number of conclusions seem reasonably certain.

1. The controls of food intake and energy expenditure in human beings are not simple; they are interdependent and are subject to many influences. It is unlikely that change in any single component can explain the major disturbances of energy balance in human beings.
2. There is a facultative component in the thermogenic responses to cold, excess caloric intake, and other stimuli of normal subjects, which originally had survival value.
3. There is a direct relationship between degree of insulin sensitivity and facultative response to overfeeding. A likely sequence is increase in effective serum insulin → central stimulation and activation of the sympathetic nervous system → increased turnover of norepinephrine → increased activity of substrate cycles, electrolyte pumping, and protein turnover, and possibly uncoupling of mitochondrial phosphorylation in brown fat.
4. The composition of the diet is important for energy balance and fat storage, independent of the total caloric content and palatability. Increase in the fraction of carbohydrate in the diet increases the dietary thermogenic response. Increase in the fraction of fat in isocaloric diets, at least in experimental animals, leads to a greater increase in body fat.
5. The various subtypes of the obese are subject to a distressingly large number of factors, genetic, metabolic, endocrine, psychological,

and, particularly in our present society, environmental, which work to perpetuate their excess energy reserves ("the demons within and without"). Many of these also once had survival value, and hence, are the more difficult to overcome.

6. In at least some subtypes of the obese and in those with non-insulin-dependent diabetes type IIB, the ability to adapt normally to a caloric excess is impaired. Such impairment is only one of many potential disturbances of the interlocking mechanisms determining energy balance and affects a relatively small proportion of the total energy expenditure.

7. When fasting, both normal persons and the obese conserve energy essentially by a reversal of the above processes. These mechanisms, however, become operative in at least some subtypes of the obese when the range of stores of energy are greater than in the normal.

8. The insulin resistance associated with obesity serves to make overt or to accentuate non-insulin-dependent diabetes, with its associated complications. The hyperinsulinemia and increased catecholamine turnover of at least some subtypes of the obese or of the physiologically obese are closely linked to hypertension. The two disorders are major contributors to development of cardiovascular disease and impairment of the quality of life. Thus considerations of energy balance in human beings are of great importance to both preventive and therapeutic medicine.

9. Research in the area of energy balance and related problems has been both costly and inefficient. A major problem is our inability to identify the diverse subtypes of the obese and to standardize basic investigative procedures. Our usual approach is to compare small groups of inadequately characterized obese subjects with a control group of normal subjects and to hope that the experiment will be blessed with the all-important significance at $p = 0.05$. If the aim were to compare horses and cows, it would be quite possible to include in the experimental group a few Percherons, burros, and jackasses, along with the Morgans and thoroughbreds and to emerge with the statistical conclusion that there really is no difference. Even if we cannot yet classify the overweight, I believe that it is now essential to refine methods of characterizing our subjects.

ACKNOWLEDGMENTS

First, to Dr. Raymond L. Zwemer, at P & S, Columbia (1938–1942), to Dr. John P. Peters and the Chemical Division of the Yale School of Medicine (1943–1950), and to Dr. Bernard R. Landau of Western Reserve University School of Medicine (1964–1965) for their contributions to my interest in metabolism, and second to the many collaborators and the volunteers in the Vermont Study of experimental obesity. The Study was supported by NIH Grant AM 10254 1-17 (EAHS) and AM 18535 (Dr. Danforth) and RR-109 (General Clinical Research Center).

REFERENCES

Abraham, S., and Nordsieck, M. (1960). The relationship of excess weight on children and adults. *Publ. Health Rep.* **75,** 263–273.

Acheson, K. J., Campbell, I. T., Edholm, O. G., Miller, D. S., and Stock, M. J. (1980). A longitudinal study of body weight and body fat changes in Antarctica. *Am. J. Clin. Nutr.* **33,** 972–977.

Acheson, K., Jequier, E., and J. Wahren (1983). Influence of beta-adrenergic blockade on glucose-induced thermogenesis in man. *J. Clin. Invest.* **72,** 981–986.

Acheson, K. J., Flatt, J. P., and E. Jequier (1982). Glycogen synthesis versus lipogenesis after a 500 gram carbohydrate meal in man. *Metabolism* **31,** 1234–1240.

Acheson, K., Schutz, Y., Bessard, E., Ravussin, E., Jequier, E., and Flatt, J. P. (1984a). Nutritional influences on lipogenesis and thermogenesis after a carbohydrate meal. *Am. J. Physiol.* **246,** E62–E70.

Acheson, K., Jequier, E., Burger, A., and Danforth, E., Jr. (1984b). Thyroid hormones and thermogenesis, the metabolic cost of food and exercise. *Metabolism* **33,** 262–265.

Acheson, K. J., Ravussin, E., Wahren, J., and Jequier, E. (1984c). Thermic effect of glucose in man. Obligatory and facultative thermogenesis. *J. Clin. Invest.* **74,** 1572–1580.

Angel, A., Hollenberg, C. H., and Roncari, D. A. K., eds. (1983). "The Adipocyte and Obesity: Cellular and Molecular Mechanisms." Raven, New York.

Astrup, A., Bulow, J., and Madsen, J. (1984). Interscapular brown adipose tissue blood flow in the rat. *Pflugers Arch.* **401,** 414–417.

Astrup, A. J., Bülow, J., Madsen, J., and Christensen, N. (1985). Contribution of BAT and skeletal muscle to thermogenesis induced by ephedrine in man. *Am J. Physiol.* **248** (*Endocrinol. Metab.* **11**), E507–E515.

Astwood, E. B. (1962). The heritage of corpulence. *Endocrinology* **71,** 337–341.

Balon, T. W., Zorzano, A., Goodman, M. N., and Ruderman, N. B. (1984). Insulin increases thermogenesis in rat skeletal muscle following exercise. *Am. J. Physiol.* **248** (*Endocrinol. Metab.* **11**), E148–E151.

Bazelmans, J., Nestel, P. J., O'Dea, K., and Esler, M. D. (1985). Blunted norepinephrine responsiveness to changing energy states in obese subjects. *Metabolism* **34,** 154–160.

Bazin, R., Planche, E., Dupuy, F., and Lavau, M. (1985). Evidence that corticosterone is not required for the emergence of obesity in Zucker *fa/fa* pups. *Int. Symp. Metab. Complicat. Hum. Obesity, Marseille.*

Benedict, F. G. (1915). A study of prolonged fasting. Publication No. 203. Carnegia Institute of Washington, D.C.

Benedict, F. G., Miles, W. R., Roth, P., and Smith, H. M. (1919). Human vitality under restricted diet. Publication No. 280. Carnegie Institute of Washington, D.C.

Bennett, W., and Gurin, J. (1982). "The Dieter's Dilemma. Eating Less and Weighing More," p. 315. Basic Books, New York.

Berchtold, P., Sims, E. A. H., and Brandau, K., eds. (1981). Obesity and hypertension. *Satellite Symp. Int. Congr. Obesity,* Florence, *3rd, Oct. 1980.* [*Int. J. Obesity* **5** (Suppl. 1)], 1–188.

Bessard, T., Schutz, Y., and Jequier, E. (1983). Energy expenditure and postprandial thermogenesis in obese women before and after weight loss. *Am. J. Clin. Nutr.* **38,** 680.

Beutler, B., Milsark, I. W., and Cerami, A. C. (1985). Passive immunization against cachectin. Tumor necrosis factor protects mice from lethal effect of endotoxin. *Science* **229,** 869–70.

Bielinski, R., Schutz Y., and Jequier, E. (1985). Energy metabolism during the postexercise recovery in man. *Am. J. Clin. Nutr.* **42,** 69–82.

Bier, D. M., Kaplan, S. L., and Havel, R. J. (1977). The Prader–Willi syndrome. Regulation of fat transport. *Diabetes* **26,** 874–881.

Billewicz, W. Z., and Thompson, A. M. (1970). Body weight in parous women. *Br. J. Soc. Prevent. Med.* **24,** 97–104.

Bisdee, J., James, W. P. T., Shaw, M. A., and Ashwell, M. (1985). Hormonal levels and changes in energy expenditure over the menstrual cycle. *Int. Symp. Metab. Complicat. Obesities, Marseilles, May 30-June 1.*

Björntorp, P. (1980). Results of conservative therapy of obesity: Correlation with adipose tissue morphology. *Am. J. Clin. Nutr.* **33,** 370–375.

Björntorp, P. (1985). Adipose tissue in obesity (Willendorf Lecture). *In* "Recent Advances in Obesity Research: IV" (J. Hirsch and T. B. Van Itallie, eds.). Libbey, London.

Björntorp, P., and Sjöström, L. (1971). Number and size of adipose tissue fat cells in relation to metabolism in human obesity. *Metabolism* **20,** 703–713.

Björntorp, P., Cairella, M., and Howard, A. N., eds. (1981). Recent advances in obesity research: III. *Proc. Int. Congr. Obesity, 3rd, Oct. 1980* pp. 1–392.

Blackburn, M. W., and Calloway, D. H. (1976a). Basal metabolic rate and work energy expenditure of mature pregnant women. *J. Am. Diet. Assoc.* **69,** 24–28.

Blackburn, M. W., and Calloway, D. H. (1976b). Energy expenditure and consumption of mature, pregnant and lactating women. *J. Am. Diet. Assoc.* **69,** 29–37.

Blaza, S., and Garrow, J. S. (1983). Thermogenic response to temperature, exercise and food stimuli in lean and obese women, studied by 24 h direct calorimetry. *Am. J. Nutr.* **49,** 171–180.

Bogardus, C., Ravussin, E., Robbins, D. R., Wolfe, R. R., Horton, E. S., and Sims, E. A. H. (1984). Effects of physical training and diet therapy on carbohydrate metabolism in patients with glucose intolerance and non-insulin-dependent diabetes milletus. *Diabetes* **33,** 311–318.

Bogardus, C., Lillioja, S., Mott, D., Zawadzki, Z., Young, A., and Abbott, W. (1985). Evidence for reduced thermic effect of insulin and glucose infusions in Pima Indians. *J. Clin. Invest.* **75,** 1264–1269.

Bouchard, C. (1985). Body composition in adopted and biological siblings. *Hum. Biol.* **57,** 61–75.

Bradfield, R. B., Paulos, J., and Grossman, L. (1971). Energy expenditure and heart rate of obese high school girls. *Am. J. Clin. Nutr.* **24,** 1482.

Bray, G. A. (1969). Effect of caloric restriction on energy expenditure in obese patients. *Lancet* **Aug. 23,** 397.

Bray, G. A. (1972). Lipogenesis in human adipose tissue: Some effects of nibbling and gorging. *J. Clin Invest.* **51,** 537.

Bray, G. A. (1984). Hypothalamic and genetic obesity: An appraisal of the autonomic hypothesis and the endocrine hypothesis. *Int. J. Obesity* **8** (Suppl. 1), 119–137.

Bray, G. A. (1986). Autonomic and endocrine factors in the regulation of energy balance. *Fed. Proc., Fed. Am. Soc. Exp. Biol.* **45,** 1404–1410.

Bray, G. A., and York, D. A. (1971). Genetically transmitted obesity in rodents. *Physiol. Rev.* **51,** 598–646.

Bray, G. A., and Nishizawa, Y. (1981). Hypothalamic obesity. The autonomic hypothesis and the lateral hypothalamus. *Diabetologia* **20,** 366–377.

Bray, G. A., and Gallagher, T. F., Jr. (1975). Manifestations of hypothalamic obesity in man: A comprehensive investigation of eight patients and a review of the literature. *Medicine (Baltimore)* **54,** 301–330.

Brook, C. G. D., Lloyd, J. K., and Wolf, O. H. (1972). Relation between age of onset of obesity and size and number of adipose cells. *Br. Med. J.* **2,** 25–27.

Brownell, K. D., and Stunkard, A. J. (1980). Physical activity in the development and control of obesity. *In* "Obesity" (A. J. Stunkard, ed.), pp. 300–324. Saunders, Toronto.

Brunzell, J. D., Schwartz, R. S., Eckel, R. H., and Goldberg, A. P. (1981). Insulin and adipose tissue lipoprotein lipase activity in humans. *Int. J. Obesity* **5,** 685–694.

Bullen, B. A., Reed, R. B., and Mayer, J. (1964). Physical activity of obese and non-obese adolescent girls appraised by motion picture sampling. *Am. J. Clin. Nutr.* **4,** 211–233.

Burse, R. L., Bynum, G. D., Pandoff, K. B., Goldman, R. F., Sims, E. A. H., and Danforth, E., Jr. (1975). Increased appetite and unchanged metabolism upon cessation of smoking with diet held constant. *Physiologist* **18,** 157.

Cahill, G. F., Jr. (1970). Starvation in man *N.E. J. Med.* **282,** 668–675.

Callaway, C. W., and Greenwood, M. R. C. (1984). Introduction to the workshop on methods for characterizing human obesity. *Int. J. Obesity* **8,** 477–480.

Cannon, W. B. (1932). "The Wisdom of the Body," pp. 198–199. Norton, New York.

Castonguay, T. W., Applegate, E. A., Upton, D. E., and Stern, J. S. (1984). Hunger and appetite: Old concepts/new distinctions. *In* "Nutrition Reviews Present Knowledge in Nutrition." The Nutrition Foundation, Washington, D.C.

Chaffee, R. R., Allen, J. R., Cassuto, Y., and Smith, R. E. (1964). Biochemistry of brown fat and liver of cold-acclimated hamsters. *Am. J. Physiol.* **207,** 1211.

Chakrabarty, K., Tauber, J. W., Sigel, B., Bombeck, C. T., and Jeffay, H. (1984). Glycerokinase activity in human adipose tissue as related to obesity. *Int. J. Obesity* **8,** 609–622.

Chirico, A.-M., and Stunkard, A. J. (1960). Physical activity and human obesity. *New Engl. J. Med.* **263,** 935–940.

Chopra, I. J., Huang, T. S., Beredo, A., Solomon, G. N., Chua Teco, and Mead, J. F. (1985). Evidence for an inhibitor of extrathryoidal conversion of thyroxine to 3,5,3′-triiodothyronine in sera of patients with nonthyroidal illnesses. *J. Clin. Endocrinol. Metab.* **60,** 666.

Christin, L., Nacht, C.-A., Vernet, O., Ravussin, E., Jequier, E., and Acheson, K. J. (1985). Insulin: Its role in the thermic effect of glucose. *J. Clin. Invest* **77,** 1747–1755.

Cincotta, A. H., and Meier, A. H. (1984). Circadian rhythms of lipogenic and hypoglycemic responses to insulin in the golden hamster (*Mesocricetus auratus*). *J. Endocrinol.* **103,** 141–146.

Cioffi, L. A., James, W. P. T., and Van Itallie, T. B. (1981). "The Body Weight Regulatory System: Normal and Disturbed Mechanisms." Raven, New York.

Clark, M. G., Bloxham, D. P., Holland, P. C., and Lardy, H. A. (1973a). Estimation of the fructose diphosphatase–phosphofructokinase substrate cycle in the flight muscle of *Bombus affinis*. *Biochem. J.* **134,** 589–597.

Clark, D. G., Rognstad, R., and Katz, J. (1973b). Isotopic evidence for futile cycles in liver cells. *Biochem. Biophys. Res. Commun.* **54,** 1141.

Clausen, T., and Kohn, P. G. (1977). The effect of insulin on the transport of sodium and potassium in rat soleus muscle. *J. Physiol. (London)* **265,** 19–42.

Cohen, M. R., Cohen, R. M., Pickar, D., and Murphy, D. L. (1985). Naloxone reduced food intake in humans. *Psychosomat. Med.* **47,** 132–8.

Copinschi, G. (1978). Simultaneous study of cortisol, growth hormone and prolactin nyctohemeral variations in normal and obese subjects. Influence of prolonged fasting in obesity. *Clin. Endocrinol.* **9,** 15–26.

Cunningham, J., Calles, J., Eisikowitz, L., Zawalich, W., and Feling, P. (1983). Increased efficiency of weight gain and altered cellularity of brown adipose tissue in rats with impaired glucose tolerance during diet-induced overfeeding. *Diabetes* **32,** 1023–1027.

Cushing, H., and Goetsch, E. (1915). Hibernation and the pituitary body. *J. Exp. Med.* **22,** 25.

Dallosso, H., and James, W. P. T. (1984a). Whole-body calorimetry studies in adult men. 2. The interaction of exercise and overfeeding on the thermic effect of a meal. *Br. J. Nutr.* **52,** 65–72.

Dallosso, H. M., and James, W. P. T. (1984b). Whole-body calorimetry studies in adult men. I. The effect of fat over-feeding on 24 h energy expenditure. *Br. J. Nutr.* **40,** 542–52.

Dallosso, M., Murgatroyd, P. R., and James, W. P. T. (1982). Feeding frequency and energy balance in adult males. *Hum. Nutr. Clin. Nutr.* **36C,** 25–39.

Danforth, E., Jr. (1983). The role of thyroid hormones and insulin in the regulation of energy metabolism. *Am. J. Clin. Nutr.* **38,** 1006–1017.

Danforth, E., Jr. (1985). Diet and obesity. *Am. J. Clin. Nutr.* **41,** 1132–1145.

Danforth, E., Jr., and Landsberg, L. (1983). Energy expenditure and its regulation. *In* "Contemporary Issues in Clinical Nutrition" (M. R. C. Greenwood, ed.), Vol. 4. Churchill Livingston, New York.

Danforth, E., Jr., and Sims, E. A. H. (1983). Thermic effect of overfeeding: Role of thyroid hormones, catecholamines, and insulin resistance. *In* "The Adipocyte and Obesity: Cellular and Molecular Mechanisms" (A. Angel, C. H. Hollenberg, and D. A. K. Roncari, eds.), pp. 271–282. Raven, New York.

Danforth, E., Jr., Horton, E. S., O'Connell, M., Sims, E. A. H., Burger, A., Ingbar, S. H., Braverman, L., and Vagenakis, A. G. (1979). Diet-induced alterations in thyroid hormone metabolism during overnutrition. *J. Clin. Invest.* **64,** 1336–1347.

Dauncey, M. J. (1980). Metabolic effects of altering the 24 hour energy intake in man, using direct and indirect calorimetry. *Br. J. Nutr.* **43,** 257–269.

DeFronzo, R. A., Thorin, D., Felber, J. P., Simmonson, D. C., Thiebaud, D., Jequier, E., and Golay, A. (1984). Effect of beta and alpha adrenergic blockade on glucose-induced thermogenesis in man. *J. Clin. Invest.* **73,** 633–639.

DeFronzo, R. A., Golay, A., and Felber, J. P. (1985). Glucose and lipid metabolism in obesity and diabetes mellitus. *In* "Substrate and Energy Metabolism in Man" (J. S. Garrow and D. Halliday, eds.), pp. 70–81. Libbey, London.

DeLuise, M., and Flier, J. S. (1985). Evidence for coordinate genetic control of Na^+,K^+-pump density in erythrocytes and lymphocytes. *Metabolism* **34,** 771–776.

DeLuise, M., Izumo, H., Grace, E. E., and Flier, J. S. (1983). Effect of diet upon the erythrocyte Na^+,K^+-pump. *J. Clin. Endocrinol. Metab.* **56,** 739–743.

Deslypere, J. P., Verdonick, L., and Vermeulen, A. (1985). Fat tissue: A steroid reservoir and site of steroid metabolism. *J. Clin. Endocrinol. Metab.* **61,** 564.

Devlin, J. T., and Horton, E. S. (1985). Effects of prior high-intensity exercise on glucose metabolism in normal and insulin-resistant men. *Diabetes* **34,** 973–79.

Digby, J. P., Raffoux, C., Pointel, J. P., Perrier, P., Drouin, P., Mejean, C., Streiff, F., and Debry, G. (1985). HLA and familial obesity: Evidence for a genetic origin. *In* "Recent Advances in Obesity Research" (J. Hirsch and T. Van Itallie, eds.), Vol. 4, pp. 171–175. Libbey, London.

Dore, C., Hesp, R., Wilkins, D., and Garrow, J. S. (1982). Prediction of energy requirements of obese patients after massive weight loss. *Hum. Nutr. Clin. Nutr.* **35C,** 41–48.

Drewnowski, A. (1984). New techniques; multidimensional analyses of taste responsiveness. *Int. J. Obesity* **8,** 599–607.

Drewnowski, A., and Greenwood, M. R. C. (1983). Cream and sugar; human preferences for high-fat foods. *Physiol. Behav.* **30,** 629–633.

Drewnowski, A., Brunzell, J. D., Sande, K., Iverius, P. H., and Greenwood, M. R. C. (1985). Sweet tooth reconsidered: Taste responsiveness in human obesity. *Physiol. Behav.* **35,** 617–622.

Dulloo, A. G., and Miller, D. S. (1985). Increased body fat due to elevated energetic efficiency following chronic administration of inhibitors of sympathetic nervous system activity. *Metabolism* **34,** 1061–1065.

Duncan, K. H., Bacon, J. A., and Weinsier, R. L. (1983). The effects of high and low energy density diets on satiety, energy intake, and eating time of obese and non-obese subjects. *Am. J. Clin. Nutr.* **37,** 763–767.

Dunn, H. G. (1968). The Prader–Labhart–Willi syndrome: Review of the literature and report of nine cases. *Acta Pediatr. Scand. Suppl.* **186.**

Durnin, J. V. G. A., and Ferro-Luzzi, A. (1983). Conducting and reporting studies on human energy intake and output: Suggested standards. *Am. J. Clin. Nutr.* **35,** 624–626.

Durnin, J. V. G. A., Edholm, O. G., Miller, D. S., and Waterlow, J. C. (1973). How much food does man require? *Nature (London)* **242,** 418.

Durrant, M. L., Royston, J. P., Wloch, R. T., and Garrow, J. S. (1982). The effect of covert changes in energy density of preloads on subsequent and libitum energy intake in lean and obese human subjects. *Hum. Nutr. Clin. Nutr.* **36C,** 297–306.

Dustan, H. P., ed. (1984). The 1984 report of the Joint National Committee on Detection, Evaluation, and Treatment of High Blood Pressure. *Arch. Intern. Med.* **144,** 1045–1057.

Edholm, O. G., Fletcher, J. G., Widdowson, E. M., and McCance, R. A. (1955). The energy expenditure and food intake of individual men. *Br. J. Nutr.* **9,** 286–300.

Elahi, D., Andersen, D. K., Muller, D. C., Tobin, J. D., Blix, P. M., Rubenstein, A. R., Unger, R. H., and Andres, R. (1984). The enteric enhancement of glucose-stimulated insulin release. The role of GIP in aging, obesity and non-insulin-dependent diabetes. *Diabetes* **33,** 950–957.

Esanu, C., Oprescu, M., Mitrache, L., Cristoveanu, A., Tache, A., and Klepsch, I. (1972). A clinical form of hypercortisolism differing from Cushing's Syndrome. *Rev. Roum. Endocrinol.* **5,** 267–286.

Esler, M. (1982). Assessment of sympathetic nervous system function in humans from norepinephrine plasma kinetics. *Clin. Sci.* **62,** 247–54.

Evans, D. J., Hoffmann, R. G., Kalkhoff, R. K., and Kissebah, A. H. (1983a). Relationship of androgenic activity to body fat topography, fat cell morphology and metabolic aberrations in premenopausal women. *J. Clin. Endocrinol. Metab.* **57,** 304–310.

Evans, D. J., Murray, R., and Kissehah, A. H. (1983b). Relationship between skeletal muscle insulin resistance, insulin-mediated glucose disposal, and insulin binding. Effects of obesity and body fat topography. *J. Clin. Invest.* **74,** 1515–1525.

Fantino, M., Hosotte, J., and Apfelbaum, M. (1986). An opioid antagonist, naltrexone, reduces the preference for sucrose in man. *Am. J. Physiol.,* in press.

Felig, P., Cunningham, J., Levitt, M., Hendler, R., and Nadel, E. (1983). Energy expenditure in obesity and fasting and postprandial state. *Am. J. Physiol.* **244,** E45–51.

Finer, N., Swan, P. C., and Mitchell, F. T. (1985). Suppression of norepinephrine-induced thermogenesis in human obesity by diet and weight loss. *Int. J. Obesity* **9,** 127–134.

Fisher, U., Hommet, U., Ziegler, M., and Michad, M. (1972). The mechanism of insulin secretion after oral glucose administration. *Diabetologia* **8,** 104–110.

Flatt, J. P. (1978). The biochemistry of energy expenditure. "Recent Advances in Obesity Research" (G. S. Bray, ed.), Vol. 2, pp. 211–228. Newmann, London.

Flatt, J. P. (1985). Energetics of intermediary metabolism. *In* "Substrate and Energy Metabolism in Man" (J. S. Garrow and J. Halliday, eds.), pp. 58–69. Libbey, London.

Flatt, J. P., Ravussin, E., Acheson, K. J., and Jequier, E. (1985). Effects of dietary fat on post-prandial substrate oxidation and on carbohydrate and fat balances. *J. Clin. Invest.* **76,** 1019–1024.

Fontaine, E., Savard, R., Tremblay, A., Despres, J. P., Poehllman, E., and Bouchard, C. (1985). Resting metabolic rate in monozygotic and dizygotic twins. *Acta Genet. Med. Gemmellol.* **34,** 41–47.

Forbes, G. (1984). Energy intake and body weight: A reexamination of two "classic" studies. *Am. J. Clin. Nutr.* **39,** 349–350.

Forbes, G. B., Kreipe, R. E., and Lipinski, B. (1982). Body composition and the energy cost of weight gain. *Hum. Nutr. Clin. Nutr.* **36C,** 485–487.

Foster, D. W. (1984). From glycogen to ketones—and back. *Diabetes* **33,** 1188–1199.

Fried, S. K., Kissileff, H. R., and Kral, J. G. (1985). Sex differences in regional distribution of fat cell size and lipoprotein lipase activity in obese patients. *Int. Symp. Metab. Complicat. Hum. Obesity, Marseille.*

Friedman, M. (1950). Hyperthermia as a manifestation of stress. *Res. Publ. Assoc. Res. Nerv. Mental Dis.* **29,** 433–444.

Garn, S. M., Cole, P. E., and Bailey, S. M. (1979). Living together as a factor in family resemblance. *Hum. Biol.* **51,** 565–587.

Garn, S. M., LaVelle, M., and Pilkington, J. J. (1984). Obesity and living together. *Marriage Family Rev.* **7,** 33–47.

Garrow, J. S. (1974, 1978). "Energy Balance and Obesity in Man." Elsevier, New York.

Garrow, J. S., and Halliday, D. (1984). "Substrate and Energy Metabolism in Man." Libbey, London.

Garrow, J. S., and Hawes, S. F. (1972). The role of amino acid oxidation in causing specific dynamic action in man. *J. Nutr.* **27,** 211–219.

Gelfand, R. A., Hutchinson-Williams, K. A., Jacob, R., Bonde, P., Castellino, P., and Sherwin, R. S. (1985). Catabolic mechanisms in thyrotoxicosis; the role of adrenergic hyperresponsiveness. *Clin. Res.* **33,** 307A.

Geary, N., and Smith, G. P. (1982). Pancreatic glucagon and postprandial satiety in the rats. *Physiol. Behav.* **28,** 313–322.

Genazzani, A. R., Facchinetti, F., Petaglia, F., Pintor, C., and Corda, R. (1986). Hyperendorphinemia in obese children and adolescents. *J. Clin Endocrinol. Metab.* **62,** 36–40.

Gerardo, T., Moore, B. J., Stern, J. S., and Hurwitz, B. A. (1985). Prolactin depresses brown fat thermogenesis while increasing food intake and white fat depots. *Fed. Proc., Fed. Am. Soc. Exp. Biol.* **44,** 1160 (Abstr. 4382).

Gibbs, J., Young, R. C., and Smith, G. B. (1979). Bombesin suppresses feeding in rats. *Nature (London)* **282,** 208–210.

Girardier, L., and Stock, W. J., eds. (1983). "Mammalian Thermogenesis." Chapman & Hall, London (U. S. Distributor, Methuen, New York).

Glauser, S. C., Galuser, E. M., Reidenberg, M. M., Rusy, B. F., and Tallarida, R. T. (1970). Metabolic changes associated with the cessation of cigarette smoking. *Arch. Environ. Health* **20,** 377.

Glick, Z., Chvartz, E., Magazanik, A., and Modan, M. (1977). Absence of increased thermogenesis during short-term overfeeding in normal and overweight women. *Am. J. Clin. Nutr.* **30,** 1026–1035.

Golay, A., Schutz, Y., Meyer, H. U., Thiebaud, D., Curchod, B., Maeder, E., Felber, J.-P., and Jequier, E. (1982). Glucose-induced thermogenesis in nondiabetic and diabetic obese subjects. *Diabetes* **31,** 1023–1028.

Goldman, R. F., Haisman, M. F., Bynum, G., Horton, E. S., and Sims, E. A. H. (1975). Experimental obesity in man: Metabolic rate in relation to dietary intake. *In* "Obesity in Perspective" (G. A. Bray, ed.), pp. 165–186. U.S. Govt Printing Office, Washington, D.C.

Goodridge, A. G., and Ball, E. G. (1970). The effect of prolactin on lipogenesis in the pigeon. *In vivo* studies. *Biochemistry* **6,** 1676–1680.

Graeber, R. C., Gatty, R., and Levine, H. (1978). Human eating behavior: Preferences, consumption patterns, and biorhythms. U.S. Army Natick Research and Development Command, Natick, MA. Tech. Report Natick/TR-78-022.

Greenwood, M. R. C. (1985). Normal and abnormal growth and maintenance of adipose tissue. *In* "Recent Advances in Obesity Research": (J. Hircsh and T. B. Van Itallie, eds, Vol. 4. Libbey, London.

Greenwood, M. R. C., and Turkenkopf, J. (1983). Genetic and metabolic aspects. *In* "Obesity" (M. R. C. Greenwood, ed.), p. 209. Churchill Livingstone, New York.

Gulick, A. (1922). A study of weight regulation in the adult human body during overnutrition. *Am. J. Physiol.* **60,** 371–395.

Gurr, M. I., Mawson, R., Rothwell, N. J., and Stock, M. J. (1980). Effects of manipulating dietary protein and energy intake on energy balance and thermogenesis in the pig. *J. Nutr.* **110,** 532–542.

Hashim, S. A., and Van Itallie, T. B. (1965). Studies in normal and obese subjects with a monitored food-dispensing service. *Ann. N.Y. Acad. Sci.* **131,** 654–661.

Hawkins, M., Whittaker, J., Wales, J. K., and Swaminathan, R. (1984). Erythrocyte sodium content, sodium transport, ouabain binding capacity and Na^+,K^+ATPase activity in lean and obese subjects. *Horm. Metab. Res.* **16,** 282–286.

Haydar, N. A., Conn, H. L., Afifi, A., Wakid, N., Ballas, S., and Fawaz, K. (1971). Severe hypermetabolism with primary abnormality of skeletal muscle mitochondria. *Ann. Intern. Med.* **74,** 548–558.

Heaton, J. M. (1972). The distribution of brown adipose tissue in the human. *J. Anat.* **112,** 35–39.

Herman, C. P., and Polivy, J. (1980). Restrained eating. *In* "Obesity" (A. J. Stunkard, ed.), pp. 208–225. Saunders, Philadelphia.

Hervey, G. R., and Tobins, G. (1983). Luxuskonsumption, diet-induced thermogenesis and brown fat: A critical review. *Clin. Sci.* **64,** 7–18.

Heymsfield, S., McManus, C., Hill, J., DiGirolamo, M., Nixon, D., Head, A., and Grossman, G. (1985). Bioenergetic studies in adult patients recovering from semi-starvation. *Int. J. Obesit.* **9,** (Suppl. 2).

Hill, J. O., Heymsfield, S. B., McMannus, C., and DiGirolamo, M. (1984). Meal size and thermic response to food in male subjects as a function of maximum aerobic capacity. *Metabolism* **33,** 743–749.

Hill, J. O., DiGirolamo, M., and Heymsfield, S. B. (1985). New approach for studying the thermic response to dietary fuels. *Am. J. Clin. Nutr.* **42,** 1290–1298.

Hilton, J., and Treharne, I. (1985). Changes in body weight in the puerperium and the relationship to lactation. *Int. J. Obesity* **8,** 380.

Himms-Hagen, J. (1984). Thermogenesis in brown adipose tissue as an energy buffer. Implications for obesity. *N. Engl. J. Med.* **311,** 154–1558.

Himms-Hagen, J. (1985a). Letter to the editor. *N. Engl. J. Med.* **312,** 1063.

Himms-Hagen, J. (1985b). Brown adipose tissue metabolism and thermogenesis. *In* "Annual Reviews" (R. E. Olson, ed.), Vol. 5. Annual Review of Nutrition, Palo Alto, CA.

Hirsch, J., and Batchelor, B. (1976). Adipose tissue cellularity in human obesity. *Clin. Endocrinol. Metab.* **5,** 299–311.

Hirsch, J., and Van Itallie, T. B. (1985). Recent advances in obesity research. *Proc. Int. Congr. Obesity, 4th* pp. 1–402.

Horton, E. S., and Terjung, R. L., eds. (1986). "Exercise, Nutrition, and Energy Metabolism." Macmillan, New York, in press.

Horton, E. S., Danforth, E. D., Jr., and Woo, R. (1985). Regulation of energy expenditure. *Satellite Symp. Int. Congr. Obesity, 4th, Sept. 30, 1983; Int. J. Obesity Suppl.* **2,** pp. 1–184.

Howard, A. N., Bray, G. A., Novin, D., Björntorp, P. (1981). *Int. J. Obesity* **5** (Suppl. 1), 11–188.

Howard, B. V., Savage, P. J., Nagulesparan, M., Bennion, L. J., Unger, R. H., and Bennett, P. H. (1979). Evidence for marked sensitivity to the antilipolytic action of insulin in obese maturity-onset diabetics. *Metabolism* **28,** 744–750.

Hue, L., and Hers, H.-G. (1974). On the use of (^{3}H, ^{14}C)-labelled glucose in the study of the so-called "futile cycles" in liver and muscle. *Biochem. Biophys. Res. Commun.* **58,** 532.

Huttunen, P., Hirvonen, J., and Kinnula, V. (1981). The occurrence of brown adipose tissue in outdoor workers. *Eur. J. Appl Physiol.* **46,** 339–345.

James, W. P. T., ed. (1977). "Research on Obesity: A Report of the DHSS/MRC Group." Her Majesty's Stationery Office, London.

James, W. P. T. (1979). Comparison of genetic models of obesity in animals with obesity in man. *In* "Animal Models of Obesity" (M. F. W. Festing, ed.), pp. 221–235. Macmillan, London.

James, W. P. T., and Shetty, P. S. (1982). Metabolic adaptation and energy requirements in developing countries. *Hum. Nutr. Clin. Nutr.* **36C** 331–336.

James, W. P. T., Davies, H. L., Bailes, J., and Dauncey, M. J. (1978). Elevated metabolic rates in obesity. *Lancet* **1,** 1122–1125.

Jayarajan, M. P., Balasubramanyam, A., and Shetty, P. S. (1985). Increased cardiovascular β-adrenoceptor responsiveness in underweight subjects. *Hum. Nutr. Clin. Nutr.* **39,** 271–277.

Jequier, E. (1984). Energy expenditure in obesity. *In* "Clinics in Endocrinology and Metabolism" (W. P. T. James, ed.), pp. 563–580. Saunders, Philadelphia.

Jequier, E., Gygax, P.-H., Pittet, Ph., and Vannotti, A. (1974). Increased thermal body insulation: Relationship to the development of obesity. *J. Appl. Physiol.* **36,** 674–678.

Jeejeebhoy, K. N. (1985). Energy metabolism in the critically ill. *In* "Substrate and Energy Metabolism in Man" (J. S. Garrow and D. Halliday, eds.), pp. 93–101. Libbey, London.

Joseph, M. M., and Meier, A. H. (1974). Circadian component in the fattening and reproductive responses to prolactin in the hamster. *Proc. Soc. Exp. Biol. Med.* **146,** 1150–1155.

Jung, R. T., Gurr, M. I., Robinson, M. P., and James, W. P. T. (1978). Does adipocyte hypercellularity in obesity exist? *Br. Med. J.* **2,** 319–321.

Jung, R. T., Shetty, P. S., Barrand, M., Callingham, B. A., and James, W. P. T. (1979). Role of catecholamines in hypotensive response to dieting. *Br. Med. J.* **1,** 12–13.

Jung, P. T., Shetty, P. S., and James, W. P. T. (1980). The effect of beta-adrenergic blockade on metabolic rate and peripheral thyroid metabolism in obesity. *Eur. J. Clin. Invest.* **10,** 179–182.

Jung, R. T., Shetty, P. S., James, P. T., Barrand, M. A., and Callingham, B. A. (1981). Caffeine: Its effect on catecholamines and metabolism in lean and obese humans. *Clin. Sci.* **60,** 527–535.

Kalkhoff, R. K., Hartz, A. H., Rupley, D., Kissebah, A. H., and Kelber, S. (1983). Relationship of body fat distribution to blood pressure, carbohydrate tolerance, and plasma lipids in healthy obese women. *J. Lab. Clin. Med.* **102,** 621–627.

Kang, B. S. (1970). Calorigenic action of norepinephrine in Korean women divers. *J. Appl. Physiol.* **29,** 6–9.

Katzeff, H. L., O'Connell, M., Horton, E. S., and Danforth, E., Jr. (1985). Metabolic studies in human obesity during over- and undernutrition: Thermogenic and hormonal responses to norepinephrine. *Metabolism,* in press.

Keesey, B. (1980). A set-point analysis of the regulation of body weight. *In* "Obesity" (A. J. Stunkard, ed.), pp. 144–181. Saunder, Philadelphia.

Kelso, T. B., Herbert, W. G., Gwazdauskas, F. C., Goss, F. L., and Hess, J. L. (1984). Exercise-thermoregulatory stress and increased plasma β-endorphin/β-lipotropin in humans. *J. Appl. Physiol. Respir. Environ. Exercise Physiol.* **57,** 444–449.

Keys, A., Brozek, J., Hanschel, A., and Michelson, O. (1950). "The Biology of Human Starvation." Univ. of Minnesota Press, Minneapolis.

Keys, A., Taylor, H. L., and Grande, F. (1973). Basal metabolism and age of adult man. *Metabolism* **22,** 579–587.

Kissebah, A. H., Vydelingum, N., Murray, D. J., Evans, D. J., Hartz, A. J., Kalkoff, R. K., and Adams, P. W. (1982). Relation of body fat distribution to metabolic consequences of obesity. *J. Clin. Endocrinol. Metab.* **54,** 254–260.

Kissileff, H. R., and Van Itallie, T. B. (1982). Physiology of food intake. *Annu. Rev. Nutr.* **2,** 371–418.

Kissilef, H. R., Pi-Sunyer, F. X., Thornton, J., and Smith, G. P. (1981). Cholecystokinin-octapeptide (CCK-8) decreases food intake in man. *Am. J. Clin. Nutr.* **34,** 154–160.

Kleiber, M. (1975). "The Fire of Life. An Introduction to Animal Energetics" (Rev. Ed.). Krieger, Huntington, New York.

Klein, P. D., James, W. P. T., Wong, W. W., Irving, C. S., Murgatroyd, P. R., Cabrera, M., Dallosso, H. M., Klein, E. R., and Nichols, B. L. (1984). Calorimetic validation of the doubly-labelled water method for determination of energy expenditure in man. *Hum. Nutr. Clin. Nutr.* **38C,** 95–106.

Klakhoff, R., and Ferrou, C. (1971). Metabolic differences between obese overweight and muscular overweight men. *N. Engl. J. Med.* **284,** 1236.

Klimes, I., Nagulesparan, M., Unger, R. H., Arnoff, S. L., and Mott, M. (1982). Reduced Na^+,K^+-ATPase activity in intact red cells and isolated membranes in obese men. *J. Clin. Endocrinol. Metab.* **54,** 721–724.

Knutson, R. (1974). Heat production and temperature regulation in eastern skunk cabbage. *Science* **186,** 746–747.

Krieger, D. T. (1984). Brain peptides *In* "Vitamins and Hormones" (G. D. Aurbach and D. B. McCormick, eds.), Vol. 41, pp. 1–275. Academic Press, New York.

Kortkiewski, M., and P. Björntorp. (1978). The effect of estrogen treatment of carcinoma of prostate on regional adipocyte size. *J. Endocrinol. Invest.* **1,** 365–366.

Krotkiewski, M., Toss, L., Björntorp, P., and Holm, G. (1981). The effect of a very low calorie diet with and without chronic exercise. *Int. J. Obesity* **5,** 287–293.

Kusaka, M. (1977). Activation of the Cori cycle by epinephrine. *Am. J. Physiol.* **232,** E145–155.

Kush, R. D., Young, J. B., Danforth, E., Jr., Garrow, J. S., Katzeff, H. L., Scheidigger, K., Ravussin, E., Howard, B. V., Sims, E. A. H., Horton, E. S., and Landsberg, L. (1986). Effect of diet on energy expenditure and plasma norepinephrine in lean and obese Pima Indians. *Metabolism,* in press.

Landsberg, L., and Young, J. B. (1978). Fasting, feeding, and the regulation of the sympathetic nervous system. *N. Engl. J. Med.* **298,** 1295–1301.

Landsberg, L., and Young, J. B. (1985). Insulin-mediated glucose metabolism in the relationship between dietary intake and sympathetic nervous system activity. *Int. J. Obesity* **9** (Suppl.), 2, 63–68.

Landsberg, L., Saville, M. E., and Young, J. B. (1984). Sympathoadrenal system and regulation of thermogenesis. *Am. J. Physiol.* **247,** E181–189.

Larsen, P. R., Silva, J. E., and Kaplan, M. M. (1981). Relationships between circulating and intracellular thyroid hormones: Physiological and clinical implications. *Endocr. Rev.* **2,** 87–102.

Lean, M. E. J., and James, W. P. T. (1983). Uncoupling protein in human brown adipose tissue mitochondria: Isolation and detection by specific antiserum. *FEBS Lett.* **163,** 235–40.

LeBlanc, J. (1985). Thermogenesis in relation to feeding and exercise training. *Int. J. Obesity* **9** (Suppl. 2), 75–79.

LeBlanc, J., and Brondel, L. (1985). Role of palatability on meal-induced thermogenesis in human subjects. *Am. J. Physiol. Endocrinol. Metab.* **11,** E333–E336.

LeBlanc, J., Cabanac, M., and Samson, P. (1984a). Reduced postprandial heat production with gavage as compared to meal feeding in man. *Am. J. Physiol. Endocrinol. Metab.* **9,** E95–E101.

LeBlanc, J., Mercier, P., and Samson, P. (1984b). Diet-induced thermogenesis with relation to training state in female subjects. *Can. J. Physiol. Pharmacol.* **62,** 334–337.

Leibel, R. L., and Hirsch, J. (1984). Diminished energy requirements in reduced-obese patients. *Metabolism* **33,** 164–170.

Leibel, R. L., and Hirsch, J. (1985). Metabolic characterization of obesity. *Ann. Intern. Med.* **103,** 1000–1002.

Leonard, J. I., Leach, C. S., and Rambaut, P. C. (1983). Quantitation of tissue loss during prolonged space flight. *Am. J. Clin. Nutr.* **38,** 667–679.

Leveille, G. A., and Hanson, R. W. (1966). Adaptive changes in enzyme activity and metabolic pathways in adipose tissue from meal-fed rats. *J. Lipid Res.* **7,** 46–55.

Lillioja, S., Bogardus, C., Mott, D. M., Kennedy, A. L., Knowler, W. C., and Howard, B. V. (1985). Relationship between insulin-mediated glucose disposal and lipid metabolism in man. *J. Clin. Invest.* **75,** 1106–1115.

Lotter, E. C., Krinsky, R., McKay, J. M., Treneer, C. M., Porte, Jr., D., and Woods, S. C. (1981). Somatostatin decreases food intake in rats and baboons. *J. Comp. Physiol. Psychol.* **95,** 278–287.

Luft, R., and Effendic, S. (1979). Low insulin response—genetic aspects and implications. *Horm. Metab. Res.* **11,** 415–423.

McCarron, D. A., Filer, L. J., and Van Itallie, T. (1982a). Current perspectives in hypertension: A symposium on food, nutrition, and health, Princeton N.J. March, 1982. *Hypertension* **4** (Part II), 1–177.

MacDonald, I. A., Bennett, T., and Fellows, I. W. (1985). Catecholamines and the control of metabolism in man. *Clin. Sci.* **68,** 613–619.

Malcolm, R., O'Neil, P. M., Sexauer, J. D., Riddle, F. E., Curry, H. S., and Counts, C. (1985). A controlled trial of naltrexone in obese humans. *Int. J. Obesity* **9,** 347–353.

Mancia, G., Ferrari, A., Gregorini, L., Leonetti, G., Parati, G., Picotti, G. B., Ravazanni, C., and Zanchetti, A. (1983). Plasma catecholamines do not invariably reflect sympathetically induced changes in blood pressure in man. *Clin. Sci.* **65,** 227–235.

Mann, G. V., Teel, K., Hayes, O., McNally, A., and Bruno, D. (1955). Exercise in the disposition of dietary calories. *N. Engl. J. Med.* **253,** 349–354.

Marin, P., Rebuffe-Scrive, M., and Björntorp, P. (1985). Intake of orally administered labelled glucose in triglycerides in different lipid depots. *Int. Symp. Metab. Complicat. Hum. Obesity, Marseille, May.*

Mayer, J. (1965a). Genetic factors in human obesity. *Ann. N.Y. Acad. Sci.* **131,** 412–421.

Mayer, J. (1965b). Inactivity as a major factor in adolescent obesity. *Ann. N.Y. Acad. Sci.* **131,** 502–518.

Meier, A. H. (1977). Prolactin, the liporegulatory hormone. *In* "Comparative Endocrinology of Prolactin" (H. D. Dellman, J. A. Johnson, and D. M. Klachko, eds.). Plenum, New York.

Meier, A. H., and co-workers (1976). Prolactin, the liporegulatory hormone. *Proc. Midwest Conf. Endocrinol. Metab., Columbia, MO,* pp. 153–171.

Meyers, A. W., and Stunkard, A. J. (1980). Food accessibility and food choice. A test of Schachter's externality hypothesis. *Arch. Gen. Psych.* **37,** 1133–1135.

Miller, D. S., and Mumford, P. (1967a). Gluttony. I. An experimental study of overeating low- or high-protein diets. *Am. J. Clin. Nutr.* **20,** 1212–1222.

Miller, D. S., and Payne, P. R. (1962). Weight maintenance and food intake. *J. Nutr.* **78,** 255–262.

Miller, D. S., Mumford, P., and Stock, M. J. (1967b). Gluttony. II. Thermogenesis in overeating man. *Am. J. Clin. Nutr.* **20,** 1223–1229.

Minaker, K. L., Rowe, J. W., Young, J. B., Sparrow, J. A., Pallotta, J. A., and Landsberg, L. (1982). Effect of age on insulin stimulation of sympathetic nervous system activity in man. *Metabolism* **31,** 1181–1184.

Moore, R. D. (1981). Stimulation of Na : H exchange by insulin. *Biophys. J.* **33,** 203–210.

Morgan, K. R., and Bartholomew, G. A. (1982). Homeothermic response to reduced ambient temperature in a scarab beetle. *Science* **216,** 1409.

Morley, J. E., and Levine, A. S. (1982). The role of the endogenous opiates as regulators of appetite. *Am. J. Clin. Nutr.* **35,** 757–761.

Mrosovsky, N. (1985). Cyclical obesity in hibernators: The search for the adjustable regulator. *In* "Recent Advances in Obesity Research" (J. Hirsch and T. B. Van Itallie, eds), pp. 45–56. Libbey, London.

Mrosovsky, N., and Powley, T. L. (1977). Set points for body weight and fat. *Behav. Biol.* **20,** 205–223.

Mueller, W. H. (1983). The genetics of human fatness. *Yearb. Phys. Anthropol.* **26,** 215–230.

Naeye, R. L., and Roode, P. (1970). The sizes and numbers of cells in visceral organs in human obesity. *Am. J. Clin. Pathol.* **54,** 251.

Nair, K. S., Halliday, D., and Garrow, J. S. (1983). Thermic response to isoenergetic protein, carbohydrate or fat meals in lean and obese subjects. *Clin. Sci.* **65,** 307–312.

Narasinga Rao, B. S. (1984). Metabolic adaptation to chronic malnutrition. *In* "Substrate and Energy Metabolism in Man" (R. S. Garrow and D. Halliday, eds.), pp. 145–154. Libbey, London.

National Diabetes Data Group (1979). Classification and diagnosis of diabetes mellitus and other categories of glucose intolerance. *Diabetes* **28,** 1039–1057.

Neel, J. V. (1962). Diabetes mellitus: A "thrifty" genotype rendered detrimental by "progress"? *Am. J. Hum. Genet.* **14,** 353–362.

Neumann, R. O. (1902). Experimentelle Beitraege zur Lehre von dem taeglichen Nahrungsbedarf des Menschen unter besonderer Beruecksichtigung der notwendigen Eiweissmenge. *Arch. Hyg.* **XLV,** 1–87.

Newgard, C. B. (1983). Studies on the mechanism by which exogenous glucose is converted into liver glycogen in the rat. *J. Biol. Chem.* **258,** 8046–8052.

Newsholme, E. A. (1976). Substrate cycles in metabolic regulation and in heat generation. *Biochem. Soc. Symp.* **41,** 61–109.

Newsholme, E. A. (1978). Substrate cycles: Their metabolic, energetic and thermic consequences in man. *Biochem. Soc. Symp.* **43,** 183–205.

Newsholme, E. A. (1980). A possible metabolic basis for the control of body weight. *N. Engl. J. Med.* **302,** 400–405.

Nichols, D., and Locke, R. (1983). Cellular mechanisms of heat dissipation. *In* "Mammalian Thermogenesis" (L. Girardier and M. J. Stock, eds.). Chapman & Hall, London.

Nicoll, C. S. (1974). Physiological actions of prolactin. *In* "Handbook of Physiology" (E. Knobil and W. H. Sawyer, eds), pp. 253–292. Williams & Wilkins, Baltimore.

Norgan, N. G., and Durnin, J. V. G. A. (1980). The effect of 6 weeks of overfeeding on the body weight, body composition, and energy metabolism of young men. *Am. J. Clin. Nutr.* **33,** 978–988.

Novin, D., Wyrwicka, W., and Bray, G. A., eds. (1976). "Hunger, Basic Mechanism and Clinical Implications." Raven, New York.

O'Connell, M., Danforth, E., Jr., Horton, E. S., Salans, L. B., and Sims, E. A. H. (1973). Experimental obesity in man. III. Adrenocortical function. *J. Clin. Endocrinol. Metab.* **36,** 323–329.

O'Dea, K. (1982). Noradrenaline turnover during under- and overeating in normal weight subjects. *Metabolism* **31,** 896–99.

O'Dea, K., Esler, M., Leonard, P., Stockigt, J. R., and Nestel, P. (1982). Noradrenaline turnover during under- and overeating in normal weight subjects. *Metabolism* **31,** 896–899.

O'Hara, W. J., Shephard, R. J., and Allen, G. (1979). Fat loss in the cold—a controlled study. *J. Appl. Physiol. Respir. Environ. Exer. Physiol.* **46,** 872–877.

Olefsky, J., Crapo, P. A., Ginsberg, H., and Reaven, G. M. (1975). Metabolic effects of increased caloric intake in man. *Metabolism* **24,** 495–503.

Oomura, Y., and Kita (1981). Insulin acting as a modulator of feeding through the hypothalamus. *Diabetologia* **20,** 290–298.

Oppenheimer, J. H. (1079). Thyroid hormone action at the cellular level. *Science* **203,** 971–979.

Oscai, L. B., Brown, M. M., and Miller, W. C. (1984). Effect of dietary fat on food intake, growth and body composition. *Growth* **48,** 415–424.

Parra-Covarrubias, A., Rivera-Rodriquez, I., and Almaraz-Ugalde, A. (1971). Cephalic phase of insulin secretion in obese adolescents. *Diabetes* **20,** 800–802.

Pasquali, R., Venturoli, S., Paradisi, R., Capelli, M., Parenti, M., and Melchionda, N. (1982). Insulin and C-peptide levels in obese patients with polycystic ovaries. *Horm. Metab. Res.* **6,** 284–286.

Pasquali, R., Malini, P. L., Strocchi, E., Casimiri, F., Melchionda, N., and Ambrosioni, E. (1984). Erythrocyte Na^+-K^+-ATPase in obese patients. *Horm. Metab. Res.* **16,** 279–282.

Perkins, M. N., Rothwell, N. J., Stock, M. J., and Stone, T. W. (1981). Activation of brown adipose tissue thermogenesis by the ventromedial hypothalamus. *Nature (London)* **289,** 401–402.

Pernick, S. B., Prince, H., and Hinkle, L. E. (1966). Fall in plasma content of free fatty acids associated with sight of food. *N. Engl. J. Med.* **275,** 416–419.

Perlmuter, R. C., Pettitt, D. J. *et al.* (1983). Excessive obesity in offspring of Pima Indian women with diabetes during pregnancy. *N. Engl. J. Med.* **5,** 242–245.

Perlmuter, R. C., Hakami, M. K., Hodgsohn, C., Ginsberg, J., Katz, J., Singer, D. E., Nathan, D. M. (1984). Decreased cognitive function in aging non-insulin dependent diabetic patients. *Am. J. Med.* **77,** 1043–1048.

Pettersson, P., Karlsson, M., and Björntorp, P. (1985). Adipocyte precursor cells in obese and nonobese humans. *Metabolism* **34,** 808–830.

Pettitt, D. J., Baird, H. R., Aleck, K. A., Bennett, P. H., and Knowler, W. C. (1983).

Excessive obesity in offspring of Pima Indian women with diabetes during pregnancy. *N. Engl. J. Med.* **308,** 242–245.

Pi-Sunyer, X., Kissileff, H. R., Thornton, J., and Smith, G. P. (1982). C-terminal octapeptide of cholecystokinin decreases food intake in obese men. *Physiol. Behav.* **29,** 627–630.

Pikalisto, O. J., Smith, P. H., and Brunzell, J. D. (1975). Determinants of human adipose tissue lipoprotein lipase; effects of diabetes and obesity on basal and diet-induced activity. *J. Clin. Invest.* **56,** 1108.

Pittet, P., Gygax, P. H., and Jequier, E. (1974). Thermic effect of glucose and amino acids in man studied by direct and indirect calorimetry. *Br. J. Nutr.* **31,** 343–349.

Pittet, P., Chappuis, P., Acheson, K., deTechtermann, F., and Jequier, E. (1976). Thermic effect of glucose in obese subjects studied by direct and indirect calorimetry. *Br. J. Nutr.* **35,** 281.

Poehlman, E. T., Despres, J.-P., Bessette, H., Fontaine, E., Tremblay, A., and Bouchard, C. (1985). The influence of caffeine on the resting metabolic rate of exercise-trained and inactive subjects. *Med. Sci. Sports Exercise* **17,** 689–694.

Poehlman, E. T., Despres, J.-P., Marcotte, M., Tremblay, A., Theriault, G., and Bouchard, C. (1986a). Genotype dependency of adaptation in adipose tissue metabolism following short-term overfeeding. *Am. J. Physiol.* **250** (*Endocrinol. Metab* **13**), E480–E485.

Poehlman, E. T., Tremblay, A., Fontaine, E., Després, J. P., Nadeau, A., Dussault, J., and Bouchard, C. (1986b). Genotype dependency of the thermic effect of a meal and associated hormonal changes following short-term overfeeding. *Metabolism* **35,** 30–36.

Pollitt, E., and P. Amante (1984). "Energy Intake and Activity," Vol. 11.

Porikos, K. P., and Pi-Sunyer, F. (1984). Regulation of food intake in human obesity: Studies with caloric dilution and exercise. *In* "Clinics in Endocrinology and Metabolism" (W. P. T. James, ed.), pp. 547–562. Saunders, Philadelphia.

Porikos, K. P., and Pi-Sunyer, F. (1984). Regulation of food intake in human obesity: Studies with caloric dilution and exercise. *In* "Clinics in Endocrinology and Metabolism" (W. P. T. James, ed.), pp. 547–562. Saunders, Philadelphia.

Porte, D., and Woods, S. C. (1981). Regulation of food intake and body weight by insulin. *Diabetologia* **20,** 274–280.

Powers, P. S., Holland, P., Miller, C., and Powers, H. P. (1982). Salivation patterns of obese and normal subjects. *Int. J. Obesity* **6,** 267–270.

Quaade, F. (1963). Insulation in leanness and obesity. *Lancet* **Aug. 31,** 429–432.

Randle, P. J., Garland, P. B., Hales, C. N., Newsholme, E. A., Denton, R. M., and Pogson, C. I. (1966). Interactions of metabolism and the physiological role of insulin. *Recent Prog. Horm. Res.* **22,** 1–48.

Ravelli, G. P., Stein, Z. A., and Susser, M. W. (1976). Obesity in young men after famine exposure *in utero* and in early infancy. *N. Engl. J. Med.* **295,** 349–490.

Ravussin, R., and Bogardus, C. (1982). Thermogenic response to insulin and glucose infusions in man: A model to evaluate the different components of the thermic effect of carbohydrate. *Life Sci.* **3,** 2011–2018.

Ravussin, E., and Bogardus, C. (1985). "Fidgeting": A significant component of 24 hour energy expenditure in man. *Jt. Conf. Obesity Non-Insulin-Depend. Diabetes, Toronto, Oct. 30.*

Ravussin, E., Burnard, B., Schutz, Y., and Jequier, E. (1982). Twenty-four-hour energy expenditure and resting metabolic rate in obese, moderately obese, and control subjects. *Am. J. Clin. Nutr.* **35,** 566–573.

Ravussin, E., Bogardus, C., Schwartz, R. S., Robbins, D. C., Wolfe, R. R., Horton, E. S., Danforth, E., and Sims, E. A. H. (1983). Thermic effect of infused glucose and insulin in man: Decreased response with increased insulin resistance in obesity and non-insulin-dependent diabetes mellitus. *J. Clin. Invest.* **72,** 893–902.

Ravussin, E., Schutz, Y., Acheson, K. J., Dusmet, M., Bourquin, L., and Jequier, E. (1985a). Short term mixed diet overfeeding in man. No evidence for luxuskonsumption. *Am. J. Physiol.* **249** (*Endocrinol. Metab.* **5**), E470–475.

Ravussin, E., Burnand, B., Schutz, Y., and Jequier, E. (1985b). Energy expenditure before and during energy restriction in obese patients. *Am. J. Clin. Nutr.* **41,** 753–759.

Ravussin, E., Acheson, K. J., Vernet, Danforth, E., Jr., and Jequier, E. (1985c). Evidence that insulin resistance is responsible for the decreased thermic effect of glucose in human obesity. *J. Clin. Invest.* **76,** 1268–1273.

Ravussin, E., Schoeller, D. A., Schutz, Y., Acheson, K. J., Baertschi, P., and Jequier, E. (1985d). Human energy expenditure measured by the doubly labelled water method: A 4-day comparison with respiratory exchange measurement. *Clin. Res.* **33,** 276A.

Reeds, P. J., Fuller, M. F., and Nicholson, B. A. (1984). Metabolic basis of energy expenditure with particular reference to protein. *In* "Substrate and Energy Metabolism in Man" (J. S. Garrow and D. Halliday, eds.), pp. 46–57. Libbey, London.

Rice, D. W., and Wolman, A. A. (1971). The life history and ecology of the gray whale (*Escherichtius robustus*). Special Publication 3, Amer. Soc. Mammalogists.

Robbins, D. C., Danforth, E., Horton, E. S., Burse, R. L., Goldman, R. F., and Sims, E. A. H. (1979). The effect of diet on thermogenesis in acquired lipodystrophy. *Metabolism* **28,** 908–916.

Robbins, D. R., Horton, E. S., Tulp, O., and Sims, E. A. H. (1982). Familial partial lipodystrophy: Complications of obesity in the non-obese. *Metabolism* **31,** 445–452.

Rodin, J. (1980). The externality theory today. *In* "Obesity" (A. J. Stunkard, ed.), pp. 226–239. Saunders, Philadelphia.

Rodin, J. (1985). Effect of insulin and glucose on feeding behavior. *Metabolism* **34,** 826–831.

Rolls, B. J., Rowe, E. A., and Rolls, E. T. (1981). Variety in a meal enhances food intake in man. *Physiol. Behav.* **26,** 215.

Roncari, D. A. K., Lau, D. C. W., and Kindler, S. (1981). Exaggerated replication in culture of adipocyte precursors from massively obese persons. *Metabolism* **30,** 425–427.

Roncari, D. A. K., Lau, D. C. W., Djian, P., Kinder, S., and Arhaud, G. (1983). Culture and cloning of adipocyte precursors from lean and obese subjects: Effects of growth factors. *In* "The Adipocyte and Obesity: Cellular and Molecular Mechanisms" A. Angel, C. H. Hollenberg, and D. A. K. Roncari, eds.), pp. 65–73. Raven, New York.

Roncari, D. A. K., Kindler, S., and Hollenberg, C. H. (1986). Excessive proliferation in culture of reverted adipocytes from massively obese persons. *Metabolism* **35,** 1–4.

Rose, G. A., and Williams, R. T. (1961). Metabolic studies on large and small eaters. *Br. J. Nutr.* **15,** 1–9.

Rothwell, N., and Stock, M. J. (1978). A paradox in the control of energy intake in the rat. *Nature (London)* **273,** 145–146.

Rothwell, N. J., and Stock, M. J. (1983). Luxuskonsumption, diet-induced thermogenesis and brown fat: The case in favour. *Clin. Sci.* **64,** 19–23.

Rothwell, N. J., Stock, M. J., and Tyzbir, R. (1983a). Energy balance and mitochondrial function in liver and brown fat of rats fed a cafeteria diets of varying protein content. *J. Nutr.* **112,** 1663–1672.

Rothwell, N. J., Stock, M. J., and Tyzbir, R. S. (1983b). Mechanisms of thermogenesis induced by low protein diets. *Metabolism* **32,** 257–261.

Rothwell, N. J., Stock, M. J., and Warwick, B. P. (1985a). Energy balance and brown fat activity in rats fed cafeteria diets of high-fat, semisynthetic diets at several levels of intake. *Metabolism* **34,** 474.

Rothwell, N. J., Stock, M. J., and Warwick, B. P. (1985b). Involvement of insulin in the acute thermogenic response to food and non-metabolizable substances. *Metabolism* **34,** 43.

Rowe, J. W., Young, J. B., Minaker, K. L., Stevens, A. L., Pallotta, J., and Landsberg, L. (1981). Effect of insulin and glucose infusions on sympathetic nervous system activity in normal man. *Diabetes* **30,** 219–225.

Rubner, M. (1902, 1968). Die Gesetze des Energie Verbrauchs bei der Ernaehrung. (R. J. T. Joy, transl.). U. S. Army Research Institute of Environmental Medicine, Natick, Massachusetts.

Ruderman, N. B., Schneider, S. H., and Berchtold, P. (1981). The "metabolically-obese" normal-weight individual. *Am. J. Clin. Nutr.* **34,** 1617–1621.

Salans, L. B., Horton, E. S., and Sims, E. A. H. (1971). Experimental obesity in man: Cellular character of the adipose tissue. *J. Clin. Invest.* **50,** 1005.

Salmon, D. M. W., and Flatt, J. P. (1986). Effect of dietary fat content on the incidence of obesity among ad libitum fed mice. *Int. J. Obesity* **9,** 443–449.

Salmonds, K. W., and Hegsted, D. M. (1978). Protein deficiency and energy restriction in young cebus monkeys. *Proc. Natl. Acad. Sci. U.S.A.* **75,** 1600–1604.

Schachter, S. (1968). Obesity and eating: Internal and external cues differentially affect the eating behaviour of obese and normal subjects. *Science* **161,** 751–856.

Scheidegger, K., O'Connell, M., Robbins, D. C., and Danforth, E., Jr. (1984). Effects of chronic β-receptor stimulation on sympathetic nervous system activity, energy expenditure, and thyroid hormones. *J. Clin. Endocrinol. Metab.* **58,** 895–903.

Schoeller, D. A. (1983). Energy expenditure from doubly labeled water: Some fundamental considerations in humans. *Am. J. Clin. Nutr.* **38,** 999–1005.

Schutz, Y., Acheson, K., Bessard, T., and Jequier, E. (1982a). Effect of a 7-day carbohydrate (CHO) hyperalimentation on energy metabolism in healthy individuals. *Clin. Nutr.* **1** (Suppl. F100).

Schutz, Y., Ravussin, E., Diethelm, R., and Jequier, E. (1982b). Spontaneous physical activity measured by radar in obese and control subjects studied in a respiration chamber. *Int. J. Obesity* **6,** 23–28.

Schutz, Y., Bessard, T., and Jequier, R. (1984a). Diet-induced thermogenesis measured over a whole day in obese and nonobese women. *Am. J. Clin. Nutr.* **40,** 542–52.

Schutz, Y., Golay, A., Felber, J.-P., and Jequier, E. (1984b). Decreased glucose-induced thermogenesis after weight loss in obese subjects: A predisposing factor for relapse of obesity? *Am. J. Clin. Nutr.* **39,** 380–387.

Schutz, Y., Acheson, K. J., and Jequier, L. F. (1985). Twenty-four hour energy expenditure and thermogenesis, response to progressive carbohydrate overfeeding in man. *Int. J. Obesity* **9** (Suppl. 2), 111–114.

Schwartz, R. S., and Brunzell, J. D. (1981). Increase of adipose tissue lipoprotein lipase activity with weight loss. *J. Clin. Invest.* **67,** 1425–1430.

Schwartz, R. S., Brunzell, J. D., and Bierman, E. L. (1979). Elevated adipose tissue lipoprotein lipase in the pathogenesis of obesity in Prader–Willi syndrome. *Trans. Assoc. Am. Phys.* **92,** 89–95.

Schwartz, R. S., Halter, J., Eckel, R. H., and Goldberg, A. P. (1983a). Reduced thermic effect of feeding in obesity: Role of triiodothyronine and norepinephrine. *Metabolism* **32,** 114.

Schwartz, R. S., Halter, J., and Bierman, E. (1983b). Reduced thermic effect of feeding in obesity: Role of norepinephrine. *Metabolism* **32,** 114–117.

Schwartz, R. S., Ravussin, E., Massari, M., O'Connell, M., and Robbins, D. C. (1985). The thermic effect of carbohydrate versus fat feeding in man. *Metabolism* **34,** 285–293.

Schwartz, R. S., Jaeger, L. F., and Veith, R. C. (1985). The thermic effect of feeding and sympathetic nervous system activity. *Int. J. Obesity* **9** (4), A93 (Abstr.).

Seaton, T. B., and Welle, S. (1985). Thermogenesis in brown adipose tissue. *N. Engl. J. Med.* **312,** 1062 (letter to the editor).

Seaton, T., Welle, S., Lilavivat, V., and Campbell, R. G. (1984). The effect of adrenergic blockade on glucose-induced thermogenesis. *Metabolism* **33,** 415–419.

Segal, K. R., and Gutin, B. (1983). Thermic effects of food and exercise in lean and obese women. *Metabolism* **32,** 581–589.

Segal, K. R., Gutin, B., Nyman, A. M., and Xavier Pi-Sunyer, F. (1985). Thermic effect of food at rest, during exercise, and postexercise in lean and obese men of similar body weight. *J. Clin. Invest.* **76,** 1107–1112.

Sharief, N. N., and Macdonald, I. (1982). Differences in dietary-induced thermogenesis with various carbohydrates in normal and overweight men. *Am. J. Clin. Nutr.* **35,** 267–272.

Sheldahl, L. M., Buskirk, E. R., Loomis, J. L., Hodgson, J. L., and Mendez, J. (1980). Effects of exercise in cool water on body weight loss. *Int. J. Obesity* **6,** 29–42.

Shetty, P. S. (1984). Adaptive changes in basal metabolic rate and lean body mass in chronic undernutrition. *Hum. Nutr. Clin. Nutr.* **38C,** 443–451.

Shetty, P. S., Jung, T. T., James, W. P. T., Barrand, M. A., and Callingham, B. C. (1981). Postprandial thermogenesis in obesity. *Clin. Sci.* **60,** 519–525.

Shulman, G. I., Rothman, D. L., Smith, D., Johnson, C. M., Blair, J. B., Shulman, R. G., and DeFronzo, A. (1985). Mechanism of liver glycogen repletion *in vivo* by nuclear magnetic resonance spectroscopy. *J. Clin. Invest.* **76,** 1229–1236.

Sims, E. A. H. (1976). Experimental obesity, dietary induced thermogenesis and their clinical implications. *Clin. Endocrinol. Metab.* **5,** 377–395.

Sims, E. A. H. (1982). Mechanisms of hypertension in the overweight. *Hypertension* **4** (Suppl. III), 43–49.

Sims, E. A. H. (1984). Effects of overnutrition and underexertion on the development of diabetes and hypertension: A growing epidemic? *In* "Malnutrition: Determinants and Consequences" (P. L. White and N. Selvey, eds.), pp. 151–163. Liss, New York.

Sims, E. A. H. (1985a). Why, oh why can't they just lose weight? *Nutrition and the MD.* **11** (5).

Sims, E. A. H. (1985b). The characterization of obesity and the importance of fat distribution. Blood pressure and physical activity in the Hanes I survey. *Int. Symp. Metab. Complicat. Hum. Obesities, Marseille May 30-June 1.*

Sims, E. A. H. (1986). Physical activity in the development and management of obesity and its complications. *In* "Exercise, Nutrition, and Energy Metabolism" (E. S. Horton and R. L. Terjung, eds.), Chap. 14., Collamore Press, New York, in press.

Sims, E. A. H., and Sims, D. F. (1986). Living with non-insulin-dependent diabetes. The interplay of physiological, cultural, and emotional factors. *In* "Clinical Diabetes" (J. Davidson, ed.), Chap. 53, Sect. 7, Part 21, in press.

Sims, E. A. H., Kelleher, P. E., Horton, E. S., Gluck, C. M., Goldman, R. F., and Rowe, D. W. (1968). Experimental obesity in man. *Trans. Am. Assoc. Phys.* **81,** 153–170.

Sims, E. A. H., Danforth, E., Jr., Horton, E. S., Bray, G. A., Glennon, J. A., and Salans, L. B. (1973). Endocrine and metabolic effects of experimental obesity in man. *Recent Prog. Horm. Res.* **29,** 457–496.

Sims, E. A. H., Weed, L. L., Hertzberg, R. Y., and Weed, C. C. (1985). Management of a data base for obesity by problem-knowledge coupling using personal computers. *In*

"Recent Advances in Obesity Research" (J. Hirsch and T. B. Van Itallie, eds.), Vol. 4, pp. 155–162. Libbey, New York.
Sjöstrom, L. (1986). Adrenergic effects of energy restriction and refeeding in obesity. *Int. Symp. Metab. Complicat. Hum. Obesity, Marseille.*
Sjöström, L., Garellick, G., Krotkiewski, M., and Luyckx, A. (1980). Peripheral insulin in response to the sight and smell of food. *Metab. Clin. Exp.* **29,** 901–909.
Smith, G. P. (1984). The therapeutic potential of cholecystokinin. *Int. J. Obesity* **8** (Suppl. 1), 35–38.
Smith, G. P., and Gibbs, J. (1984). Gut peptides and postprandial satiety. *Symp. Am. Soc. Pharmacol. Exp. Ther., Chicago, April 12, 1983.*
Smith, R. E., and Hoijer, D. J. (1962). Metabolism and cellular function in cold acclimation. *Physiol. Rev.* **42,** 60–142.
Smith, T. J., and Edelman, I. S. (1979). The role of sodium transport in thyroid thermogenesis. *Fed. Proc., Fed. Soc. Exp. Biol.* **38,** 2150–2153.
Solomon, S. J., Kurzer, M. S., and Calloway, D. H. (1982). Menstrual cycle and basal metabolic rate in women. *Am. J. Clin. Nutr.* **36,** 611–616.
Stirling, J. M., and Stock, M. J. (1968). Metabolic origins of thermogenesis induced by diet. *Nature (London)* **220,** 801–02.
Stricker, E. M., and Zigmond, M. J. (1984). Brain catecholamines and the central control of food intake. *Int. J. Obesity* **8** (Suppl. 1), 39–50.
Stunkard, A. J., and McLaren-Hume, M. (1959). The results of treatment for obesity. *Arch. Intern. Med.* **103,** 79–85.
Sullivan, A. C., and Garattini, S., eds. (1984). Novel approaches and drugs for obesity. *Proc. Satellite Symp. Int. Congr. Obesity, 4th,* New York, *3-5 Oct., 1983 (Int. J. Obesity (Suppl.)* **8,** 1–248.
Sundin, U., Mills, I., and Fain, J. N. (1984). Thyroid–catecholamine interactions in isolated rat brown adipocytes. *Metabolism* **33,** 1028.
Thiebaud, D., Schutz, Y., Acheson, K., Jacot, E., DeFronzo, R. A., and Jequier, E. (1983). Energy cost of glucose storage in human subjects during glucose-insulin infusion. *Am. J. Physiol.* **244,** E216–E221.
Thorin, D., Golay, A., Simonson, D. C., Jequier, E., Felber, J. P., and DeFronzo, R. A. (1986). The effect of selective beta adrenergic blockade on glucose-induced thermogenesis in man. *Metabolism* **35,** 524–528.
Torbay, N., Bracco, E. F., Geliebter, A., Stewart, I. M., and Hashim, S. A. (1985). Insulin increases body fat despite control of food intake and physical activity. *Am. J. Physiol.* **248** (*Reg. Comp. Physiol.* **17**), R120–124.
Torti, F. M., Dieckmann, B., Beutler, B., Cerami, A., and Ringold, G. M. (1985). A macrophage factor inhibits adipocyte gene expression: An *in vitro* model of cachexia. *Science* **229,** 867–68.
Tulp, O. L. (1981). The development of brown adipose tissue during experimental overnutrition in rats. *Int. J. Obesity* **5,** 579–591.
Tyzbir, R. S., and Williamson, J. A. (1985). Diet alters brown adipose tissue (BAT) mitochondrial function during postnatal development in rats. *Nutr. Rep. Int.* **31,** 219–228.
Tyzbir, R. S., Kunin, A. S., Sims, N. M., and Danforth, E., Jr. (1981). Influence of diet composition on serum triiodothyronine (T_3) concentration, hepatic mitochondrial metabolism and shuttle system activity in rats. *J. Nutr.* **111,** 252–259.
Vague, J., and Björntorp, P. eds. (1985). *Int. Symp. Metab. Complicat. Hum. Obesities, Marseille, May 30-June 1.*
Vague, J., Bjorntorp, P., Guy-Grand, B., and Vague, J., eds. (1985). Metabolic Complica-

tions of Human Obesities. *Proc. 6th Int. Meeting, Marseille May 30–June 1, 1985. Int. Congr. Ser.* 68. Excerpta Medica, Amsterdam, New York, Oxford.

Vernet, O., Christin, L., Schutz, Y., Danforth, E., Jr., and Jequier, E. (1986a). β-Adrenergic blockade and intravenous nutrient induced thermogenesis in lean and obese women, in press.

Vernet, O., Christin, L., Schutz, Y., Danforth, E., Jr., and Jequier, E. (1986b). Enteral versus parenteral nutrition: Comparison of energy metabolism in lean and moderately obese women. *Am. J. Clin. Nutr.* **43,** 194–209.

Voit, C. (1881). Physiologie des Stoffwechsels. *Hermann's Handb. Physiol.* **6,** 209.

Wack, J. T., and Rodin, J. (1982). Smoking and its effects on body weight and the systems of caloric regulation. *Am. J. Clin. Nutr.* **35,** 366–380.

Webb, P. (1981). Energy expenditure and fat-free mass in men and women. *Am. J. Clin. Nutr.* **34,** 1816–1826.

Webb, P., and Annis, J. F. (1982). Adaptation to overeating in lean and overweight men and women. *Hum. Nutr. Clin. Nutr.* **37,** 117–131.

Welle, S. (1985). Evidence that sympathetic nervous system does not regulate dietary thermogenesis in humans. *Int. J. Obesity* **9** (Suppl. 2), 115–122.

Welle, S., and Campbell, R. (1983a). Stimulation of thermogenesis by carbohydrate overfeeding: Evidence against sympathetic nervous system mediation. *J. Clin. Invest.* **71,** 916–925.

Welle, S. L., and Campbell, R. G. (1983b). Normal thermic effect of glucose in obese women. *Am. J. Clin. Nutr.* **37,** 87–92.

Welle, S., Lilavivat, U., Hana, R., and Campbell, R. G. (1981). Thermic effect of feeding in man. Increasing plasma norepinephrine levels following glucose but not protein or fat consumption. *Metab. Clin. Exp.* **30,** 953–958.

Welle, S. L., Amatruda, J. M., Forbes, G. B., and Lockwood, D. H. (1984). Resting metabolic rates of obese women after rapid weight loss. *J. Clin. Endocrinol. Metab.* **59,** 41–44.

Wirtshafter, D., and Davis, J. D. (1977). Set points, settling points, and the control of body weight. *Physiol. Behav.* **19,** 75–78.

Withers, R. F. J. (1964). Problems in the genetics of human obesity. *Eugen. Rev.* **56,** 81–90.

Wolkowitz, O. M., Doran, A. R., Cohen, M. R., Cohen, R. M., Wise, T. N., and Pickar, D. (1985). Effect of naloxodone on food consumption in obesity. *N Engl. J. Med.* **313,** 327.

Woo, R., and Pi-Sunyer, F. X. (1985). Effect of increased physical activity on voluntary intake in lean women. *Metabolism* **34,** 836–841.

Woo, R., Garrow, J. S., and Pi-Sunyer, F. X. (1982). Voluntary food intake during prolonged exercise in obese women. *Am. J. Clin. Nutr.* **36,** 478–484.

Woo, R., O'Connell, M., Horton, E. S., and Danforth, E., Jr. (1985). Changes in resting metabolism with increased intake and exercise. *Clin. Res.* **33,** 712A (Abstr.).

Woods, S. C., West, D. B., Stein, L. J., McKay, L. D., Lotter, E. C., Porte, S. G., Kenney, N. J., and Porte, D., Jr. (1981). Peptides and the control of meal size. *Diebetologia* **20,** 305–313.

Wurtman, R. J., Hefti, F., and Melamed, E. (1981). Precursor control of neurotransmitter synthesis. *Pharmacol. Rev.* **32,** 315–335.

Yen, T. T., McKee, M. M., and Stamm, N. B. (1984). Thermogenesis and weight control. *Int. J. Obesity* **8** (Suppl. 1), 65–78.

Yitzhak, F., Braham, J., and Cohen, B. E. (1974). The Kleine–Levin syndrome. *Am. J. Dis. Child.* **127,** 412.

Young, R. A. (1976). Fat, energy, and mammalian survival. *Am. Zool.* **17,** 699–710.

Young, R. A., Salans, L. B., and Sims, E. A. H. (1982). Adipose tissue cellularity in woodchucks: Effects of season and captivity at an early age. *J. Lipid Res.* **23,** 887–892.

Yukimura, Y., Bray, G. A., and Wolfsen, A. R. (1978). Some effects of adrenalectomy in the fatty rat. *Endocrinology* **103,** 1924–28.

Zahorska-Markiewicz, B. (1980). Thermic effects of food and exercise in obesity. *Eur. J. Appl. Physiol.* **44,** 231–235.

Zed, C., and James, W. P. T. (1980). Post-prandial thermogenesis (PPT) in obese subjects after either protein or carbohydrate. *Alim. Nutr. Metab.* **1,** 385.

Zed, C., and James, W. P. T. (1981). Thermic response to fat feeding in lean and obese subjects. *Proc. Nutr. Soc.* **41,** 32A.

Zierler, K. L., and Rabinovitz, D. (1964). Effect of very small concentrations of insulin on forearm metabolism. Persistence of its action on potassium and free fatty acids without its effects on glucose. *J. Clin. Invest.* **43,** 450–462.

Zinder, O., Hamosh, M., Fleck, T. R. C., and Scow, R. O. (1974). Effect of prolactin on lipoprotein lipase in mammary gland and adipose tissue of rats. *Am. J. Physiol.* **226,** 744–748.

Zwillich, C., Martin, B., Hofeldt, F., Charles, A., Subryan, V., and Birman, K. (1981). Lack of effects of beta sympathetic blockade on the metabolic and respiratory responses to carbohydrate feeding. *Metabolism* **30,** 451–55.

Note Added in Proof

Some further developments in this field are summarized in a paper written in collaboration with Dr. Elliot Danforth, Jr., "Energy Expenditure in Man (Perspective Article)." *J. Clin. Invest.,* in press.

VITAMINS AND HORMONES, VOL. 43

Genetic Defects in Vitamin Utilization. Part I: General Aspects and Fat-Solumbe Vitamins

LOUIS J. ELSAS AND DONALD B. McCORMICK

Departments of Biochemistry and Pediatrics (Medical Genetics), Emory University School of Medicine, Atlanta, Georgia 30322

I. Introduction

A. Genetic Perspective and Inherited Metabolic Disorders

Geneticists approach the general subject of nutrition and the specific requirement for vitamins with the view that there are no generalized standards by which minimum or recommended daily allowances (RDA) for essential nutrients can be established for everyone. Rather, there is a continuum within a population of genetically determined variations in requirements extending over a wide range. This concept arose historically from two older scientific disciplines: human biochemical genetics and vitamin research. The former discipline originated with Sir Archibald Garrod's Croonian lectures of 1908. Garrod defined four "inborn errors of metabolism" as blocks in metabolic processes. Biochemical and clinical expression of these metabolic blocks revealed patterns of inheritance consistent with Gregor Mendel's predictions for transmission of single genes with large effect on the phenotype. Thus arose the concept that genes controlled metabolism and that disease states were produced by accumulated precursors and deficient products in sequences of biochemical reactions. Today, we recognize that "inborn errors" are discontinuous traits attributable to variation in structure and function of enzymes or other protein molecules which in turn are controlled by DNA sequences of genes. Over 3000 monogenic human disorders were catalogued in 1983, and of these, about 250 were defined biochemically (McKusick, 1983). The extent of normal variation in genes controlling enzyme activity suggests that about 30% of our population is heterozygous for common alleles (Harris, 1980). Within this continuous diversity, mutations produce discontinuous, relatively rare traits expressed as disease under normal environmental conditions. Mutant gene frequencies vary in populations; for example, mitochondrial branched-chain α-ketoacid dehydrogenase deficiency (maple syrup urine disease) occurs in one of every 250,000 newborns on a worldwide basis, but one in 176 in an inbred Mennonite population (Naylor and Flores, 1983; Marshall and DiGeorge, 1981). The mutation produces extreme toxicity to accumulated branched-chain α-ketoacids if affected newborns are fed the recommended daily allowance of branched-chain amino acids. However, normal growth and development are possible upon restriction of dietary leucine, isoleucine, and valine to 20–40% of the recommended daily allowance (RDA), depending on the degree of enzyme impairment (Elsas *et al.*, 1981; Acosta and Elsas, 1976). There is considerable human variation in the activity of this and many other enzymes involved in the catabolism of essential amino acids, but only a few are so impaired that ingestion of RDA amount creates severe disease. Dietary intervention is now applied at a public health level to at least five rare inborn errors in which screening of the newborn predicts genetic susceptibility to a normal diet (Elsas, 1982; Elsas *et al.*, 1983). By contrast to these relatively rare inborn errors, the human species lacks the enzyme that converts L-gulonolactone to ascorbic acid, but scurvy does not occur provided sufficient vitamin C is ingested and absorbed (Burns, 1959). Thus, the frequency of genetic susceptibility to a "normal" diet ranges from rare to common and extends to the metabolic flow of vitamins and their products, *viz.* active cofactors.

B. Vitamin Deficiency

This brings us to the second discipline, that of modern vitamin research. While Garrod's followers documented hundreds of inherited metabolic disorders, Frederick G. Hopkins began to study "accessory food substances" (Needham, 1962). His studies of 1912 demonstrated that rats fed a synthetic diet required small amounts of "accessory factor" from milk. In 1915 McCollum and Davis recognized that both water-soluble and fat-soluble "accessory factors" were required for normal growth in rats.

The Polish scientist Casimir Funk investigated man and described a beriberi-curing substance and coined the term *vitamine* (Funk, 1922). He postulated "vitamine" deficiency as a cause of several human disorders including not only beriberi, but also pellegra, rickets, and scurvy. In 1929 Hopkins and Funk were awarded Nobel Prizes for their work.

By the mid-1930s, the molecular structure of several "vitamines" had been established and the *e* dropped because, although all were essential to life, many were not amines. Thus, the concept of human disease caused by vitamin deficiency was clearly established.

C. Vitamin Dependencies

Today we define vitamins as organic compounds required in trace amounts (micrograms to milligrams per day) in the diet for health, growth, and reproduction of one or more species. It is commonly understood that vitamins are natural materials that can be isolated from organisms capable of synthesizing these compounds. Only small amounts of vitamins are required for the functional, often catalytic (coenzymatic) roles their products serve in contrast to the relatively large amounts of macronutrients such as protein, lipid, and carbohydrate which constitute the bulk of the ingesta and serve primarily as sources for energy and reconstitution of body mass. Hence, it is inappropriate to consider inositol or choline as vitaminic substances when they are utilized in sizable quantities largely for incorporation into such constitutive material as phospholipids. However, some compounds such as carnitine, lipoic acid, and biopterin, although apparently synthesized in sufficient quantities by the "normal" human, fulfill this definition under conditions produced by developmental or genetic variation.

Historically, two disorders initiated the concepts of vitamin dependency. In 1937, Albright and his colleagues found that a 16-year-old boy with hypophosphatemia and rickets improved upon treatment with vitamin D given orally in doses over 1000 times that necessary to prevent deficiency (Albright *et al.,* 1937). The disorder, "vitamin D-resistant rickets" or "familial hypophosphatemic rickets," was found through pedigree analyses to be caused by a single, dominant, mutant gene located on the X chromosome (Winters *et al.,* 1958). The second example of inherited excessive requirement for a specific vitamin was seizures in the newborn specifically cured by administration of pyridoxine in doses 10 times that normally required for health. Affected siblings responded specifically to intravenous pyridoxine but not to routine anticonvulsant therapy. Hunt coined the term *vitamin dependence,* meaning the control of seizures depended on large doses of pyridoxine, to differentiate this phenomenon from *deficiency* (Hunt *et al.,* 1954).

From these two early reports, "vitamin dependency disorders" were defined with four important points to differentiate them from vitamin deficiency. First, vitamin-dependent disorders were *inherited* and caused by mutant genes of large effect. Deficiency states were caused by nutritional or environmental lack of vitamins rather than an inherited etiology. Second, vitamin dependency was *specific* for one vitamin as compared to generalized lack of vitamins attendant upon nutritional deficiency. As the mechanisms producing the vitamin dependency states were determined, this concept of "specificity" extended to the unique biochemical reactions yielding the active cofactor from the vitamin. By contrast, many generalized reactions would be impaired by deficiency of a vitamin where different cofactor products of the vitamin are involved. This "specificity" issue required reinterpretation when genetic causes such as mutations producing malabsorption or biological unavailability of specific vitamins were discovered. Thus, a third point or caveat was made to include those vitamin dependency states caused by genetically impaired bioavailability. Vitamin dependency states may require a different route (e.g., parenteral) of administration to correct the clinical signs attendant on the lack of a specific vitamin. Finally, vitamin dependency states usually require larger than RDA doses to correct and prevent clinical expression of disease. *Supraphysiological* doses and/or *alternate routes* of vitamin administration are used to treat these inherited vitamin-dependent disorders. In Table I are summarized the recommended daily intake of vitamins required to prevent vitamin deficiency. By contrast, in Table II are given the ranges of daily requirements to control disease in inherited

TABLE I
RECOMMENDED ORAL INTAKE PER DAY TO PREVENT VITAMIN DEFICIENCY[a]

Vitamin[b]	Units	Infant (0–1 year)	Child (1–10 years)	Adolescent (9–17 years)	Adult
Retinols (A)	μg	400	400–700	1000	1000
Calciferols (D)	μg	10	10	10	7.3–5
2-Methylnaphthoquinones (K)	μg	12	15–40	30–60	70–140
Tocopherols (E)	mg	4	5–7	8	10
Thiamin (B_1)	mg	0.4	0.8	1.4	1.2
Riboflavin (B_2)	mg	0.4	1.3	2	1.7
Niacin	mg	6	14	22	19
Pyridoxine (B_6)	mg	0.4	1	2	2
Pantothenate	mg	3	4	4–7	4–7
L-Carnitine (B_T)[c]	mg	10–30	0	0	0
Biotin (H)	μg	35–50	65–120	100–200	100–200
Folacin	μg	30–45	100–300	400	400
Cobalamin (B_{12})	μg	2.5	2.5	5	5
Ascorbate (C)	mg	30–100	45	60	60

[a] Modified from Pennington and Church (1983) and Committee on Dietary Allowances (1980).

[b] Common chemical name of the vitamin is followed by the alphabetical letter given to it at discovery.

[c] Calculated from Borum (1981) and Brenner (1983).

TABLE II
DOSE AND ROUTE OF VITAMINS USED TO TREAT INHERITED VITAMIN DEPENDENCY DISORDERS

Vitamin[a]	Units/day	Route[b]	Dosage range
Retinol (A)	μg	p.o., im	7,500–25,000
Cholecalciferol (D_3)	μg	p.o., im	1,250–5,000
2-Methylnaphthoquinones (K)	μg	p.o., im, iv	1,000–6,000
α-Tocopherol (E)	mg	p.o.	200–2,000
Lipoic Acid	mg	p.o.	200
Thiamin (B_1)	mg	p.o., iv	10–1,000
Riboflavin (B_2)	mg	p.o.	20–300
Niacin	mg	p.o.	40–200
Pyridoxine (B_6)	mg	p.o.	10–1,000
Pantothenic Acid	mg	p.o.	100–1,000
L-Carnitine (B_T)	mg	p.o., iv	1,000–2,000
Biotin (H)	μg	p.o.	10,000
Folacin	μg	p.o.	200–10,000
Cobalamin (B_{12})	μg	p.o., im	5–500
Ascorbate (C)	mg	p.o.	1,000–10,000

[a] Actual forms administered depend upon route; e.g., a retinyl ester is given im or menadione is given iv.
[b] Route symbols: p.o., per os; im, intramuscular; iv, intravenous.

vitamin-dependency syndromes. Various interactions between genes, environment, and development in man alter normal requirements for vitamins. For instance, acquired or inherited disorders impairing bile secretion may cause malabsorption of fat-soluble vitamins and a requirement for parenteral administration of vitamins A, D, E, and K. Some pharmacological agents can alter vitamin requirements. For instance, anticonvulsants such as dilantin and phenobarbital enhance the degradation of vitamin D through induction of microsomal enzymes. In children so treated the vitamin D requirement to prevent rickets is increased (Hahn *et al.*, 1972). The antituberculosis drug isoniazide competitively inhibits pyridoxal kinase, reducing the conversion of pyridoxine to pyridoxal phosphate, and, consequently, increasing requirements for vitamin B_6 (Vilter, 1964). In the genetically determined "slow inactivator" of isoniazide the concentration of the drug increases more rapidly in the body than in persons characterized genetically as "fast inactivators." This emphasizes the complexity of environment, genetic susceptibility, and clinical condition in determining a recommended dietary allowance for a given vitamin in a given patient.

Age also is a factor determining vitamin requirements. Many enzymes under developmental control are not fully active in the newborn. A good example is the inability of the newborn to synthesize carnitine. (Hahn, 1981; Brenner, 1983). The enzyme γ-butyrobetaine hydroxylase increases gradually from 12 to 100% of normal by age 15; this emphasizes the essentiality of carnitine in the pediatric age group (Rebouche and Engel, 1980; Borum, 1981). Transient neonatal tyrosinemia is cured by giving 25 mg/kg of vitamin C orally to premature infants, whereas only 1 mg/kg is needed by older children. This added need for vitamin C is caused by the unique substrate susceptibility in the newborn of the rate-limiting enzyme in tyrosine catabolism *p*-hydroxyphenylpyruvic acid oxidase, which must be reduced by vitamin C for stability (Scriver, 1973). This age-related vitamin dependency, although common, may also be genetically controlled as suggested by discontinuous incidence data. Vitamin C-responsive tyrosinemia is found in 33% of premature and 0.005% of full-term infants (Scriver, 1973). Many excellent reviews of these concepts have been published over the last 15 years (Frimpter *et al.*, 1969; Rosenberg, 1969, 1970, 1973, 1974, 1976; Mudd 1971, 1974, 1982; Scriver 1973; Fernhoff *et al.*, 1980) and were used extensively in this review.

D. Mechanisms Producing Vitamin Dependency

Disorders of vitamin dependency provide insight into the normal processing of vitamins to active cofactors and modes of salvage for reutilization. Moreover, these experiments of nature indicate how a genetic defect can alter individual requirements. Even though the RDA is attained through oral consumption, it in no way ensures that in a given individual the vitamin will be absorbed, transported, processed, and conserved in quantities sufficient to catalyze its specific enzymatic reaction(s). Each vitamin acts within a distinct metabolic step, and a consideration of current mechanisms reported to produce vitamin dependency provides a conceptual framework for further classification. Table III summarizes some of these inherited mechanisms. The fat-soluble vitamins (A, D, E, K) are emulsifiable with bile salts, thus enhancing their uptake by mucosal cells of the small intestine and facilitating hydrolysis of esterified forms such as retinyl esters by pancreatic ester hydrolases (Hegsted *et al.*, 1976). Several heritable disorders decrease bile formation, causing fat malabsorption, impaired fat uptake by intestinal mucosal cells, restricted formation of chylomicrons, and diminished transfer of fat-soluble vitamins to the lymphatic system. Abetalipoproteinemia represents a mutation preventing pro-

TABLE III
MECHANISMS PRODUCING INHERITED VITAMIN DEPENDENCY SYNDROMES

1. Intestinal malabsorption
   a. Reduced availability of lipid emulsants
   b. Defective intrinsic factors
   c. Impaired active transepithelial transport
   d. Impaired cleavage from natural protein
2. Impaired transport by blood protein or lymphatic chylomicrons
3. Defective plasma membrane uptake
4. Defective release from cytosolic transfer protein
5. Impaired production of active cofactors (coenzyme)
6. Impaired covalent bonding of vitamin to apoenzyme
7. Defective noncovalent binding of coenzyme to apoenzyme
8. Rapid degradation of holoenzyme
9. Slowed recycling of covalently bound vitamin
10. Rapid excretion

duction of apoprotein B with consequent loss of capacity to synthesize low-density lipoproteins (Gotto *et al.,* 1971). Acanthocytosis, ataxia neuropathy, and pigmentary retinopathy are the well-recognized clinical results. Although the pathogenesis of this condition is not fully understood, a lack of the antioxidant effects of the tocopherols (vitamin E) was considered. The hypothesis is supported by the observation that large amounts (100 mg/kg) of administered vitamin E prevented these signs from occurring in younger siblings affected by this autosomal recessive trait (Mueller and Lloyd, 1982).

Among the water-soluble vitamins, the processing of vitamin B_{12} (cobalamin) to its two coenzyme forms has contributed to our current understanding that at least 12 different proteins under separate genetic control are required to form a holoenzyme which contains one of the active cobalamin cofactors. These include gastric intrinsic factors, ileal transporter proteins, transcobalamin I (TCI), transcobalamin II (TCII), B_{12}-specific plasma membrane transporters, TCII-B_{12} lysosomal hydrolases, at least two anaerobic cobalamin reductases, deoxyadenosyltransferase, cobalamin I methylase, and binding sites on the apoenzymes of methylmalonyl-CoA mutase and homocysteine methyltransferase. Human heritable defects in most of these vitamin-processing functions have been identified through the clinical response to parenteral administration of supraphysiological doses of B_{12} and biochemical or complementation analysis (Rosenberg, 1983; Rosenblatt *et al.,* 1985). Thus, inborn errors expressing vitamin B_{12} dependency are caused by many of the genetic mechanisms outlined in Table III.

Holoenzyme metabolism is a problem in at least two vitamin-dependency disorders in which the biological half-life of the enzyme is prolonged if the vitamin product or coenzyme binding sites are saturated. Vitamin B_1-dependent forms of maple syrup urine disease (deficient branched-chain α-ketoacid dehydrogenase) and B_6-dependent forms of homocystinuria (impaired cystathionine β-synthase) represent examples of this type. Saturation of coenzyme binding sites prolongs the biological half-life of mutant apoenzymes (Kim and Rosenberg, 1974; Longhi *et al.*, 1977; Elsas and Danner, 1982; Hefflefinger *et al.*, 1984).

Recent studies of biotin-dependent carboxylase deficiencies have provided insight into two more mechanisms producing vitamin dependency. The first involves synthesis in which covalent linkage of biotin to its apoprotein is impaired (mechanism 6, Table III). The second involves impaired cleavage, and thus, bioavailability through absorption and recycling of biotin when it is ingested or degraded after covalent binding to protein (mechanism 9, Table III) (Wolf *et al.*, 1980, 1983, 1985). These disorders produce multiple carboxylase deficiencies and are characterized by severe metabolic acidosis in the newborn with excretion of unusual urinary organic acids including β-methylcrotonylglycine and 3-hydroxypropionate. It was discovered that the biotin-dependent enzymes, 3-methylcrotonyl-CoA carboxylase, and propionyl-CoA carboxylase are not biotinylated when normal amounts of biotin are ingested, but that when 2500-fold higher intakes of biotin are administered enzyme function returns (Saunders *et al.*, 1982). The apoenzymes are normal, but the holocarboxylase synthetase, an enzyme responsible for covalently linking biotin to its apoenzyme, is defective. A late-onset form of multiple carboxylase deficiency is also dependent on massive amounts of orally administered biotin. The mechanism here is impairment of the enzyme biotinidase (EC 3.5.1.12) (Wolf *et al.*, 1983; Wastell *et al.*, 1984). This enzyme cleaves biotin from its covalent linkage at the ε-amino terminus of lysyl residues. Bioavailability of biotin for recycling into active holoenzymes requires that it be cleaved from both endogenous enzymatic proteins and from exogenous dietary proteins. This form of multiple carboxylase deficiency is characterized by onset at age 6 months of hair loss, dermatitis, organic aciduria, and loss of function of four biotin-dependent enzymes. All enzyme defects are corrected by large amounts of ingested biotin, and biotinidase is undetectable in tissues and physiological fluids. Thus, another mechanism producing vitamin dependency was defined to include genetically defective enzymes which recycle covalently bound vitamins.

This recycling process *in vivo* may also include renal tubular reabsorption (mechanism 10, Table III). For instance, in normal man, carnitine is lost mainly by urinary excretion, 10–20 μmol/kg body weight each day. This represents about 8% of the total body pool (Brenner, 1983). Renal carnitine losses were found and corrected in several patients with autosomal recessive forms of systemic carnitine deficiency syndromes (Engel *et al.,* 1981; Rebouche and Engel, 1983). There are still further heritable mechanisms yet to be discovered whereby vitamin requirements are altered by genes controlling vitamin-regulating proteins and functions. For each vitamin and active cofactor form there is a unique set of processing, recycling, and enzymatic steps required for function. We will, therefore, discuss separately each vitamin and the recognized genetic defects in its utilization.

E. Toxicity to Vitamins

At the onset of this discussion of genetic defects in vitamin utilization, a word of caution and dissociation from the indiscriminate use of megadose vitamins is indicated. Historically, the use of vitamins progressed from the identification of vitamin deficiency to our present use of increased vitamin dosage for uniquely altered metabolic sequences. More recently, a nonscientific but popular "orthomolecular" megadosage approach arose. This popularity began in the early 1970s, probably as a misinterpretation by the press of vitamin dependency (Hodges, 1982; Rudman and Williams, 1983). However, the use of 20- to 600-fold excesses of all vitamins is meant to treat neither deficiency nor dependency but to "saturate various apoenzymes and maximize catalytic processes by mass action." Gram quantities of vitamin C are said to cure infections, prevent colds, prevent colon cancer, and increase mental alertness. Yet, none of these claims has been substantiated in controlled studies, nor have they clear scientific bases. From these misjudgments, considerable new information regarding vitamin C toxicity has evolved. For instance, hyperoxaluria with nephrolithiasis is now a clearly associated toxic effect (Swartz *et al.,* 1984), and "rebound scurvy" in adults and in the infants of mothers who used megadosage vitamin C therapy has been described (DiPalma and Ritchie, 1977; Alhadeff *et al.,* 1984). Additionally, excessive vitamin C may interact and alter the requirements for other vitamins. It decreases B_{12} absorption (Herbert and Jacob, 1974) while increasing iron absorption (Cook and Monsen, 1977). Excessive vitamin C may also interfere with the anticoagulation properties of warfarin and shorten prothrombin time (Stockley, 1981). Thus, even this presumably harmless, water-soluble vitamin has potentially hazardous side effects when taken in supraphysiological amounts. Large amounts should not be ingested without a clear and rational purpose; both physician and patient must be aware of potential toxicity.

Normal physiology and biochemistry of each of the four lipid-soluble vitamins (A, D, K, E) will be discussed in the next section. In the next volume we will discuss nine water-soluble vitamins (B_1, B_2, niacin, B_6, pantothenic acid, biotin, folacin, B_{12}, C) and two recently defined human "vitamins" (lipoic acid, carnitine). Genetic diseases and developmental conditions which produce a specific vitamin dependency state will be defined. The toxic effects of each substance will be discussed not only to dissuade the orthomolecular, megadose fadist, but also to allow patients and physicians who use supraphysiological doses to weigh the benefits and potential costs of this unique therapy for vitamin-dependent inherited metabolic disorders.

II. Fat-Soluble Vitamins

A. Vitamin A

It is historically appropriate to begin a discussion of inherited vitamin dependency syndromes with the "fat-soluble A" which was the first essential, lipid-soluble substance of foods discovered (McCollum and Davis, 1913). Early nomenclature differentiated lipid-soluble factors from the "water-soluble B" complex which was essential for growth in rats. Later investigators subdivided "fat-soluble A" which shared the chemical characteristic of extractibility into organic solvents into vitamins A, D, E, and K. Vitamin A and its derived retinoids are now recognized as specifically required for vision, reproduction, maintenance of epithelial cell differentiation, and mucus secretion (Moore, 1957). Several extensive reviews have recently been published (Sporn *et al.,* 1984; Goodman, 1984; Tielsch and Sommer, 1984).

1. *Chemistry, Physiology, and Functions*

The two natural forms of vitamin A, *retinol* (A_1) and *3-dehydroretinol* (A_2), are C_{15} isoprenoid alcohols containing substituted β-ionone and 3-dehydro-β-ionone rings, respectively (Fig. 1). These compounds are yellowish oils that are practically insoluble in water. The vitamin is sensitive to oxygen and ultraviolet light, which induces a greenish fluorescence. The more common A_1 predominates, especially as long-chain fatty acid esters, in mammalian liver and in salt-water fish i.e., cod liver oil, whereas the less active A_2 derives from freshwater fish oils. Although man cannot biosynthesize the β-ionone-type

R = CH_2OH for retinols, CHO for retinals, CO_2H for retinoic acids:

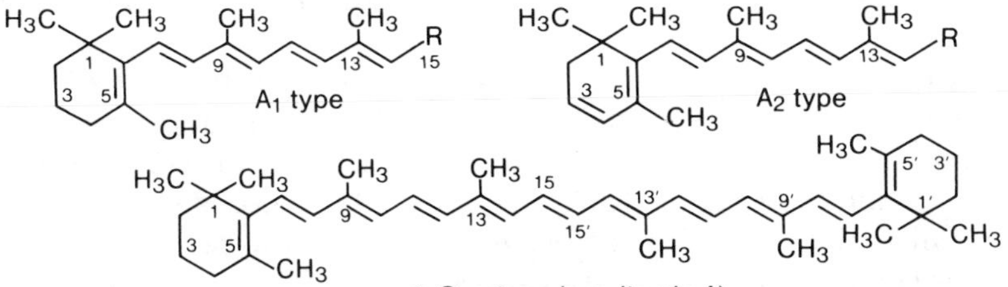

A_1 type

A_2 type

β-Carotene (provitamin A)

FIG 1. Structures of vitamin A and provitamin A.

ring structure, he can derive the aldehyde retinol from intestinal dioxygenase-catalyzed cleavage of plant-derived carotenes which serve as provitamins. Retinal is then reversibly reduced by pyridine nucleotide-dependent enzymes to retinol.

The structure for the most common and effective provitamin A, *β-carotene,* is also given in Fig. 1. Although carotenoid compounds, which constitute the yellow-to-orange pigments of most vegetables and fruits, show considerable variation in the availability to the human, they often comprise the main dietary source of what ultimately becomes vitamin A. On the basis of structure alone, it has been estimated that the number of provitamin A precursors would be between 50 and 60 known carotenoid and apocarotenoid compounds (Simpson and Chichester, 1981).

In the intestinal lumen, free provitamin and vitamin A forms are emulsified by bile salts to micelles which enable uptake by mucosal cells of the small intestine. This micelle formation facilitates hydrolysis of dietary retinyl esters by pancreatic and brush border retinyl ester hydrolase. Dietary carotenoids are cleaved by the cellular dioxygenase system, converted to retinal, and reduced to retinol. Cellular free retinol is reesterified with long-chain fatty acids, predominantly palmitic and stearic, within the mucosal cell. Retinyl esters in association with chylomicrons then pass via the lymphatic system to the liver. Hepatic uptake of chylomicron remnants involves apoliprotein E (Sherril *et al.,* 1980). Parenchymal cells again hydrolyze chylomicron-associated retinyl esters to retinol. Intrahepatic retinol-binding proteins bind retinol which, when adequately supplied, is reesterified by acyl-CoAs, mainly palmitoyl, stearyl, and oleyl, and stored in a lipoglycoprotein complex. Esteratic release of retinol from this complex allows association with plasma retinol-binding protein synthesized by rough endoplasmic reticulum. Hepatocytes via secretory vesicles release holo-retinol-binding protein (21,000 MW), which then associates with circulating prealbumin (55,000 MW) to form a molecular aggregate in blood which is of sufficient size to avoid loss by glomerular filtration.

Retinol mobilization from liver and delivery to peripheral tissues are regulated by rates of hepatic synthesis and secretion of these circulating transporter proteins, and their production in turn is regulated by the availability of retinol (Sporn *et al.*, 1984). There is some evidence that delivery of this circulating retinol complex to peripheral target cells involves specific cell-surface receptors. Within the target tissue, there are specific intracellular binding proteins both for retinol and retinoic acid with different tissue specificities (Chytil, 1982; Adachi *et al.*, 1981; Ong *et al.*, 1982). At least one kind of retinol-binding protein (type 2) is found in high levels in the gut mucosal cells, where absorption of the vitamin is facilitated (Crow and Ong, 1985). It has been suggested that these intracellular proteins may also be important in the biological action of vitamin A.

Retinol is degraded by a series of chain-shortening steps to biologically inactive products. Little is known about these reactions or their function in controlling vitamin A action. However, they do affect hepatic stores and daily requirements for vitamin A.

Among physiological functions of vitamin A, the best understood is the participation of retinal in vision (Wald, 1968). The predominant circulating form of vitamin A is all-*trans*-retinol. After uptake into retinal cells the compound is isomerized to 11-*cis*-alcohol which is reversibly dehydrogenated to 11-*cis*-retinal (Fig. 2). This sterically hindered geometrical isomer of the aldehyde combines as a lysyl-linked

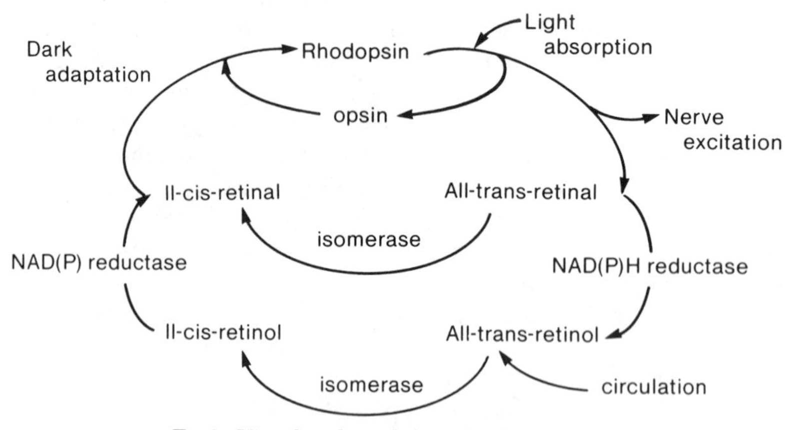

FIG 2. Visual cycle and the role of vitamin A.

Schiff base with suitable proteins, e.g., opsin, to generate photosensitive pigments, e.g., rhodopsin. Illumination of such pigments cause photoisomerization and release of all-*trans*-retinal plus the protein opsin, a process which couples the large conformational change to ion flux and optic nerve transmission. The all-*trans*-retinal is isomerized to the 11-*cis* isomer, which again combines with the liberated opsin to reconstitute the photopigment in a visual cycle shown in Fig. 2. The pyridine nucleotide-dependent dehydrogenase (reductase) can also reduce the all-*trans*-retinal to all-*trans*-retinol.

Other broader functions of A are in reproduction and growth. Systemic effects that reflect an optimal level of A are the stabilization of cellular and intracellular membranes and the synthesis of glycoproteins. All-*trans*-retinyl-1β-phospho-D-mannose is formed from retinyl phosphate and UDP mannose and is a good donor *in vitro* of mannose to certain glycoproteins. Thus, one molecular mechanism proposed for vitamin A action is to maintain glycoprotein synthesis in a manner similar to dolichol conversion to dolichyl glycosides. Another postulated mechanism is that retinoids alter gene expression analogous to effects of steroid hormones. This hypothesis does not require retinol or retinoic binding protein complexes to interact with genomic DNA through nuclear binding sites. The ability of natural and synthetic retinoids to alter cell differentiation and prevent some forms of neoplastic transformation offers credence and importance to this mechanism (Goodman, 1984).

2. *Requirements and Deficiency*

Adult man requires approximately 1000 μg of retinol, or twice as much β-carotene, to maintain an adequate blood concentration and to prevent deficiency symptoms (Table I). Greater intakes are necessary to produce significant liver storage. Recommended allowances (RDAs) for adult females may be slightly less at 800 retinol equivalents, where 1 equivalent = 1 μg retinol or 6 μg β-carotene or 12 μg of other provitamin A carotenoids. In terms of international units (IU), 1 retinol equivalent = 3.33 IU of retinol or 10 IU of β-carotene. The RDA for infants, based on content and volume of human milk, is 420 retinol equivalents until 6 months and 400 from then to the first year. Higher amounts are recommended to satisfy growth needs for children and adolescents. Supplements of 200 retinol equivalents is recommended for pregnant women and 400 retinol equivalents for lactating women. A comprehensive review of the A requirements of the human, including the effects of exercise, stress, and genetic defects, has been published (Rodriguez and Irwin, 1980).

Degenerative changes in eyes and skin are always observed in vitamin A deficiency. Poor dark adaptation or night blindness (nyctalopia) is an early symptom, followed by degenerative changes in the retina. Vitamin A deficiency causes mucus formation with generalized drying of the eye (xerophthalmia). Small gray plaques with foamy surfaces (Bitot's spots) may develop on the sclera. These lesions are reversible with vitamin A administration. More serious and nonreversible effects of deficiency are known as kerotomalacia and cause ulceration and necrosis of the cornea, which leads to perforation, endophthalmitis, and blindness. Usually, skin changes are associated including dryness, roughness, papular eruptions, and follicular hyperkeratosis. There is, in general, an atrophy of specialized epithelia followed by metaplastic hyperkeratinization which is expressed not only in the eye, but also in lung, sweat glands, and gastrointestinal tract.

Xerophthalmia is worldwide and common, with 500,000 new cases of active corneal degeneration reported yearly in India, Bangladesh, Indonesia, and the Philipines. It is most common in those areas where leafy vegetables containing β-carotene are not consumed. This is the leading cause of childhood blindness, probably because neither human nor cow's milk contains sufficient vitamin A to meet the needs of growing children.

Two epidemiological studies reported that low serum retinol concentrations were associated with increased cancer risk, but a third study refuted this finding (Wald *et al.*, 1980; Kark *et al.*, 1981; Willet *et al.*, 1984). There has been no attempt to determine genetic susceptibility in these classical case-control studies (Sporn and Roberts, 1983).

3. *Inherited Disorders Producing Dependency*

From a cursory view of known mechanisms producing vitamin dependency syndromes (Table III) and the many proteins involved in vitamin A uptake, processing, and cellular regulation (lipoproteins, transport proteins, esterases, retinol-binding proteins, intracellular binding proteins, degrading proteins), one could postulate many causes for vitamin A dependency. To date, only two heritable conditions are specifically treatable by administering supraphysiological amounts of Vitamin A. One is congenital biliary stenosis with cirrhosis. The second is abetalipoproteinemia, an inherited disorder of apoprotein B and consequent chylomicron production (Herbert *et al.*, 1983; Herlong *et al.*, 1981). In biliary cirrhosis, night blindness is a commonly associated symptom. It is reversible by giving 25,000 μg vitamin A orally per day. The true therapeutic range has not been established. Because evidence of cirrhosis is usually present, mechanisms involving liver processing of vitamin A, such as hepatic synthesis or release of retinol-binding proteins, have been postulated (Walt *et al.,* 1984). In familial abetalipoproteinemia, the heritable deficiency of chylomicrons restricts the transport of retinyl esters from intestinal epithelium through the lymphatics to the liver and reduces the liver stores. Oral administration of 25,000 μg vitamin A/day restores liver stores and reverses peripheral neuropathy and retinal regeneration (Bieri *et al.,* 1984). Pretreatment of affected siblings before these manifestations develop is preventative (Mueller *et al.,* 1977; Illingworth *et al.,* 1980). In all cases, however, other fat-soluble vitamins, particularly vitamin E, were given as well.

4. *Toxicity*

Hypervitaminosis A develops from ingestion of excess vitamin or as a side effect of inappropriate therapy. One of the most important factors is the form of vitamin A administered (Sporn *et al.,* 1984). Symptoms can appear at earlier times with administration of aqueous emulsions rather than oily solutions (Korner and Vollm, 1974). Hypervitaminosis A occurs after liver storage of retinol and its esters exceeds 10,000 IU/g tissue, a level 10 times the estimated normal. Toxicity develops as the capacity of circulating retinol-binding protein to transport retinol is exceeded (Smith and Goodman, 1976). Acute toxicity from a single massive dose is reflected by abdominal pain, nausea, vomiting, severe headache, dizziness, sluggishness, and irritability followed within a few days by desquamation of the skin and recovery. Chronic toxicity with moderately high doses taken for protracted periods is characterized by bone and joint pain, hair loss, dryness and fissures of the lips, anorexia, and benign intracranial hypertension, weight loss, hepatomegaly, and sometimes hypercalcemia. Chronic excessive intake of carotene-rich foods, principally carrots, leads to carotenemia benign yellowing of skin; the excess carotene is deposited rather than converted to excess A.

Congenital malformations are also caused by excessive retinol taken during pregnancy. These teratogenic effects are presumably caused by disruption of cell migration (Fernhoff and Lammer, 1984). In children, hypercalcemia and bone pain with periosteal resorption is described as a toxicity syndrome to vitamin A (Frame *et al.,* 1974). In adults, gouty arthritis is another toxic effect (Mawson, 1984). These toxic effects are also produced by the analog, isoretinoin, given to treat acne at 40–80 mg per day, orally.

B. Vitamin D

1. *Chemistry, Physiology, and Functions*

Advances in separation and analysis of vitamin D precursors, products, and interacting proteins now allow better categorization of vitamin D dependency disorders. Many excellent reviews on this topic have been published over the last 5 years (Norman *et al.*, 1982; Avioli and Haddad, 1984; DeLuca, 1979; Bikle, 1982, 1985; Fraser, 1980; Marx *et al.*, 1983), but a brief coverage will be presented here.

The two forms of dietary vitamin D are *ergocalciferol* (D_2), a vegetable form, and *cholecalciferol* (D_3), an animal form. D_2 is produced by ultraviolet irradiation of the naturally occurring plant sterol, ergosterol. Light causes ring cleavage to yield an intermediate preergocalciferol which thermally rearranges to ergocalciferol (Fig. 3). D_3 is derived from irradiation of provitamin 7-dehydrocholesterol in skin to produce, via thermal arrangement of precholecalciferol, the natural cholecalciferol. As shown by structures in Fig. 3, the only chemical difference between the two vitamin and provitamin forms is in the side chain. There are at least 10 compounds known to yield vitamin D-active compounds on irradiation. Most differ only in the side chain at C_{17} of the sterol nucleus. Both forms of vitamin D are also efficiently absorbed from the gastrointestinal tract unless there is fat malabsorption caused by lack of bile salts, pancreatic insufficiency, or a defect of intestinal mucosal function. After uptake, the vitamin is bound directly to chylomicrons and transported initially via the lymphatics. To exert its biological activity, vitamin D is hydroxylated sequentially at

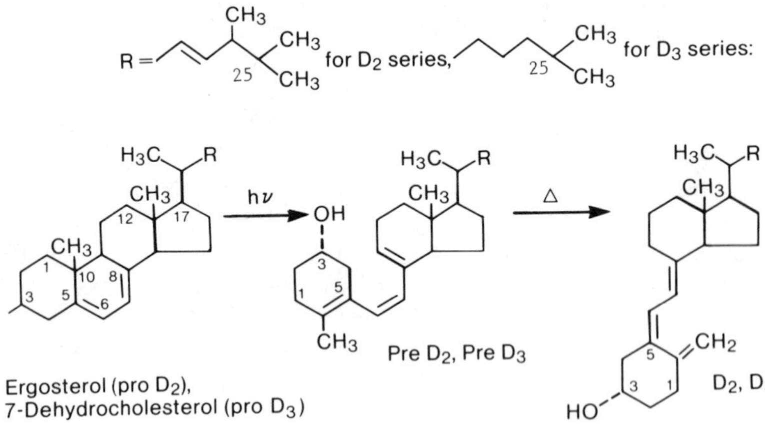

Fig 3. Conversion of previtamin forms of D to vitamin D.

position 25 and the position 1. Much of the prohormone-like vitamin initially supplied to the liver is hydroxylated at the terminal side-chain position to yield 25-hydroxy-D. This process involves molecular oxygen and a pyridine nucleotide-dependent, microsomal, mixed-function oxidase system. There is little, if any, regulation of this reaction. The 25-hydroxycholecalciferol, which represents the major metabolite of D_3 in plasma, circulates bound to D-binding α-globulin (52,000 MW).

In kidneys, the second hydroxylation occurs at the 1α-position by cytochrome P-450-mediated, mixed-function oxidase located on the inner mitochondrial membrane. There is considerable regulation at this step. Normally, the kidney 1α-hydroxylase is stimulated by increased 25-hydroxy-vitamin D, parathyroid hormone (PTH), and low serum phosphate (DeLuca, 1981; Haussler *et al.*, 1982). The kidney can also direct formation of 24,25-dihydroxy-D (an inactive catabolite) at normal concentrations of calcium and phosphate rather than toward the 1α,25-dihydroxy-D at decreased blood Ca^{2+}, which leads to parathormone release, cyclic AMP formation, renal loss of phosphate, and stimulation of the 1α-hydroxylase. The 1,25-dihydroxycholecalciferol formed in the kidney complexes with the D-binding protein for transfer via blood to target tissues, e.g., small intestine, bone, skin, placenta, and parathyroid. In the intestinal mucosal cell, the hormonally active 1α,25-dihydrocholecalciferol binds to a cytosolic receptor protein (45,000 MW) before entrance into the nucleus in association with a chromatin receptor. A prime effect may be on DNA-dependent RNA polymerase II to mediate synthesis of a specific calcium-binding protein which, in turn, increases calcium absorption (Symposium, 1982). An outline of the transport, activation, and catabolism of vitamin D is given in Fig. 4.

2. *Requirements and Deficiency*

It has been determined that 2.5 μg (100 IU) of precursor vitamin D per day is required to prevent rickets in the young, but 10 μg (400 IU) promotes better calcium absorption and optimal growth (Table I). Therefore, the higher amount is recommended from infancy through

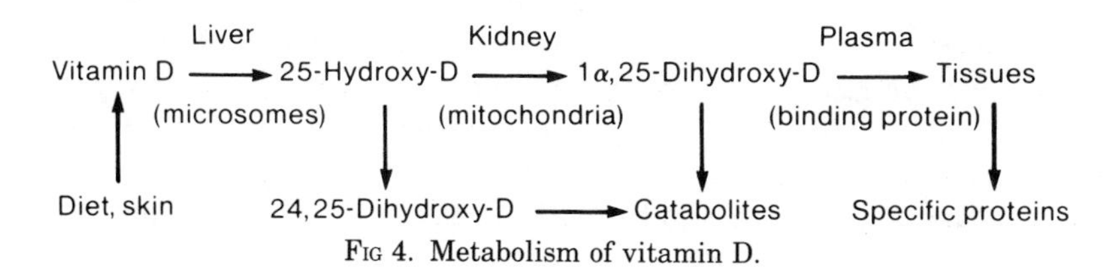

FIG 4. Metabolism of vitamin D.

age 18 years. As the rate of skeletal growth and calcium needs decrease, the daily allowances are reduced to 7.3 μg during the ages 19–22 years and to 5 μg thereafter. An additional 5 μg/day (i.e., 10 μg/day) is recommended for pregnant and lactating women.

The extent to which ultraviolet irradiation of 7-dehydrocholesterol in skin contributes to production of vitamin D_3 is quite variable and depends upon seasonal variation in sunlight, clothing, degree of skin pigmentation, etc. Availability and consumption of such D_3-containing animal foods as fatty fish, eggs, liver, and butter also are variable. Hence, widespread fortification of food with vitamin D has been adopted to ensure a more secure supply. Both cow and human breast milk are deficient in vitamin D. Cows' milk and infant formulas are now routinely marketed to contain 10 μg (400 IU) of added vitamin D per quart. Both ergocalciferol and cholecalciferol are about equally converted in the human to hormonally active dihydroxy forms.

Recently, 1,25-dihydroxy-D or calcitriol has become commercially available for medical usage, and its circulating concentrations have been measured and used as a probe for diagnosis and management of metabolic bone disease (Haussler *et al.,* 1982; Manolagos *et al.,* 1982; Gray *et al.,* 1982; Rosen and Chesney, 1983). Normal ranges of 1,25-dihydroxy-D are 19–70 and 15–40 pg/ml in children and adults, respectively. The calcidiols, i.e., 25-hydroxy-D_2 and 25-hydroxy-D_3, circulate at thousand-fold higher ranges, 2–8, and 8–45 ng/ml, respectively. Normal replacement is 0.1–1.0 μg/day of dihydroxy-D orally.

Vitamin D requirements increase in vitamin D deficiency (insufficient sunlight or inadequate dietary sources), malabsorption, inherited or acquired diseases with impaired conversion of vitamin D to its active metabolite (Tables III and IV), and the dihydroxy vitamin D receptor defects (Marx *et al.,* 1983). All of these disorders cause defective mineralization expressed as rickets in childhood as osteomalacia in adults (Bikle, 1985).

3. *Inherited Disorders Producing Dependency*

Since neonatal and childhood requirements for vitamin D supplements have been defined and provided, vitamin D deficiency states have become less common, but inherited variations in vitamin D metabolism have gained attention. The mechanisms producing these genetically determined, increased requirements have become defined by advances in methods for determining 25-hydroxy-D, 1,25-dihydroxy-D, their catabolic products, and the cellular binding protein (Manolagos *et al.,* 1982; Gray *et al.,* 1982).

The X-linked hypophosphatemic rickets in children or osteomalacia in adults is the prototypic vitamin D-resistant disease in humans (Albright *et al.,* 1937; Winters *et al.,* 1958). However, it was soon found that treatment with high doses of D_3 alone did not improve skeletal growth or rickets without producing hypercalcemia and hypercalciuria. The underlying genetic defect was determined to be phosphate malabsorption by kidney and intestine, but phosphate replacement alone did not restore skeletal mineralization and this regimen often led to secondary hyperparathyroidism (Scriver, 1974). With the advent of vitamin D metabolite assays, plasma 25-hydroxy-D was found to be normal in these patients, but 1,25-dihydroxy-D was low. By contrast, the normal response to phosphorus depletion is to increase 1,25-dihydroxy-D (Haddad *et al.,* 1973; Dominquez *et al.,* 1976; Rosen and Chesney, 1983). Several long-term studies show that treatment with high doses of 1,25-dihydroxy-D, 3 μg per day, is effective (Drezner *et al.,* 1980). Thus, studies on this prototypic D-dependency syndrome show not only a defect in phosphate transport, but also a regulatory defect in kidney 25-hydroxy-D-1α-hydroxylase response to stimulation by low blood phosphate (Table IV). In several other inherited renal disorders with renal phosphate wasting there may also be reduced 25-hydroxy-D-1α-hydroxylase responses due to generalized renal damage. These include Fanconi syndrome, cystinosis, Lowe's syndrome, and Wilson's disease among others. They are not listed in Table IV.

Lack of response to PTH is found in pseudohypoparathyroidism (Drezner *et al.,* 1976; Lambert *et al.,* 1980). Control of this enzyme in producing the active cofactor of vitamin D has also been implicated in the pathogenesis of senile osteoporosis (Tsai *et al.,* 1984). Regulation at this critical step in producing 1,25-dihydroxy-D was also found defective in mild rickets with reduced serum phosphate, mimicking vitamin deficiency, but circulating 25-hydroxy-D is normal, 1,25-dihydroxy-D is low, and there is poor response to physiological doses of vitamin D (Fraser and Scriver, 1976). This autosomal recessive trait was called vitamin D-dependent rickets type I (VDDR-I) and it responded clinically to small amounts of 1,25-dihydroxy-D (Delvin *et al.,* 1981) (Table IV). Type I was then differentiated from type II vitamin D-dependent rickets (VDDR-II) by more severe clinical presentation in the latter which included alopecia, enamel hypoplasia, seizures, refractory hypocalcemia, and elevated concentration of 1,25-dihydroxy-D. VDDR-II became the prototype for end-organ resistance to the active vitamin D metabolite 1,25-dihydroxy-D; defective nuclear uptake of tritiated 1,25-dihydroxy-D by cultured skin fibroblasts was demonstrated (Eil *et al.,* 1981; Marx *et al.,* 1983). With assays for this receptor, this disorder

TABLE IV
INHERITED DISORDERS OF VITAMIN D METABOLISM

Condition	Inheritance	Clinical features	Biochemical mechanism	Treatment
Melanotic skin	Polygenic	Rickets, poor growth, breast feeding, geophagia	Lack of UV conversion of ergosterol to D_3	Sunlight; D supplements
Familial hypophosphatemic rickets (FHPR)	X-linked dominant Autosomal dominant	Rickets and growth restriction; low serum phosphate, normal calcium, and PTH	Renal and intestinal phosphate malabsorption Impaired 25(OH)D-1α-hydroxylase response to hypophosphatemia	Oral phosphate supplements; 50,000–100,000 IU D_3 or 1–3 μg/day $1,25(OH)_2D$
Vitamin D-dependent rickets type I (VDDR-1)	Autosomal recessive	Rickets, poor growth, normal 25(OH)D, low $1,25(OH)_2D$	Impaired 25(OH)D-1α-hydroxylase	1 μg/day $1,25(OH)_2D$
Vitamin D-dependent rickets type II (VDDR-II)	Autosomal recessive	Severe rickets, alopecia, enamel hypoplasia, seizures, hypocalcemia, increased plasma $1,25(OH)_2D$	End organ resistance to $1,25(OH)_2D$ with kinetically altered intracellular binding proteins	3–5 μg/day $1,25(OH)_2D$; oral calcium

Pseudophypoparathyroidism	X-linked dominant Autosomal dominant Autosomal recessive Multifactorial	Skeletal anomalies, hypocalcemia, low $1,25(OH)_2D$, short stature, metatarsals, and metacarpals	PTH receptor defect; failure of renal $25(OH)D$-1α-hydroxylase to respond to PTH	1–3 μg/day $1,25(OH)_2D$
Hereditary hypophosphatemic rickets with hypercalciuria (absorptive hypercalciuria)	Autosomal dominant	Hypercalciuria with renal stones; elevated plasma and $1,25(OH)_2D$; low PTH	Phosphate malabsorption with overactivity of renal $25(OH)D$-1α-hydroxylase	Oral phosphate
Tumoral calcinosis	Autosomal dominant	Calcific tumor masses, dental anomalies, elevated $1,25(OH)_2D$ and serum phosphate	Overproduction of $1,25(OH)_2D$	Genetic counseling
Osteopetrosis	Autosomal recessive	Osteosclerotic bones	Defective osteoclast response to $1,25(OH)_2D$	High dose $1,25(OH)_2D$ (32 μg/day)
Williams syndrome	Sporadic, polygenic	Mental retardation, eflin face, aortic stenosis ± hypercalcemia	Hypersensitivity to D with increased 25-OH-D and/or $1,25(OH)_2D$	Restrict vitamin D and calcium

became recognized as heterogeneous, with different degrees of impaired 1,25-dihydroxy-D binding to intracellular protein. These mutations apparently impair the binding domain of the protein rather than through gene deletion (Pike *et al.,* 1984). Even 5 μg/day of oral 1,25-dihydroxy-D caused no increase in calcium uptake (Rosen *et al.,* 1979; Tsuchiya *et al.,* 1980; Devlin *et al.,* 1981).

Another family of inherited diseases associated with end-organ resistance by osteoclasts to 1,25-dihydroxy-D causes osteopetrosis. Recent use of extremely high 1,25-dihydroxy-D (32 μg/day) enhanced bone resorption in one patient (Key *et al.,* 1984). The differential genetic control of osteoclasts to resorb bone calcium and intestinal epithelial cells to transport dietary calcium is exemplified by these phenotypically distinct inborn errors of vitamin D metabolism. Interestingly, one complication of X-linked hypophosphatemic rickets with low phosphate and 1,25-dihydroxy-D is calcification of entheses (Polisson *et al.,* 1985).

Another group of inherited diseases of D metabolism may develop from overproduction or sensitivity to 1,25-dihydroxy-D at the end organ (Table IV). Tumoral calcinosis (Lyles *et al.,* 1985), hereditary hypophosphatemic rickets with absorptive hypercalcuria (Tieder *et al.,* 1985), and Williams syndrome are three examples. In the absorptive hypercalciuria syndromes, oral phosphate supplements have been used to reduce 1,25-dihydroxy-D overproduction and hyperabsorption of calcium (Broadus *et al.,* 1984; Tieder *et al.,* 1985). There is conflicting information concerning regulation of 25-hydroxy-D and 1,25-dihydroxy-D in Williams syndrome (Taylor *et al.,* 1982; Garabedian *et al.,* 1985). In carefully controlled studies of children during the hypercalcemic phase, 1,25-dihydroxy-D was elevated, while in the normocalcemic phase, excessive conversion of 25-hydroxy-D to 1,25-dihydroxy-D under loading conditions was alleviated.

For completeness, it is useful to list drugs and other disorders that increase vitamin D requirements. In senile osteoporosis, intestinal malabsorption, and liver disease, there is decreased vitamin D absorption and conversion to active metabolites. Anticonvulsants, particularly dilantin, impair conversion of D_3 to 25-hydroxy-D by liver and secondarily impair calcium uptake by intestine (Haussler and McCain, 1977). Hypophosphatemia due to decreases in phosphate absorption from gut (aluminum hydroxide gels), kidney (nephrotic syndrome), or phosphaturic peptides (epidermal nervus syndrome) (Aschinberg *et al.,* 1977) also causes decreased conversion of 25-hydroxy-D to 1,25-dihydroxy-D, with resultant rickets and increased requirements for orally administered, active biological products of vitamin D (DeLuca, 1981).

4. *Toxicity*

It is now generally accepted that intoxication with vitamin D is caused by excessive production in liver of 25-hydroxy-D rather than excessive 1,25-dihydroxy-D production in kidney. This concept was derived from clinical observations that the hypercalcemia of overzealous vitamin D usage produced bone demineralization with calcium deposition in soft tissue and that anephric patients with elevated blood phosphate became hypercalcemic upon ingestion of excess D_3. 25-Hydroxy-D normally circulates at 1000 times the concentration of 1,25-dihydroxy-D. The monohydroxy-D stimulates production of intestinal calcium transporter protein and mobilizes bone at concentrations 100 times that of 1,25-dihydroxy-D. Furthermore, the production of 25-hydroxy-D from D_3 by liver is unregulated and the biological clearance is measured in days as compared to hours for 1,25-dihydroxy-D (Haussler and McCain, 1977).

Accumulated 25-hydroxy-D is the probable cause of intoxication with D_3, but excessive 1,25-dihydroxy-D also causes toxicity (Chan *et al.*, 1983) manifested by sudden episodes of hypercalcemia and progressive loss of renal function due to nephrocalcinosis. A related type of hypercalcemia is produced in certain diseases characterized by formation of granulomatous tissues (e.g., sarcoidosis) which aberrently produce extrarenally excess amounts of 1,25-dihydroxy D (Bell *et al.*, 1979).

C. Vitamin E

1. *Chemistry, Physiology, and Functions*

Vitamin E was discovered in 1922 by Evans and Bishop as a fat-soluble factor essential for normal reproduction by the rat (Evans and Bishop, 1922). The word *tocopherol,* the main chemical group which comprises vitamin E, is Greek and means "to bear offspring." The most potent form of vitamin E is d-α-tocopherol. Eight related natural compounds in this group are biosynthesized in plants; thus, these compounds are especially abundant in vegetable oils (Janiszowska and Pennock, 1976). As shown by structures in Fig. 5, all bear a 6-chromanol nucleus substituted with methyl groups at postions 2 and 8 and further, with a branched isoprenoid chain at 2 that is saturated (phytyl) for tocopherols or unsaturated at positions 3′, 7′, and 11′ for tocotrienols. The Greek letter prefixes signify methylation at positions 5 and/or 7. The vitamin E group are viscous oils at room temperature.

Vitamin E absorption from the small intestine is facilitated by bile.

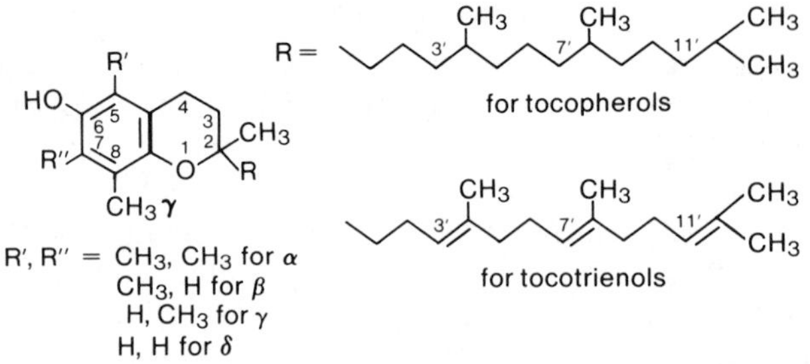

FIG 5. Structures of vitamin E and related compounds.

Most of tocopherol enters the blood stream via lymph where it is associated with chylomicrons and very-low-density lipoproteins. The vitamin is stored in most tissues with the largest amount in adipose tissue. Vitamin E metabolism differs from vitamin A in that E is not stored primarily in the liver and is not bound to specific blood transporter proteins in the circulation. Vitamin E is deposited and associated with lipoproteins in cellular membranes. Tocopherol exchanges rapidly between erythrocyte membranes and plasma lipoproteins. A small fraction of physiological doses appears in urine as the quinoid tocopheronic acid and the β-glucuronide conjugates of the hydroquinoid form (Simoin *et al.*, 1956). Some of the dynamics of metabolism undoubtedly are reflected in the relative biological activity of tocopherols. For example, the less active γ-vitamer is taken up as effectively as the α form but is turned over more rapidly (Hegsted *et al.*, 1976).

The best defined role for vitamin E is as an antioxidant for unsaturated fatty acyl moieties of lipids within membranes. Polyunsaturated fatty acyl moieties of membrane phospholipids are damaged oxidatively by hydrogen peroxide produced through flavoprotein oxidases. Concurrent free radical damage can ensue. Interactions among vitamin E, selenium, and sulfur amino acids have been rationalized on the basis that, while E is oxidized in lieu of unsaturated fatty acyl functions, the Se-containing glutathione peroxidase helps reduce lipid peroxides, thereby decreasing peroxidative autocatalysis (Hegsted *et al.*, 1976).

In mammals there is no proof that any enzyme reaction is specifically affected by E, though decreases in liver microsomal drug hydroxylation (Carpenter and Howard, 1974) and increases in net synthesis of xanthine oxidase (Catigani *et al.*, 1974) have been found in E-deficient animals. At present, the only direct evidence for participation of E-like compounds is in the anaerobic rumen bacterium *Butyrivibrio fibrisolvens,* where *cis*-9, *trans*-11-octadecanoate is hydrogenated by a system coupled to α-tocopherolquinol to form α-tocopherolquinone and *trans*-11-octadecenoate (Hughes and Tove, 1980).

2. *Requirements and Deficiency*

The requirement for vitamin E is related to the polyunsaturated fatty acid content of cellular structure and, therefore, depends upon the nature and quantity of dietary fat which affects such composition. Hence, the minimum requirement of E for adults is not certain, but it is probably no more than 3–4 mg (4.5–6 IU) of d-α-tocopherol per day for infants ingesting a diet containing the minimum for essential fatty acids, i.e., 3% of calories (Table I). Since vitamin E activity derives from a series of tocopherols and tocotrienols in usual mixed diets, requirements are based on abundance and activity relative to the biologically most active d-α-tocopherol. Mass in milligrams of β-tocopherol is to be multiplied by 0.5, γ-tocopherol by 0.1, and α-tocotrienol by 0.3. This sum plus milligrams of α-tocopherol represents mass of α-tocopherol equivalents. It has been estimated that a range of 7–13 mg of α-tocopherol equivalents (10–20 IU) is required in balanced adult diets supplying 1800–3000 kcal. This intake maintains plasma concentrations of total tocopherols in a normal range of 0.5–1.2 mg/dl, which also ensures an adequate concentration in all tissues (Bieri and Evarts, 1975).

Recommended daily dietary allowances based on the foregoing considerations are 10 mg α-tocopherol equivalents for adult males and 8 mg for males 11–14 years old and adult females. The increased caloric intake during pregnancy and lactation calls for 2- and 3-mg increases to compensate for amounts deposited in the fetus and secreted in milk, respectively. It is recommended that infants be given 3 mg during the first half-year, since the E-content of human milk averages no more than this, yet is sufficient to raise blood tocopherols to the adult level in 2 or 3 weeks. Increases from 4 to 8 mg/day are suggested for children.

Until recently, no isolated deficiency state for vitamin E was described in man because E deficiency was always accompanied by lack of other fat-soluble vitamins. Deficiency syndromes in newborns and adults were postulated. Premature and low-birth-weight infants are susceptible to development of vitamin E deficiency, since placental transfer is poor and there is limited adipose tissue for storage (Winnick, 1983). A deficiency syndrome of the newborn was described which included irritability, edema, and hemolytic anemia. The anemia reflected a shortened life span of erythrocytes with fragile membranes, and did not respond to iron therapy, which aggravated the condition. Deficiency symptoms rarely develop in children or adults except in cases of severe fat malabsorption. In cases in which low blood content of vitamin E was detected, however, symptoms were not corrected with E therapy alone. In adults with long-standing inability to absorb fat, the deficiency syndrome included fragility of erythrocytes, increased urinary excretion of creatine including muscle loss, and deposition of ceroid pigment in the musculature of the small intestine (Binder *et al.*, 1965).

3. *Inherited Disorders Producing Dependency*

The importance of vitamin E in neurological function was brought into focus by disorders involving prolonged fat malabsorption with resultant deficiency of E (Binder *et al.*, 1965; Muller *et al.*, 1977; Elias and Muller, 1983; Sokol *et al.*, 1984). The recent identification of selective malabsorption of vitamin E confirmed a unique degeneration of spinocerebellar function specifically associated with tocopherol deficiency (Harding *et al.*, 1985) (Table V). In abetalipoproteinemia (lack of apoprotein B) there is deficient formation of chylomicrons, low-density lipoproteins, and very-low-density lipoproteins. Thus, from birth, fat-soluble vitamins in general are malabsorbed, affecting vitamin E in particular, because there is low storage capacity for it and it is not transported to peripheral tissues. It is undetectable in serum and cellular membranes. From early childhood, steatorrhea, progressive ataxia, and pigmentary retinopathy develop. Supraphysiological doses of vitamin E are required to prevent these signs and lipoproteins are uniquely required to transport E to the peripheral tissues (Muller *et al.*, 1977). Eight patients were treated with 100 mg/kg/day of vitamin E orally; this treatment led to either prevention, regression, or stabilization of these devastating neurological signs (Muller and Lloyd, 1982).

Recent findings confirmed this neurological pathology in a 23-year-old woman without fat malabsorption who suffered progressive spinocerebellar degeneration with ataxia, areflexia, and loss of proprioception. Serum vitamin E was undetectable. Heterozygotes within the family were identified by lower than normal vitamin E to cholesterol ratios in serum. Oral loading with 2 g of α-tocopheryl acetate produced normal serum vitamin E content within 4 hours, and this was maintained for 24 hours. Selective vitamin E malabsorption was postulated since there was no further neurological deterioration after 15 months treatment with 800 mg daily of vitamin E. Vitamin E in serum returned to normal. It is believed that vitamin E prevents or reverses

TABLE V

INHERITED DISORDERS EXPRESSING DEPENDENCY ON VITAMIN E

Disorder	Pattern	Expression	Pathophysiology	Therapeutic dose
Abetalipoproteinemia	Autosomal recessive	Peripheral neuropathy, spinocerebellar degeneration, pigmentary retinopathy, myopathy	Failure to transfer to chylomicrons	100 mg/kg per day, orally
Selective vitamin E malabsorption	Autosomal recessive	Spinocerebellar degeneration	Impaired intestinal transporter	20 mg/kg per day, p.o.
Cystic fibrosis	Autosomal recessive	Steatorrhea progressive pulmonary disease, sterility, axonal dystrophy	Fat malabsorption with impaired uptake	50 mg/kg per day
Erythrocyte glucose-6-phosphate dehydrogenase dificiency	X-linked	Hemolytic anemia	Insufficient antioxidant to provide membrane stabilization	1000 mg per day
Erythrocyte glutathione synthetase deficiency	Autosomal recessive	Hemolytic anemia	Insufficient antioxidant to stabilize erythrocyte membrane	1000 mg per day
Sickle cell	Autosomal recessive	Hemolytic anemia	Increased need to decrease irreversibly sickled cells	10000 mg per day
Newborn retrolental fibroplasia	Polygenic	Retinal oxygen toxicity	Increased need for antioxidant protection of membranes	100 mg/kg per day, orally

this pathology by reacting with free radicals produced by a number of oxidative metabolic processes. In the absence of this isoprenoid, these free radicals attack polyunsaturated fatty acids of peripheral and myelinated nerve membranes, and produce peroxidative decomposition of membrane lipids and consequent cellular damage. Vitamin E prevents and reverses this sequel.

In the newborn, supplemental amounts of vitamin E are necessary to prevent retrolental hyperplasia, hemolytic anemia, and neonatal hyperbilirubinemia in preterm infants who receive oxygen (Bieri *et al.*, 1983). The use of excess amounts of vitamin E may protect mature red cell membranes which are incapable of *de novo* lipid synthesis and of coping with oxidative stresses where inherited disorders produce defective reducing enzymes (Table V). Thus, the disorders of glucose-6-phosphate dehydrogenase and glutathione synthetase deficiencies are associated with chronic hemolysis, which is improved with large oral doses of vitamin E (Spielberg *et al.*, 1979; Corash, 1980; Bieri *et al.*, 1983). Decreased concentrations of vitamin E in serum are found in various inherited disorders with chronic hemolytic anemia including sickle disease (Natta *et al.*, 1980). The administration of excess vitamin E produced an increase in red cell glutathione peroxidase and a reduction in percentage of irreversibly sickled cells (Natta *et al.*, 1980; Chiu and Lubin, 1979).

Many medical conditions are putatively dependent on vitamin E, but there is poor substantiation. They include intermittent claudication, angina with low HDL, menopausal symptoms, infertility, and diabetes (Bieri *et al.*, 1983).

4. *Toxicity*

Although reports of adverse symptoms caused by large doses of vitamin E abound in the literature, most represent mild subjective gastrointestinal complaints (Oski, 1980). Two areas of clinical concern are the side effects of potentiation of warfarin anticoagulation and impairment of bactericidal capacity of leukocytes. At concentrations above 100 μmol/liter of plasma (normal range 11.5–35.0 mol/liter), vitamin E may antagonize the vitamin K-dependent carboxylation reaction and interfere with coagulation processes. In premature infants given high doses of vitamin E, a higher incidence of necrotizing colitis has been found (Sobel *et al.*, 1982).

In normal adults, increases in vitamin E content to twice normal in plasma have not produced toxicity. Since there is no evidence that concentrations greater than 70 μmol/liter produce any benefit, it is recommended that, based on the individuals genetic constitution, doses be adjusted so as not to exceed this concentration and that serum concentrations be monitored.

D. Vitamin K

1. *Chemistry, Physiology, and Functions*

Vitamin K ("Koagulations" vitamin) was discovered as an essential, fat-soluble factor of chick feed, deficiency of which caused loss of functional prothrombin and consequent hemorrhage (Dam and Doisy, 1964). Dam and Doisy shared the Nobel Prize in 1943 for isolating and characterizing vitamins K_1 and K_2. Compounds in the vitamin K series are 2-methyl-1,4-naphthoquinones which are substituted with side chains at carbon 3. The two principal natural classes, as shown in Fig. 6, are the *phylloquinones* (K_1 type) synthesized in plants and the *menaquinones* (K_2 type) of bacterial origin. Most commonly, vitamin K_1 bears a saturated, phytyl, 20-carbon side chain derived from four isoprenoid units; K_2 shows greater variation, but an all-*trans*-farnesylgeranylgeranyl, 35-carbon chain of 7 isoprenoid units is typical. Several synthetic analogs and derivatives have been used. Most are derived from *menadione* (K_3) which lacks a side-chain substituent at position 3. In a sense, the menadione-type compound is a synthetic provitamin, since K_3 is converted to menaquinone, e.g., K_2, by addition of the side chain in the liver. The K vitamins are insoluble in water, but dissolve in organic fat solvents. They are destroyed by alkaline solutions and reducing agents and are sensitive to ultraviolet light.

The absorption of natural vitamin K from the small intestine is facilitated by bile with efficiency of absorption varying from 15 to 65%

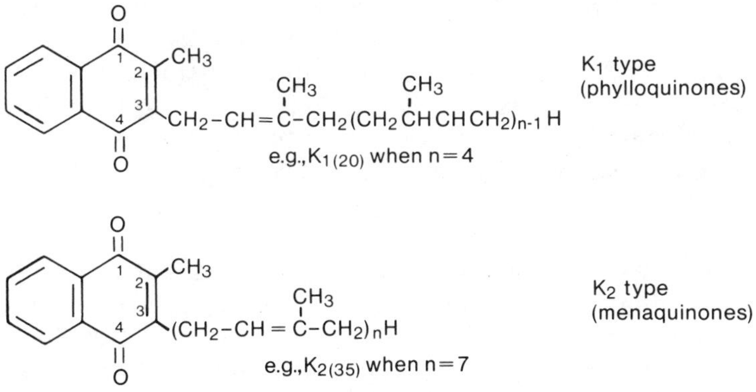

Fig 6. Structures of vitamin K.

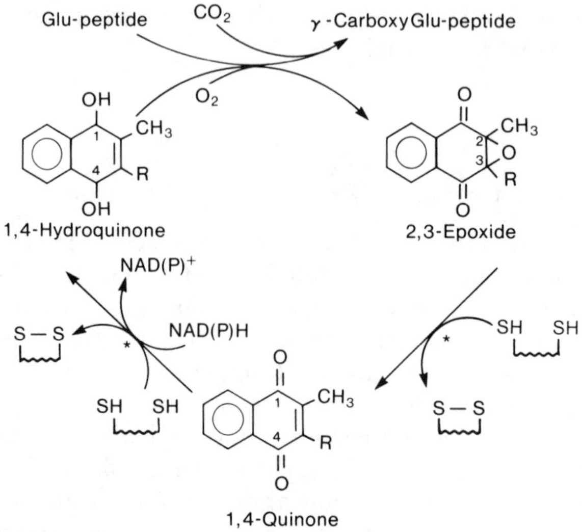

FIG 7. Vitamin K cycle and the production of γ-carboxyglutamic acid peptides. (*), Inhibited by coumarin anticoagulants.

as reflected by recovery in lymph within 24 hours. Vitamin K_1 and K_2 are bound to chylomicrons for transport from mucosal cells to the liver. Menadione (K_3), on the other hand, is more rapidly and completely absorbed before entering the portal blood. In liver, intracellular distribution is mostly in the microsomal fraction where prenylation of menadione to form K_2 occurs. Release of K_2 to the bloodstream allows association with circulating β-lipoproteins for transport to other tissues. Significant levels of K have been noted in spleen and skeletal muscle.

A microsomal vitamin K cycle exists within metabolically active and K-utilizing tissues, especially liver (Hauschka *et al.,* 1978; Suttie, 1979) (Fig. 7). The 1,4-quinone of vitamin K is reduced by an NADH-dependent and thiol-sensitive flavoprotein system to the dihydroxyquinone K, which then can participate in the oxygen- and carbon dioxide-utilizing γ-carboxylation of glutamyl residues on specific proteins (clotting factors and osteocalcin) (Gallop *et al.,* 1980). The concomitantly formed 2,3-epoxide of K is then reduced to the starting 1,4-quinones of vitamin K, a process that is antagonized by warfarin. Only traces of urinary metabolites of K_1 and K_2 appear in urine, but a considerable portion of K_3 (menadione) is conjugated at the hydroquinone level to form the β-glucuronide and sulfate esters, which are excreted.

Initially, the function of vitamin K was recognized as a dietary antihemorrhagic factor. It is necessary for liver syntheses of plasma clotting factors II (prothrombin) as well as VII (proconvertin), IX (plasma thromboplastin component), and X (Stuart factor). The latter three are also called autoprothrombin I, II, and III, respectively. These and other factors, including Ca^{2+}, initiate a process whereby an aggregate of several proteins with prothrombin, calcium ion, and phosphatide react to form thrombin which catalyzes proteolytic conversion of fibrinogen ultimately to polymerized fibrin clot. The reduced dihydroxyquinone K participates in the oxygen-dependent incorporation of CO_2 into the γ-methylene of specific L-glutamyl residues of prothrombin and other plasma proteins (Suttie, 1979) (Fig. 7).

The search for γ-carboxyglutamyl (Gla)-containing proteins has led to the realization that the vitamin K-dependent formation of such Ca^{2+}-binding proteins also includes bone Gla protein or osteocalcin which serves as a regulatory function in mineralization. The synthesis of this protein is regulated by 1,25-dihydroxy-D and acts by virtue of its specific ability to bind to hydroxyapatite (McCormick and Wright, 1971; Price and Baukol, 1980, 1981; Price and Williamson 1981; Price 1985). The occurrence of Gla-containing, Ca^{2+}-binding proteins has also been noted in kidney, urine, and renal stones (Olson and Suttie, 1977; Hauschka *et al.,* 1978).

Bis(4-Hydroxycoumarin), or dicoumarol, the anticlotting compound from spoiled sweet clover, and synthetic 4-hydroxycoumarins such as warfarin have found use as anticoagulants and have expedited the understanding of the metabolic cycling of vitamin K (Hauschka *et al.,* 1978; Wessler and Gitel, 1984). These anticoagulants interfere with the reductase-catalyzed conversion of epoxide to quinone forms of K as well as reduction of the latter to the functional dihydroxyquinone (Fig. 7). Hence, 4-hydroxycoumarins can suppress the formation of prothrombin and other K-dependent Ca^{2+}-binding proteins.

2. *Requirements and Deficiency*

No specific RDAs are presently given for vitamin K, since intestinal bacteria in normal individuals synthesize the menaquinones which are partially absorbed. However, because the sufficiency of this source of K is uncertain over long periods, an estimated adequate range of dietary intake has been suggested (Table I). The lower levels of K are based on the assumption that about half of the requirement, estimated to be 2 μg/kg body weight, is contributed by intestinal synthesis and the other half by diet (Olson, 1973). This is reasonable, as analyses of human liver indicate half of the K is of bacterial menaquinone type and the other half of plant-derived phylloquinones. The upper levels assume all the requirement is of dietary origin. The intake suggested for adults, then, is 70–140 μg/day, which is easily supplied by an average mixed diet estimated to provide 300–500 μg of K daily (Olson, 1973). The intake suggested for infants, 12 μg/day, is based on the assumption that intestinal synthesis is nil, but is within the range supplied by mature breast milk.

Hemorrhagic disease of the newborn can develop readily, since the menaquinone-synthesizing intestinal flora are established over the first week of life and early breast milk is low in vitamin K. Prothrombin content during this period is only about 25% of the adult level. The use of antibiotics in the newborn readily exacerbate the situation, so that prothrombin levels can drop below 5% of the adult with consequent hemorrhagic diathesis (Sutherland *et al.,* 1967; Oski and Naiman, 1982). Overt K deficiency may develop in adults with reduced intake, antibiotic inhibition of intestinal microflora, or 4-hydroxycoumarin-type anticoagulant therapy. Deficiency is relatively uncommon and found in patients with chronic fat malabsorption or long-term antibiotic or anticoagulant treatments (Wilson, 1982). Defective blood coagulation is, at present, the only well-established sign of K deficiency.

Conventional assessment of vitamin K status relies on blood clotting tests as reflected by prothrombin time. In this procedure, it is usual to add tissue thromboplastin (often in crude form from rabbit brain) to recalcified plasma and determine the time for clot formation, using normal plasma as a normal control. When the prothrombin concentration declines below 30% of normal, prothrombin times rise above 30 seconds. Deficiency of K can be distinguished from hypoprothrombinemia of liver disease by measurement of the noncarboxylated prothrombin precursor that accumulates in plasma in vitamin K deficiency. If K deficiency exists, administration of the vitamin should promptly correct abnormal prothrombin or clotting time.

3. *Inherited Disorders Producing Dependency*

The concept of genetically determined variation in requirements for vitamin K came first from clinical research into mechanisms producing hereditary resistance to warfarin. One patient required high doses of coumarin to reduce prothrombin time. When given a diet deficient in vitamin K, prothrombin time became prolonged after 14 days, whereas normal controls continued for weeks without abnormal prothrombin times. Repletion to normal prothrombin times required 8 μg vitamin K, intravenously. It was hypothesized that there was an altered vitamin K receptor site with reduced affinity for both the vitamin and coumarin (O'Reilly, 1971). It is probable that variable requirements of vitamin K in the newborn are also a manifestation of genetically impaired vitamin K binding sites on microsomal reductase for conversion of the 1,4-quinone to the active 1,4-dihydroquinone derivative (Fig. 7) (Gallop *et al.*, 1980). One child with bleeding at birth required 1 mg of vitamin K intravenously to cure diathesis. She was deficient in all four vitamin K-dependent clotting factors (Chung *et al.*, 1979). With high doses of vitamin K intramuscularly (5 mg/week), clotting functions improved but remained prolonged to three to four times normal. Interestingly, even with high doses of vitamin K the urine contained only 20% of normal γ-carboxyglutamyl peptides, which suggests that the genetic defect caused a marked decrease in vitamin K-binding proteins (1,4-hydroquinone reductases) (Gallop *et al.*, 1980).

The coagulation scheme is quite complex and includes several vitamin K-dependent proteins which inactivate already activated coagulation factors V and VIII (Davie and Ratnoff, 1964) and may stimulate fibrinolysis (Comp and Esmon, 1981). The principal deterrants to pathological thrombus formation are these plasma coagulation inhibitors and plasmin fibrinolytic systems (Mander, 1984). One such factor called protein C limits coagulation and promotes fibrinolysis (Comp and Esmon, 1981; Kisiel *et al.*, 1977). This protein (MW approximately 56,000) is a heterodimer of light and heavy chains. The amino-terminus of the light chain is vitamin K dependent and contains 11 γ-carboxyglutamic acid residues. Several families with protein C deficiency have expressed thrombotic episodes, some of which were responsive to vitamin K when given in large quantities (McGhee *et al.*, 1984; Vicente *et al.*, 1984; Seligson *et al.*, 1984; Bertina *et al.*, 1984). It is clear that heterogeneity exists in the types of expressed protein C deficiency. Autosomal dominant inheritance is defined for a trait characterized by an unexpected coagulopathy on initiating coumadin therapy (McGhee *et al.*, 1984). This paradoxical complication of anticoagulation therapy is corrected by intravenous vitamin K administration in some but not all patients. These patients are probably heterozygous for a mutation involving either the γ-carboxyglutamyl peptide or the K-dependent carboxylase. The rare homozygote may develop massive venous thrombosis in infancy (Seligson *et al.*, 1984).

Several new classes of vitamin K-dependent, calcium-binding proteins are defined that all have γ-carboxyglutamic acid residues arising through catalysis by vitamin K-dependent carboxylases (Fig. 7). They are unique and highly specialized proteins that promote protein–phospholipid interaction for functions such as coagulation, anticoagulation, calcium transport, calcium deposition, and the conversion of proenzymes to enzymes. Metabolic bone diseases such as postmenopausal osteoporosis have been associated with calcium loss and a postulated rapid degradation of the γ-carboxylated protein osteocalcin (Gallop *et al.*, 1980). In one study, calcium loss was reduced by daily treatment with high doses of vitamin K_2 (Tomita, 1971). It is probable that a number of inherited variations in the requirement of vitamin K will emerge. Each genetic variation will probably require a different vitamin K intake to optimize the production of these γ-carboxyglutamyl peptides and confer upon them appropriate calcium binding properties (Suttie, 1983).

4. *Toxicity*

Oral or intramuscular use of high doses of naturally occurring vitamin K (K_1 and K_2) cause no untoward effects. However, treatment with the water-soluble forms of menadione (K_3) can lead to cytoplasmic inclusions known as Heinz bodies, hemolytic anemia, and kernicterus in the newborn (Briggs, 1981). Intravenous doses greater than 1 mg per day over several days can produce this vitamin K toxicity syndrome.

REFERENCES

Acosta, P. B., and Elsas, L. J. (1976). Dietary management of inherited metabolic diseases: Phenylketonuria, galactosemia, tyrosinemia, homocystinuria, and maple syrup urine disease. CELMU Publishers, Atlanta, Georgia.

Adachi, N., Smith, J. E., Sklan, D., and Goodman, D. S. (1981). Radioimmunoassay studies of the tissue distribution and subcellular localization ocellular retinol-binding protein in rats. *J. Biol. Chem.* **256,** 9471–9476.

Albright, F., Butler, A. M., and Bloomberg, E. (1937). Rickets resistant to vitamin D therapy. *Am. J. Dis. Child.* **54,** 529–547.

Alhadeff, L., Gualtieri, C. L., and Lipton, M. (1984). Toxic effects of water soluble vitamins. *Nutr. Rev.* **42,** 33–40.

Alpan, G., Avital, A., Peleg, O., and Ogani, Y. (1984). Late presentation of hemorrhagic disease of the newborn. *Lancet* **1,** 482–483.

Anonymous (1983). Megavitamin E supplementation and vitamin K-dependent carboxylation. *Nutr. Rev.* **41,** 268–270.

Aschinberg, L. C., Solomon, L. M., Zeis, P. M., Justice, P., and Rosenthal, I. M. (1977). Vitamin-D resistant rickets associated with epidermal nevus syndrome: Demonstration of a phosphaturic substance in the dermal lesions. *J. Pediatr.* **91,** 56–60.

Avioli, L. V., and Haddad, J. G. (1984). Editorial retrospective. The vitamin D family revisited. *N. Engl. J. Med.* **311,** 47–49.

Bell, N. H., Stern, P. H., Pantzer, E., Sinha, T. K., and DeLuca, H. F. (1979). Evidence that increased circulating 1-alpha,25-dihydroxy vitamin D is the probable cause for abnormal calcium metabolism in sarcoidosis. *J. Clin. Invest.* **64,** 218–225.

Bertina, R. M., Broekmans, A. W., Krommenhoek, Van Es, C., and Van Wijngaardden, A. (1984). The use of a functional and immunological assay for plasma protein C in the study of the heterogeneity of cogenital protein C deficiency. *Thromb. Haemostasis (Stuttgart)* **57,** 1–5.

Bieri, J. G., and Evarts, R. P. (1975). Tocopherols and polyunsaturated fatty acids in human tissues. *Am. J. Clin. Nutr.* **28,** 717–723.
Bieri, J. G., Corash, L., and Hubbard, V. S. (1983). Medical uses of vitamin E. *N. Engl. J. Med.* **308,** 1063–1071.
Bieri, J. G., Hoeg, J. M., Schaefer, E. J., Zech, L. A., and Brewer, H. B. (1984). Vitamin A and vitamin E replacement in abetalipoproteinemia. *Ann. Intern. Med.* **100,** 238–239.
Bikle, D. D. (1982). The vitamin D endocrine system. *Adv. Intern. Med.* **27,** 42–75.
Bikle, D. D. (1985). Osteomalacia and rickets. *In* "Cecil, Textbook of Medicine" (J. B. Wyngaarden and L. H. Smith, eds.), pp. 1425–1431. Saunders, Philadelphia.
Binder, H. J., Hertig, D. C., Hurst, V., Finch, S. C., and Spiro, H. C. (1965). Tocopherol deficiency in man. *N. Engl. J. Med.* **273,** 1289–1292.
Borum, P. R. (1981). Possible carnitine requirements of the newborn and the effect of genetic disease on the carnitine requirement. *Nutr. Rev.* **39,** 385–390.
Brenner, J. (1983). Carnitine—metabolism and functions. *Physiol. Rev.* **63,** 1420–1480.
Briggs, M. (1981). "Vitamins in Human Biology and Medicine." CRC Press, Boca Raton, Florida.
Broadus, A., Insogna, K. L., Lang, R., Ellison, A. F., and Dreyer, B. (1984). Evidence for disordered control of 1,25-dihydroxy-vitamin D production in absorptive hypercalciuria. *N. Engl. J. Med.* **311,** 73–83.
Burns, J. J. (1959). Biosynthesis of L-ascorbic acid; basic defect in scurvy. *Am. J. Med.* **26,** 740–748.
Carpenter, M. P., and Howard, C. N. (1974). Vitamin E, steroids, and liver microsomal hydroxylations. *Am. J. Clin. Nutr.* **27,** 966–971.
Catigani, G. L., Chytil, F., and Darby, W. J. (1974). Vitamin E deficiency: Immunochemical evidence for increased accumulation of liver xanthine oxidase. *Proc. Natl. Acad. Sci. U.S.A.* **71,** 1966–1972.
Chan, J. C. M., Young, R., Alon, U., and Mamunes, P. (1983). Hypercalcemia in children with disorders of calcium and phosphate metabolism during long term 1,25-dihydroxy-vitamin D_3. *Pediatrics* **72,** 225–233.
Chiu, D., and Lubin, B. (1979). Abnormal vitamin E and glutathione peroxidase levels in sickle cell anemia: Evidence for increased susceptibility to lipid to lipid peroxidation *in vivo*. *J. Lab. Clin. Med.* **94,** 542–548.
Chung, K., Bezeaud, A., Goldsmith, J. C., McMillan, C. W., Menache, D., and Roberts, H. R. (1979). Congenital deficiency of blood clotting factors II, VII, IX, and X. *Blood* **53,** 776–787.
Chytil, F. (1982). Liver and cellular vitamin A binding proteins. *Hepatology* **2,** 282–287.
Committee on Dietary Allowances, Food and Nutrition Board, Division of Biological Sciences, Assembly of Life Sciences, National Academy of Sciences (1980). "Recommended Dietary Allowances," 9th Ed., Washington, DC.
Comp, P. C., and Esmon, C. T. (1981). Generation of fibrinolytic activity by infusion of activated protein C into dogs. *J. Clin. Invest.* **68,** 1221–1228.
Cook, J. D., and Monsen, E. R. (1977). The common cold and iron absorption. *Am. J. Clin. Nutr.* **30,** 235–241.
Corash, L. (1980). Vitamin E and the erythrocyte. *Ann. Intern. Med.* **93,** 340–341.
Crow, J. A., and Ong, D. E. (1985). Cell-specific immunohistochemical localization of a cellular retinol-binding protein (type two) in the small intestine of rat. *Proc. Natl. Acad. Sci. U.S.A.* **82,** 4707–4711.
Dam, H., and Doisy, E. A. (1964). *In* "Nobel Lectures: Physiology or Medicine, 1942–1962." Elsevier, New York.

Davie, E. W., and Ratnoff, O. D. (1964). Waterfall sequence for intrinsic blood clotting. *Science* **145,** 1310–1312.

Deluca, H. F. (1979). The vitamin D system in the regulation of calcium and phosphorus metabolism. *Nutr. Rev.* **37,** 161–195.

Deluca, H. F. (1981). Recent advances in the metabolism of vitamin D. *In* "Annual Review of Physiology" (I. S. Edelman and S. G. Schultz, eds.), pp. 199–252. Annual Reviews, Palo Alto, California.

Devlin, E., Glorieux, F., Marie, P., and Pettifor, J. (1981). Vitamin D dependency; replacement therapy with calcitriol. *J. Pediatr.* **99,** 26–30.

DiPalma, J. R., and Ritchie, D. M. (1977). Vitamin toxicity. *Annu. Rev. Pharmacol. Toxicol.* **17,** 133–150.

Dominquez, J., Gray, R., and Lemann, J. (1976). Dietary phosphate deprivation in women and men: Effects on mineral and acid balances, PTH, and the metabolism of 25-OHD. *J. Clin. Endocrinol. Metab.* **43,** 1056–1065.

Drezner, M., Nelson, F., Haussler, H., McPherson, H., and Lebovitz, H. (1976). 1,25-$(OH)_2$ D_3 deficiency: The probably cause of hypocalcemia and metabolic bone disease in pseudohypoparathyroidism. *J. Clin. Endocrinol. Metab.* **42,** 62–73.

Drezner, M. K., Lyles, K. W., Haussler, M. R., and Harrelson, J. M. (1980). Evaluation of a role for 1,25-dihydroxy vitamin D_3 in the pathogenesis and treatment of X-linked hypophosphatemic rickets and osteomalacia. *J. Clin. Invest.* **66,** 1020–1032.

Eil, C., Liberman, V. A., Rosen, J. F., and Marx, S. J. (1981). A cellular defect in hereditary vitamin D-dependent rickets, type II: Defective nuclear uptake of 1,25-dihydroxyvitamin D in cultured skin fibroblasts. *N. Engl. J. Med.* **304,** 1588–1591.

Elias, E., and Muller, D. P. R. (1983). The use of vitamin E for prevention and treatment of spinocerebellar disorders. *Compr. Ther.* **9,** 56–60.

Elsas, L. J. (1982). Newborn screening. *In* "Pediatrics" (A. M. Rudolph, ed.), 17th Ed., Appleton, New York.

Elsas, L. J., and Danner, D. J. (1982). The role of thiamin in maple syrup urine disease. *Ann. N.Y. Acad. Sci.* **378,** 404–421.

Elsas, L., Danner, D., Lubitz, P., Fernhoff, P., and Dembure, P. (1981). Metabolic consequences of inherited defects in branched chain α-ketoacid dehydrogenase: Mechanism of thiamine action. *In* "Metabolism and Clinical Implications of Branched Chain Amino and Ketoacids" (M. Walser and J. Williamson, eds.). Elsevier, New York.

Elsas, L., Brown, A., and Fernhoff, P. (1983a). Newborn screening for metabolic disorders in the State of Georgia. *In* "Neonatal Screening" (H. Naruse and M. Irie, eds.). Excerpta Medica, Amsterdam.

Elsas, L. J., Fernhoff, P. M., Dembure, P., and Danner, D. J. (1983b). Thiamine responsive maple syrup urine disease. "*In* Neonatal Screening: Proceedings of the International Symposium on Neonatal Screening for Inborn Errors of Metabolism" (H. Naruse, and M. Irie, eds.). Excerpta Medica, Tokyo.

Engel, A. G., Rebouche, C. J., Wilson, D. M., Glasgow, A. M., Romshe, C. A., and Cruse, R. P. (1981). Primary systemic carnitine deficiency. II. Renal handing of carnitine. *Neurology* **31,** 819–825.

Evans, H. M., and Bishop, K. S. (1922). On the existence of a hitherto unrecognized dietary factor essential for reproduction. *Science* **56,** 650–651.

Fernhoff, P. M., and Lammer, E. J. (1984). Craniofacial features of isoretinoin embryopathy. *J. Pediatr.* **105,** 595–597.

Fernhoff, P. M., Danner, D. J., and Elsas, L. J. (1980). Vitamin-responsive disorders. *In* "Human Nutrition, Clinical and Biochemical Aspects" (P. J. Garry and V. S. Marcum, eds.), pp. 219–238. American Association for Clinical Chemistry, Washington, D.C.

Frame, B., Jackson, C., Reynolds, W., and Umphrey, J. (1974). Hypercalcimia and skeletal effects in chronic hypervitaminosis A. *Ann. Intern. Med.* **80,** 44–48.

Fraser, D. R. (1980). Regulation of the metabolism of vitamin D. *Physiol. Rev.* **60,** 551–579.

Fraser, D., and Scriver, C. R. (1976). Familial forms of vitamin D resistant rickets revisited: X-linked hypophosphatemia and autosomal recessive vitamin D dependency. *Am. J Clin. Nutr.* **29,** 1315–1321.

Frimpter, G. W., Andelman, R. J., and George, W. F. (1969). Vitamin B_6-dependency syndromes. New horizons in nutrition. *Am. J. Clin. Nutr.* **22,** 794–806.

Funk, C. (1922). "The Vitamins." Williams & Wilkins, Baltimore.

Gallop, P. M., Lian, J. B., and Hauschka, P. V. (1980). Carboxylated calcium-binding proteins and vitamin-K. *N. Engl. J. Med.* **202,** 1460–1466.

Garabédian, M., Jacqx, E., Guillozo, H., Grimberg, R., Guillot, M., Gagnadoux, M.-F., Broyer, M., Lenoir, G. and Balsan, S. (1985). Elevated plasma 1,25-dihydroxy-vitamin D concentrations in infants with hypercalcemia and an elfin facies. *N. Engl. J. Med.* **312,** 948–952.

Garrod, A. E. (1908). Inborn errors of metabolism (Croonian lectures). *Lancet* **2,** 1–7, 73–79, 142–148, 214–220.

Goodman, D. S. (1984). Vitamin A and retinoids in health and disease. *N. Engl. J. Med.* **310,** 1023–1031.

Gotto, A. M., Levy, R. I., John, K., and Fredrickson, D. S. (1971). On the nature of the protein defect in abetalipoproteinemia. *N. Engl. J. Med.* **284,** 813–818.

Gray, T. K., McAdoo, T., Pool, D., Williams, M. E., Lester, G. E., and Thierry-Palmer, M. (1982). The development and application of a radioimmunoassay for 1,25-dihydroxycholecalciferol. *N. Engl. J. Med.* **302,** 763–767.

Haddad, J., Chyu, K., Hahn, T., and Stamp, T. C. B. (1973). Serum concentrations of 25-OHD in sex linked hypophosphatemic vitamin D-resistant rickets. *J. Lab. Clin. Med.* **81,** 22–28.

Hahn, P. (1981). The development of carnitine synthesis from gamma-butyrobetaine in the rat. *Life Sci.* **28,** 1057–1060.

Hahn, T. J., Hendin, B. A., Scharp, C. R., and Haddadd, J. G. (1972). Effect of chronic anticonvulsant therapy on serum 25-hydroxycalciferol levels in adults. *N. Engl. J. Med.* **287,** 900–905.

Harding, A. E., Matthews, S., Jones, S., Ellis, C. J. K., Booth, I. W., and Muller, D. P. R. (1985). Spinocerebellar degeneration associated with a selective defect of vitamin E malabsorption. *N. Engl. J. Med.* **313,** 32–35.

Harris, H. (1980). "The Principles of Human Biochemical Genetics," 3rd Ed. North-Holland Publ., Amsterdam.

Hauschka, P. V., Lian, J. B., and Gallop, P. M. (1978). Vitamin K and mineralization. *Trends Biochem. Sci.* **3,** 75–78.

Haussler, M. R., and McCain, T. A. (1977). Basic and clinical concepts related to vitamin D metabolism and action. *N. Engl. J. Med.* **297,** 974–983, 1041–1050.

Haussler, M. R., Kokoh, S., and Deftos, L. J. (1982). Calcidiol and calcitriol: New ultrasensitive and accurate assays in vitamin D: Chemical, biochemical, and clinical endocrinology of calcium metabolism. (A. W. Norman, K. Schaefer, D. V. Herrathy, and H. G. Gringoleit, eds.), pp. 743–749. DeGruyter, New York.

Hefflefinger, S. C., Sewell, E. T., Elsas, L. J., and Danner, D. J. (1984). Direct physical evidence for stabilization of branched chain α-ketoacid dehydrogenase by thiaminpyrophosphate. *Am. J. Hum. Genet.* **37,** 802–807.

Hegsted, D. M. *et al.*, eds. (1976). "Present Knowledge in Nutrition," 4th Ed. Nutrition Foundation, Washington, D.C.

Herbert, P. M., Assman, G., Gotto, A. M., and Fredrickson, D. S. (1983). Familial lipoprotein deficiency: Abetalipoproteinemia, hypobetalipoproteinemia, and Tangier disease. *In* "The Metabolic Basis of Inherited Disease" (J. B. Stanbury *et al.*, eds.), 5th Ed., pp. 589–621. McGraw Hill, New York.

Herbert, V., and Jacob, E. (1974). Destruction of vitamin B_{12} by ascorbic acid. *J. Am. Med. Assoc.* **230,** 241–242.

Herlong, H. F., Russell, R. M., and Maddsey, W. C. (1981). Vitamin A and zinc therapy in primary biliary cirrhosis. *Hepatology* **1,** 348–351.

Hodges, R. E. (1982). Megavitamin therapy. *Primary Care* **9,** 605–619.

Hughes, P. E., and Tove, S. B. (1980). Identification of an endogenous electron donor for biohydrogenation as α-tocopherolquinol. *J. Biol. Chem.* **255,** 4447–4452.

Hunt, A. D., Stokes, J., Jr., McCrory, V. W., and Stroud, H. H. (1954). Pyridoxine dependency: Report of a case of intractable convulsions in an infant controlled by pyridoxine. *Pediatrics* **13,** 140.

Illingworth, D. R., Conner, W. E., and Miller, R. G. (1980). Abetalipoproteinemia. Report of two cases and review of therapy. *Arch. Neurol.* **37,** 659–663.

Janiszowska, W., and Pennock, J. F. (1976). The biochemistry of vitamin E in plants. *In* "Vitamins and Hormones" (P. L. Munson *et al.,* eds.), pp. 77–105. Academic Press, New York.

Kark, J. D., Smith, A. H., Switzer, B. R., and Hames, C. G. (1981). Serum vitamin A (retinol) and cancer incidence in Evans County, Georgia. *J. Natl. Cancer Inst.* **66,** 7–16.

Key, L., Carnes, D., Cole, S., Holtrop, M., Bar-Shavit, Z., Shapiro, F., Arceci, R., Steinberg, J., Gundberg, C., Kahn, A., Teitelbaum, S., and Anast, C. (1984). Treatment of congenital osteoporosis with high dose calcitriol. *N. Engl. J. Med.* **310,** 409–415.

Kim, Y. J., and Rosenberg, L. E. (1974). On the mechanism of pyridoxine responsive homocystinuria. II. Properties of normal and mutant cystathione β-synthase from cultured fibroblasts. *Proc. Natl. Acad. Aci. U.S.A.* **71,** 4821–4825.

Kisiel, W., Canfield, W., Ericsson, L. H., and Davie, E. W. (1977). Anticoagulant properties of bovine plasma protein C following activation by thrombin. *Biochemistry* **16,** 5824–5831.

Korner, W. F., and Vollm, J. (1974). New aspects of the tolerance of retinol in humans. *Int. J. Vitam. Nutr. Res.* **45,** 363–370.

Lambert, P. W., Hollis, B. W., Bell, N. H., and Epstein, S. (1980). Demonstration of a lack of change in serum 1α,25-dihydroxy-vitamin D in response to parathormone extract in pseudohypoparathyroidism. *J. Clin. Invest.* **66,** 782–791.

Longhi, R. C., Fleisher, L. D., Tallan, H. H., and Gaul, G. E. (1977). Cystathionine β-synthase deficiency: A qualitative abnormality of the deficient enzyme modified by vitamin B_6 therapy. *Pediatr. Res.* **11,** 100–103.

Lyles, K. W., Burkes, E. J., Ellis, G. J., Lucas, K. J., Dolan, E. A., and Drezner, M. K. (1985). Genetic transmission of tumoral calcinosis: Autosomal dominant with variable clinical expressivity. *J. Clin. Endocrinol. Metab.* **60,** 1093–1096.

McCollum, E. V., and Davis, M. (1913). The necessity of certain lipids in the diet during growth. *J. Biol. Chem.* **15,** 167–175.

McCormick, D. B., and Wright, L. D., eds. (1971). "Vitamin and Coenzymes Methods in Enzymology," Vol. 18, Part C. Academic Press, New York.

McGhee, W. G., Klotz, T. A., Epstein, D. J., and Rapaport, S. I. (1984). Coumarin necrosis associated with hereditary protein C. *Ann Intern. Med.* **100,** 59–60.

McKusick, V. A. (1983). "Medelian Inheritance in Man: Catalogs of Autosomal Dominant Recessive, and X-Linked Phenotypes," 6th Ed. Johns Hopkins Univ. Press, Baltimore.

Mander, J. (1984). Molecular bad actors and thrombosis. *N. Engl. J. Med.* **310,** 588–589.

Manolagos, S. C., Howard, J. E., Abare, J. M., Culler, F. I., Brickman, A. S., and Deftos, L. J. (1982). Cytoreceptor assay for 1,25$(OH)_2D_3$: A convenient method and its application to clinical studies. *In* "Vitamin D: Chemical, Biochemical, and Clinical Endocrinology of Calcium Metabolism" (A. W. Norman *et al.,* eds.), pp. 769–771. DeGruyter, New York.

Marshall, L., and DiGeorge, A. (1981). Maple syrup urine disease (branched chain ketoaciduria). *Am. J. Hum. Genet.* **33,** 138A.

Mawson, A. R. (1984). Hypervitaminosis: A toxicity and gout. *Lancet* **1,** 1181.

Marx, S. J., Liberman, U. A., and Eil, C. (1983). Calciferols: Actions and deficiencies in action. *Vitam. Horm.* **40,** 235–308.

Moore, T. (1957). "Vitamin A." Elsevier, New York.

Mudd, S. H. (1971). Pyridoxine-responsive genetic disease. *Fed. Proc., Fed. Am. Soc. Exp. Biol.* **30,** 970–976.

Mudd, S. H. (1974). Inborn errors of metabolism vitamin-responsive genetic disease. *J. Clin. Pathol.* **27,** (Suppl. Royal Coll. Pathol.), **8,** 38–47.

Mudd, S. H. (1982). Vitamin-responsive genetic abnormalities. *Adv. Nutr. Res.* **4,** 1–34.

Muller, D. P. R., and Lloyd, J. K. (1982). Effect of large oral doses of vitamin E on the neurological sequelae of patients with abetalipoproteinemia. *Ann. N.Y. Acad. Sci.* **393,** 133–142.

Muller, D. P. R., Lloyd, J. K., and Bird, A. C. (1977). Long-term management of abetalipoproteinemia: Possible role for vitamin E. *Arch. Dis. Child.* **52,** 209–214.

Natta, C. L., Machlin, L. J., and Brin, M. (1980). A decrease in irreversibly sickled erythrocytes in sickle cell anemia patients given vitamin E. *Am. J. Clin. Nutr.* **33,** 968–971.

Naylor, E. W., and Flores, N. E. (1983). Evaluation of neonatal screening for maple syrup urine disease. *In* "Neonatal Screening" (H. Naruse and M. Irie, eds.). Excerpta Medica, Amsterdam.

Needham, J. (1962). Frederick Gowland Hopkins. *Perspect. Biol. Med.* **6,** 2–10.

Norman, A. W., Roth, J., and Orci, L. (1982). The vitamin D endocrine system, steroid metabolism, hormone receptors, and biological response (calcium binding proteins). *Endocr. Rev.* **3,** 331–366.

Olson, R. E. (1973). Vitamin K. *In* "Modern Nutrition in Health and Disease" R. S. Goodhart and M. E. Shils, eds.), pp. 166–182. Lea & Febiger, Philadelphia.

Olson, R. E., and Suttie, J. W. (1977). Vitamin K and γ-carboxyglutamate biosynthesis. *Vitam. Horm.* **35,** 57–70.

Ong, D. E., Crow, J. A., and Chytil, F. (1982). Radioimmunochemical determination of cellular retinol- and cellular retinoic acid-binding proteins in cytosols of rat tissues. *J. Biol. Chem.* **257,** 13385–13389.

O'Reilly, R. A. (1971). Vitamin K in hereditary resistance to oral anticoagulant drugs. *Am. J. Physiol.* **211,** 1327–1330.

Oski, F. A. (1980). Vitamin E: A radical defense. *N. Engl. J. Med.* **303,** 454–455.

Oski, F. A., and Naiman, J. L. (1982). "Hematologic Problems in the Newborn," 3rd Ed., pp. 161–190. Saunders, Philadelphia.

Pennington, J. A. T., and Church, H. N. (1983). "Bowes and Church's Food Values of Portions Commonly Used," 14th Ed. Lippincott, Philadelphia.

Pike, J. W., Dokoh, S., Haussler, M. R., Lieberman, U. A., Marx, S. J., and Eil, C. (1984). Vitamin D_3 resistant fibroblasts have immunoassayable 1,25-dihydroxy-vitamin D_3 receptors. *Science* **224,** 879–881.

Polisson, R. P., Martinez, S., Kjoury, M., Harrell, R. M., Lyles, K. W., Friedman, N.,

Harrelson, J. M., Reisner, E., and Drezner, M. K. (1985). Calcification of entheses associated with X-linked hypophosphatemic osteomalacia. *N. Engl. J. Med.* **313,** 1–6.

Price, P. A. (1985). Vitamin K-dependent formation of bone GLA protein (osteocalcin) and its function. *Vitam. Horm.* **42,** 65–108.

Price, P. A., and Baukol, S. A. (1980). 1,25-Dihydroxy D_3 increases synthesis of the vitamin K-dependent bone protein by osteosarcoma cells. *J. Biol. Chem.* **255,** 11660–11664.

Price, P. A., and Baukol, S. A. (1981). 1,25-Dihydroxy D_3 increases serum levels of the vitamin K-dependent bone protein. *Biochem. Biophys. Res. Commun.* **99,** 928–930.

Price, A., and Williamson, M. K. (1981). Effects of warfarin on bone. Studies on the vitamin K-dependent bone protein found in plasma and its clearance by kidney and bone. *J. Biol. Chem.* **256,** 12760–12765.

Price, P. A., Baukol, S. A., and Williamson, M. D. (1981). 1,25-Dihydroxyvitamin D_3 regulates the synthesis of the vitamin K-dependent bone protein. *Calcif. Tissue. Int.* **33,** 341–345.

Rebouche, C. J., and Engel, A. G. (1980). Tissue distribution of carnitine biosynthetic enzymes in man. *Biochim. Biophys. Acta* **630,** 22–29.

Rodriguez, M. S., and Irwin, M. I. (1980). Vitamin A requirements of man. *In* "Nutritional Requirements of Man" (M. I. Irwin, ed.), pp. 75–110. Nutrition Foundation, Washington, D.C.

Rosen, J. F., and Chesney, R. W. (1983). Circulating calcitriol concentrations in health and disease. *J. Pediatr.* **103,** 1–17.

Rosen, J., Fleischman, A., Finberg, L., Hamstra, A., and DeLuca, H. (1979). Rickets with alopecia. An inborn error of vitamin D metabolism. *J. Pediatr.* **94,** 729–734.

Rosenberg, L. E. (1969). Inherited aminoacidopathies demonstrating vitamin dependency. *N. Engl. J. Med.* **281,** 145–153.

Rosenberg, L. E. (1970). Vitamin dependent genetic disease. *Hospital Pract.* **5,** 59–67.

Rosenberg, L. E. (1973). Vitamin dependent genetic disease. *In* "Medical Genetics" (V. A. McKusick and R. Claborne, eds.), pp. 73–83. H. P. Publishers, New York.

Rosenberg, L. E. (1974). Vitamin responsive inherited diseases affecting the nervous system. *In* "Brain Dysfunction in Metabolic Disorders" (F. Plum, ed.), pp. 263–272. Raven, New York.

Rosenberg, L. E. (1976). Vitamin responsive inherited metabolic disorders. *In* "Advances in Human Genetics" (H. Harris and J. Hirschorn, eds.), Vol. 6, pp. 1–69. Plenum, New York.

Rosenberg, L. E. (1983). Disorders of propionate and methylmalonate metabolism. *In* "The Metabolic Basis of Inherited Disease" (J. B. Stanbury *et al.,* eds.), 5th Ed., pp. 474–497. McGraw Hill, New York.

Rosenblatt, D. S., Hosack, A., Matiaszuk, N. V., Cooper, B., and Laframboise, R. (1985). Defect in B_{12} release from lysosomes: Newly described inborn error of B_{12} metabolism. *Science* **228,** 1319–1321.

Rudman, D., and Williams, P. J. (1983). Megadose vitamins use and misuse. *N. Engl. J. Med.* **309,** 488–490.

Saunders, M. E., Sherwood, W. G., Duthie, M., Surk, L., and Gravel, R. (1982). Evidence for a defect of holocarboxylase synthetase activity in cultured lymophoblasts from a patient with biotin responsive multiple carboxylase deficiency. *Am. J. Hum. Genet.* **34,** 590–601.

Scriver, C. R. (1973). Progress in endocrinology and metabolism. Vitamin-responsive inborn erros of metabolism. *Metab. Clin. Exp.* **22,** 1319–1344.

Scriver, C. R. (1974). Rickets and the pathogenesis of impaired tubular transport of phosphate and other solutes. *Am. J. Med.* **57,** 43–56.

Scriver, C. R., and Rosenberg, L. E. (1973). The vitamin-responsive aminoacidopathies. *In* "Amino Acid Metabolism and Its Disorders," pp. 453–478. Saunders, Philadelphia.

Seligson, V., Berger, A., Abend, M., Rubin, L., Attias, D., Zivelin, A., and Rappaport, S. I. (1984). Homozygous protein C deficiency manifested by massive venous thrombosis in the newborn. *N. Engl. J. Med.* **310,** 559–562.

Sherrill, B. C., Inneriarity, T. L., and Mahley, R. W. (1980). Rapid hepatic clearance of the canine lipoproteins containing only the E apoprotein by a high affinity receptor: Identity with the chylomicron remnant transport process. *J. Biol. Chem.* **255,** 1804–1807.

Simoin, E. J., Eisengart, A., Sundheim, L., and Milhorat, A. T. (1956). The Metabolism of vitamin E. II. Purification and characterization of urinary metabolites of α-tocopherol. *J. Biol Chem.* **221,** 807–812.

Simpson, K. L., and Chichester, C. O. (1981). Metabolism and nutritional significance of carotenoids. *In* "Annual Review of Nutrition" (W. J. Darby, H. P. Broquist, and R. E. Olson, eds.), Vol. 1, pp. 351–375. Annual Reviews, Palo Alto, California.

Smith, R. F., and Goodman, D. S. (1976). Vitamin A transport in human vitamin A toxicity. *N. Engl. J. Med.* **294,** 805–808.

Sobel, S., Gueriguian, J., Troendle, G., and Nevius, E. (1982). Vitamin E in retrolental fibroplasia. *N. Engl. J. Med.* **306,** 867–869.

Sokol, R. J., Heubi, J. E., Iannaccone, S. T., Bove, K. E., and Balistreri, W. F. (1984). Vitamin E deficiency with normal serum vitamin E concentrations in children with chronic cholestasis. *N. Engl. J. Med.* **310,** 1209–1212.

Spielberg, S. P., Boxer, L. A., Oliver, J. M., Allen, J. M., and Schulman, J. M. (1979). Oxidative damage to neutrophilsin glutathione synthetase deficiency. *Br. J. Haematol.* **42,** 215–223.

Sporn, M. B., and Roberts, A. B. (1983). The role of retinoids in differentiation and carcinogenesis. *Cancer Res.* **43,** 3034–3040.

Sporn, M. D., Roberts, A. B., and Goodman, D. S., eds. (1984). "The Retinoids." Academic Press, New York.

Stenflo, J. (1984). The structure and function of protein-C. *Semina. Thromb. Hemostasis* **10,** 109–121.

Stockley, I. (1981). "Drug Interactions." Blackwell, Oxford.

Sutherland, J. M., Glueck, H. I., and Glesser, G. (1967). Hemorrhagic disease of the newborn. Breast feeding as a necessary factor in the pathogenesis. *Am. J. Dis. Child.* **113,** 524–533.

Suttie, J. W., ed. (1979). "Vitamin K Metabolism and Vitamin K-Dependent Proteins." Univ. Park Press, Baltimore.

Suttie, J. W. (1983). Current concepts of the mechanism of action of vitamin K and its antagonists. *In* "Nutrition in Hematology" (J. Lindenbaum, ed.), Vol. 5, pp. 245–270. Churchill Livingstone, New York.

Symposium on Vitamin D and Membrane Structure and Function (1982). *Fed. Proc., Fed. Am. Soc. Exp. Biol.* **41,** 60–98.

Taylor, A. B., Stern, P. H., Bell, N. H. (1982). Abnormal regulation of circulating 25-hydroxyvitamin D in the Williams syndrome. *N. Engl. J. Med.* **306,** 972–975.

Tieder, M., Modai, D., Samuel, R., Arie, R., Halabe, A., Bab, I., Gabizon, D., and Liberman, U. (1985). Hereditary hypophosphatemic rickets with hypercalciuria. *N. Engl. J. Med.* **312,** 611–617.

Tielsch, J. M., and Sommer, A. (1984). The epidemiology of vitamin A deficiency and xerophthalmia. *Annu. Rev. Nutr.* **4,** 183–205.

Tomita, A. (1971). Post-menopausal osteoporosis ^{47}Ca study with vitamin K_2. *Clin. Endocrinol.* **19,** 731–736.

Tsai, K.-S., Heath, H., Kumar, R., and Riggs, B. L. (1984). Impaired vitamin D metabolism with aging women. Possible role in pathogenesis of senile osteoporosis. *J. Clin. Invest.* **73,** 1668–1672.

Tsuchiya, Y., Matsuo, N., Cho, H., Kumagai, M., Yasaka, A., Suda, T., Orimo, H., and Shiraki, M. (1980). An unusual form of vitamin D-dependent rickets in a child. Alopecia and marked end-organ hyposensitivity to biologically active vitamin D. *J. Clin. Endocrinol. Metab.* **57,** 686–687.

Vark, J. D., Smith, A. H., Switzer, B. R., and Hames, G. G. (1981). Serum vitamin A (retinol) and cancer incidence in Evans County, Georgia. *J. Natl. Cancer Inst.* **66,** 7–16.

Vincente, V., Maria, R., Alberca, I., Tamagnini, G. P. T., and Borrasca, A. L. (1984). Congenital deficiency of vitamin K-dependent coagulation factors and protein C. *Thromb. Haemostasis (Stuttgart)* **57,** 343–346.

Vilter, R. W. (1964). Vitamin B_6-hydrazide relationships. *Vitam. Horm.* **22,** 77–89.

Wald, G. (1968). Molecular basis of visual excitation. *Science* **162,** 230–239.

Wald, N., Idle, M., Boreham, J., and Bailey, A. (1980). Low serum-vitamin A and subsequent risk of cancer: Preliminary results of a prospective study. *Lancet* **2,** 813–815.

Walt, R. P., Kemp, C. M., Lyness, L., Bird, A. C., and Sherlocks, S. (1984). Vitamin A treatment for night blindness in primary biliary cirrhosis. *Br. Med. J.* **288,** 1029–1031.

Wastell, H., Dale, G., and Bartlett, K. (1984). A sensitive fluorimetric rate assay for biotinidase using a new derivative of biotin, biotinyl-6-aminoquinoline. *Anal. Biochem.* **140,** 69–73.

Wessler, S., and Gitel, S. N. (1984). Warfarin from bedside to bench. *N. Engl. J. Med.* **311,** 645–652.

Willett, W. C., Polk, B. F., Underwood, B. A., *et al.* (1984). Relation of serum vitamin A, E, and carotenoids to the risk of cancer. *N. Engl. J. Med.* **310,** 430–434.

Wilson, J. A. (1982). Disorders of vitamin deficiency excess, and errors of metabolism. *In* "Harrisons Principles of Internal Medicine" (R. G. Petersdorf *et al.,* eds), Chap. 83, 10th Ed. McGraw-Hill, New York.

Winnick, H. (1980). "Nutrition in Health and Disease," Chaps. 8, 9. Wiley, New York.

Winters, R. W., Graham, J. B., Williams, T. F., McFalls, V. W., and Burnett, C. H. (1958). A genetic study of familial hypophosphatemia and vitamin D resistant rickets with a review of the literature. *Medicine* **37,** 97–142.

Wolf, G. (1978). A historical note on the mode of administration of vitamin A for the cure of night blindness. *Am. J. Clin. Nutr.* **31,** 290–292.

Wolf, B. (1980). Molecular basis for genetic complementation in propionylCoA carboxylase deficiency. *Exp. Cell Res.* **125,** 502–507.

Wolf, B., Grier, R. E., Parker, W. D., Goodman, S. I., and Allen, R. (1983). Deficient biotinidase activity in late onset multiple carboxylase deficiency. *N. Engl. J. Med.* **308,** 161–167.

Wolf, B., Grier, R. E., McVoy, J. R. S., and Heard, G. S. (1985). Biotinidase deficiency: A novel vitamin recycling defect. *J. Inherit. Metab. Dis.* **8,** 53–58.

VITAMINS AND HORMONES, VOL. 43

Hormonal Control of Sexual Development

FREDRICK W. GEORGE

Department of Cell Biology and Anatomy,
The University of Texas Health Science Center at Dallas,
Southwestern Medical School,
Dallas, Texas 75235

JEAN D. WILSON

Department of Internal Medicine,
The University of Texas Health Science Center at Dallas,
Southwestern Medical School,
Dallas, Texas 75235

I. Introduction

An endocrine theory of sexual differentiation was proposed early in this century (Bouin and Ancel, 1903; Lillie, 1916), and the studies of Alfred Jost (1953, 1961, 1972) established that development of the sexual phenotypes in the eutherian mammal is mediated by gonadal hormones. Jost formulated the paradigm that sexual differentiation is a sequential process beginning with the establishment of chromosomal (genetic) sex at fertilization, followed by the appearance of gonadal sex, and culminating in development of the sexual phenotypes (Fig. 1). This formulation was based upon the observation that the castrated mammalian embryo develops as a female; male development is induced in the embryo only in the presence of specific hormonal signals arising from the fetal testis. Each step in this sequential process is dependent on the preceding one, and under normal circumstances chromosomal sex agrees with phenotypic sex. On occasion, most often related to abnormal chromosomal complement or defective hormone formation or action, gonadal development or sexual phenotypic development is abnormal. Studies of such abnormalities have provided insight into gonadal differentiation, the mechanisms by which the gonads dictate phenotypic sexual development and the molecular processes by which the gonadal hormones act within target cells. The analyses of single-gene mutations that impair sexual development (Wilson and Goldstein, 1975; Bardin *et al.*, 1973) have been particularly informative in defining molecular and genetic determinants involved in this process.

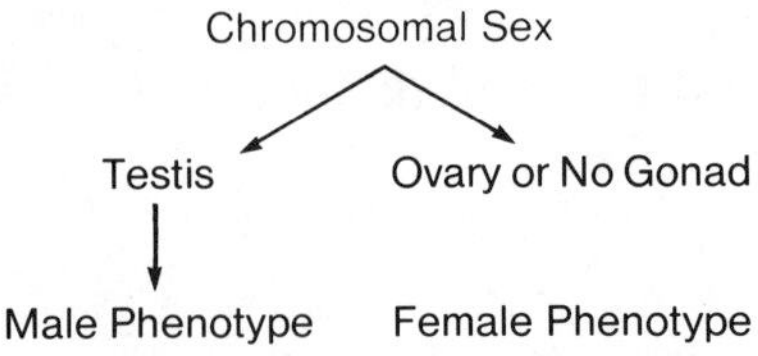

FIG. 1. Schematic representation of the Jost castration experiments. Reprinted with permission from Wilson *et al.* (1984).

In this review we consider some of the physiological (and pathophysiological) actions of hormones in controlling the development of the sexual phenotypes of eutherian mammals, the American opossum, and the chicken. In so doing we emphasize the importance of steroid metabolites formed in extraglandular tissues to overall sexual development.

II. FORMATION AND METABOLISM OF GONADAL STEROIDS IN MALES

The principal androgen in male plasma is the testicular hormone testosterone. Although testosterone itself exerts some direct actions, it also serves as the precursor (prohormone) for two other potent hormones, 5α-dihydrotestosterone and estradiol (Fig. 2). 5α-Dihydrotestosterone is the active intracellular androgen in many tissues, and it

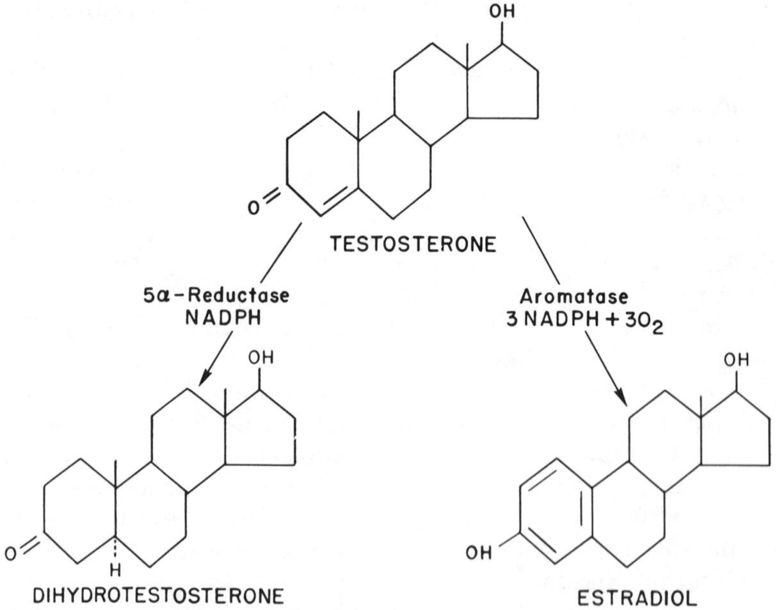

OH
O
TESTOSTERONE
5α-Reductase
NADPH
Aromatase
3 NADPH + 3O_2
OH
O
H
DIHYDROTESTOSTERONE
OH
OH
ESTRADIOL

FIG. 2. Two hormonal metabolites of testosterone.

also circulates in blood. The circulating hormone is derived primarily by conversion from testosterone in extragonadal tissues and to a lesser extent by direct secretion into the circulation by the testes. The concentration of 5α-dihydrotestosterone in plasma is about one-tenth that of testosterone (Wilson, 1975). The function of estrogen in normal men is uncertain (Marcus and Korenman, 1976), although the hormone may play a role in male sexual drive (Baum and Vreeburg, 1973; Larsson *et al.,* 1973). Excess estrogen, either relative or absolute, causes profound feminization in men; breast enlargement (gynecomastia) is the most characteristic feature of such feminizing states (Wilson *et al.,* 1980). In addition, disorders that cause an alteration in estrogen–androgen balance are frequently associated with changes in the sexual phenotype. For these reasons it is useful to review briefly the dynamics of estrogen and androgen production and metabolism in the male.

In normal men the production rates of estradiol and estrone average about 45 and 65 μg/day, respectively, whereas the plasma production rates of testosterone and androstenedione average 6000 and 3000 μg/day, respectively. Thus, the normal ratio of the production rate of testosterone to estradiol is about 100 to 1 (MacDonald *et al.,* 1979). Most (>85%) of the estradiol and estrone is derived from peripheral (extragonadal) conversion from androstenedione or testosterone, and only about 15% of the estrogens originate directly from testicular secretion (MacDonald *et al.,* 1979; Kelch *et al.,* 1972; Weinstein *et al.,* 1974). However, when human chorionic gonadotropin is administered to normal men (or if the plasma luteinizing hormone levels become pathologically elevated) direct secretion of estrogens by the testis may become significant (Weinstein *et al.,* 1974).

Feminization of men develops when the normal 100-fold excess of androgen to estrogen is diminished either by an increase in estrogen production or by a decrease in testosterone formation (or action) under circumstances in which estrogen production remains appreciable.

III. Anatomical Aspects of Mammalian Sexual Differentiation

A. Establishment of Chromosomal Sex

Chromosomal sex is established at fertilization. In mammals, the homogametic XX zygote is female and the heterogametic XY genotype is male. The Y chromosome is believed to contain genetic determinants essential for male development; without the Y chromosome female development is brought about through expression of genes on the X chromosomes and on the autosomes (Stern, 1961). Analyses of clinical disorders due to nondisjunctions of either the X or Y chromosomes have substantiated the fundamental validity of this view. For example, regardless of the number of X chromosomes, a single Y chromosome (as in 47,XXY or 48,XXXY humans) is sufficient to cause testicular differentiation and the development of a predominantly male phenotype [although males with additional X chromosomes are usually infertile (Ferguson-Smith, 1961)]. Furthermore, in the human and the mouse, the XO individual shows a female phenotype (Ford *et al.*, 1959; Russell *et al.*, 1959; Welshons and Russell, 1959). Thus, the principal function of the Y chromosome of mammals is to serve as the repository for male-determining genes.

However, the Y chromosome is not the sole determinant of male development. Indeed, genes essential for male development are located on the X chromosome (Lyon and Hawkes, 1970; Meyer *et al.*, 1975; Ohno, 1979), and genes essential to the development of both the male and female phenotypes are located on autosomes (Wilson and Goldstein, 1975). Some of these genes are important for secondary events of sexual differentiation (coding for enzymes required for steroid hormone biosynthesis or for the receptor proteins that enable a tissue to respond to a hormonal stimulus). Others are essential for differentiation of the gonads themselves. For example, at least seven sibships with familial 46,XX pure gonadal dysgenesis (defined by the presence of streak gonads despite a normal female karyotype) have been described in which the pattern of inheritance is consistent with autosomal recessive transmission, implying that at least one autosomal gene is essential for ovarian development (Josso *et al.*, 1963; Simpson *et al.*, 1971). Furthermore, several pedigrees of familial 46,XY pure gonadal dysgenesis (a disorder in which genetic men differentiate as women with streak gonads) have been identified in which the mutation involves an X-linked gene (Chemke *et al.*, 1970; Cohen and Shaw, 1965; Espiner *et al.*, 1970; Sternberg *et al.*, 1968). In short, the genetic determinants that regulate normal gonadal differentiation and development of the male and female phenotypes are complex (Simpson *et al.*, 1981) and cannot be explained by the composition of the sex chromosomes alone.

B. Establishment of Gonadal Sex

The primordium of the gonad develops as a stratification of the coelomic epithelium on the medial aspect of the mesonephric kidney (the urogenital ridge) and is initially devoid of germ cells. As are other cells of the embryo proper, the germ cells are descendants of the primitive ectodermal cells that make up the inner cell mass (Gardner *et al.*,

1985), but they are first identifiable in the endoderm of the yolk sac near the allantoic evagination (Mintz and Russell, 1957; Fujimoto *et al.*, 1977), from which they migrate through the gut mesentery to the gonadal ridge. During this migration the germ cells undergo several rounds of cell division. After migration is completed, the primitive ("indifferent") gonad is composed of three distinct cell types: (1) germ cells, (2) supporting cells of the coelomic epithelium of the gonadal ridge that differentiate into the Sertoli cells of the testis or granulosa cells of the ovary, and (3) stromal (interstitial) cells derived from the mesenchyme of the gonadal ridge.

The first morphological sign of sexual dimorphism in the gonads is the appearance of spermatogenic cords in the fetal testis. In the human this occurs between 6 and 7 weeks of gestational development. Histological differentiation of the fetal ovary commences later than that of the testis and in the human embryo is not apparent before the sixth month of gestation when primitive granulosa cells organize around the dividing oocytes to form the primary ovarian follicle (Gilman, 1948).

The mechanisms that control the differentiation of the indifferent gonad into an ovary or a testis are poorly understood. However the identification of a male-specific transplantation (H-Y) antigen in mice by Eichwald and Silmser in 1955 and subsequent investigations of this antigen have provided a working model to explain how the Y chromosome dictates testicular development (Ohno, 1979; Wachtel, 1983). H-Y antigen is expressed by virtually all tissues of the male (Gasser and Silvers, 1972) in response, directly (Wolf, 1981) or indirectly, to determinants on the Y chromosome (Silvers and Wachtel, 1977; Ohno, 1978; Wachtel, 1983). Consequently, most individuals who are Y-chromosome positive also have serologically detectable H-Y antigen, and the presence of H-Y antigen correlates with testicular formation in mammals (reviewed by Wachtel, 1983).

Evidence that the H-Y antigen induces testicular development has been provided from *in vitro* reorganization experiments with rodent gonadal cells (Ohno *et al.*, 1978; Zenzes *et al.*, 1978). Enzymatically dissociated testicular cells spontaneously reassociate in rotation culture to form tubular structures characteristic of the testis, whereas incubation of dissociated testicular cells with an antibody to the H-Y antigen blocks testicular reorganization. If H-Y antigen is involved in organizing the cytoarchitecture of the testis it is reasonable to assume that it acts at the cell surface. Indeed it is believed that H-Y antigen is anchored in the cell membrane by association with β_2-microglobulin (Beutler *et al.*, 1978). Cells of the developing ovary and testis, but not those of other tissues, are postulated to have specific receptors for H-Y antigen that are distinct from this membrane anchorage site (Müller *et al.,* 1978, 1979). Consequently, H-Y antigen in the male is believed to act via these receptors to cause organization of the fetal testis into a characteristic tubular structure.

Despite the overall attractiveness of this model, several unresolved issues preclude acceptance of H-Y antigen as the sole initiator of testicular differentiation. For example, the male-specific transplantation antigen (H-Y) originally described by Eichwald and Silmser is probably not the same antigen that is detected in the serological assay, raising the possibility that several male-specific antigens exist (Silvers *et al.,* 1982). Furthermore, in many instances the H-Y antigen phenotype is at variance with the genotype and/or the gonadal phenotype (Silvers *et al.,* 1982; Jones *et al.,* 1979; Wolfe and Goodfellow, 1985). Therefore, until the various male-specific antigens are analyzed in greater detail, it is not possible to conclude that any is the testis inducer or whether these antigens are merely closely linked to the testis determining locus on the Y chromosome.

Regardless of the mechanisms involved in the transformation of the indifferent gonad into an ovary or a testis, it is through the action of the gonads as endocrine organs that phenotypic differentiation is accomplished. In the human fetus, enzymatic differentiation of the gonad becomes apparent at 8–10 weeks of gestation when the testis acquires the capacity to synthesize testosterone (Siiteri and Wilson, 1974) and the fetal ovary acquires the enzymatic capacity to form estrogens from androgens (George and Wilson, 1978a). The onset of testosterone synthesis in the fetal testis heralds the beginning of virilization. It occurs after organization of the spermatogenic cords and correlates temporally with the histological differentiation of the primitive interstitial cells into mature Leydig cells (Catt *et al.,* 1975; Gondos, 1980). However, endocrine differentiation of the testis is independent of morphological organization of the primitive Sertoli cells into spermatogenic cords (Magre and Jost, 1984; Patsavoudi *et al.,* 1985). In contrast to the testis, estrogen synthesis by the ovary begins before organization of the primary follicles can be recognized. To date the earliest recognizable change in the developing ovary that correlates with the onset of estrogen synthesis is the accumulation of lipid in the primitive granulosa cells (Gondos *et al.,* 1983).

C. Establishment of Phenotypic Sex

In mammals, the embryogenesis of the urogenital tract is initially identical in both sexes. During this so-called "indifferent" stage of sexual development, the urogenital tract consists of two components:

(1) a dual duct system (wolffian and mullerian) that develops in the mesonephros and constitutes the anlagen of the internal accessory organs of reproduction (Fig. 3), and (2) the urogenital sinus and tubercle, the anlagen of the external genitalia (Fig. 4). It is only after the onset of endocrine function of the testis that anatomic and physiological development of male and female embryos diverge.

1. *Male Development*

The first sign of male differentiation of the urogenital tract is degeneration of the mullerian ducts adjacent to the testes, a process that commences just after formation of the spermatogenic cords in the testis. Shortly thereafter, testosterone synthesis is initiated in the Leydig cells of the fetal testis, and growth and differentiation of the wolffian duct into the epididymis, vas deferens, and seminal vesicle begins (Fig. 3). The prostate arises as a series of endodermal buds off of the male urethra (Lowsley, 1912; Kellokumpo-Lehtinen *et al.,* 1980). Development of the external genitalia of the male (Fig. 4) commences shortly after virilization of the wolffian duct and urogenital sinus. The genital

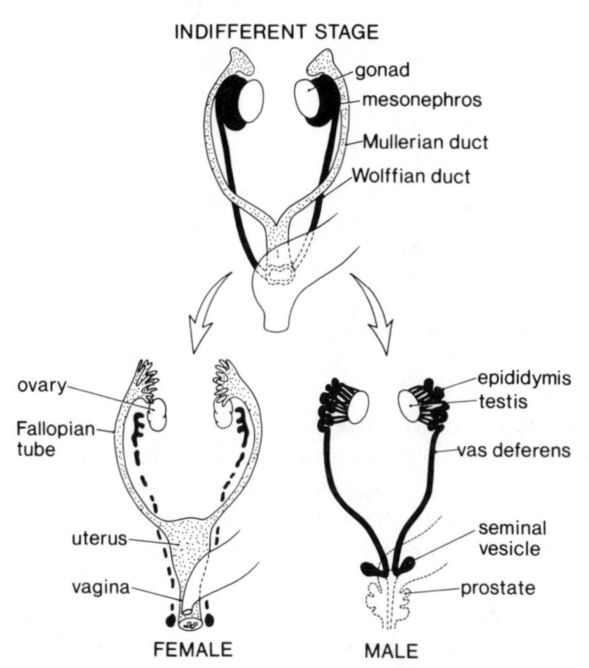

FIG. 3. Differentiation of the internal genitalia. Reprinted with permission from Wilson *et al.* (1979b).

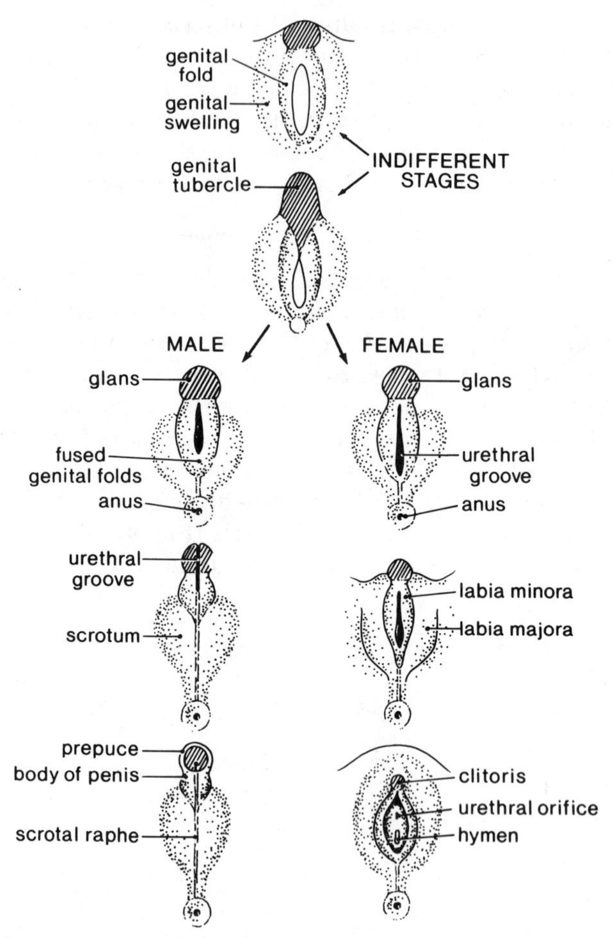

FIG. 4. Differentiation of the external genitalia. Reprinted with permission from Wilson (1979b).

tubercle elongates, and the urethral folds begin to fuse over the urethral groove from posterior to anterior. This fusion joins the two urogenital swellings into a single structure, the scrotum, leading to the formation of the penile urethra. These events are completed relatively early in fetal development (at the end of the first trimester in the human).

Two androgen-dependent events in male phenotypic development take place later, namely, descent of the testes and differential growth of the genitalia in the male. At the time of completion of the male urethra the phallus is approximately the same size in the male and female. However, under the influence of androgens from the fetal testis, the male phallus grows during the latter two-thirds of gestation and by the time of birth is much larger than in the female.

Testicular descent (Fig. 5) is a complex, poorly understood process which begins shortly after differentiation of the testis and is not completed in most species until after birth (Gier and Marion, 1969). Testicular descent can be considered as taking place in three phases. The first phase (transabdominal movement) probably involves, at a minimum, degeneration of the portion of the peritoneal fold that anchors the cranial part of the gonad to the abdominal wall, shortening of the caudal gonadal ligament (gubernaculum), and rapid growth of the abdominal–pelvic region of the fetus. As a result, the testis comes to rest against the anterior abdominal wall in the inguinal region. The second phase of testicular descent involves formation of the processus vaginalis and development of the inguinal canal and scrotum. Increasing intraabdominal pressure is believed to cause a herniation in the abdominal wall (the processus vaginalis) along the course of the inguinal portion of the gubernaculum. Continued pressure causes enlargement of the processus vaginalis around the gubernaculum and formation of

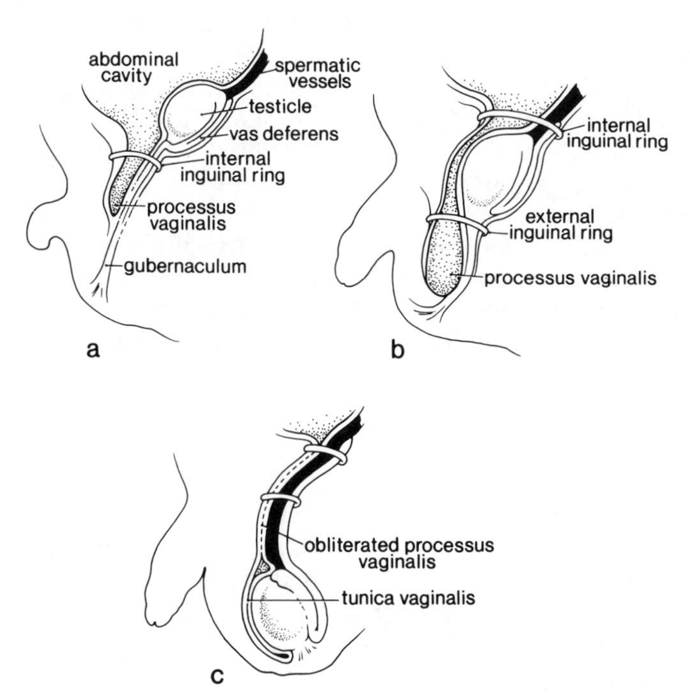

FIG. 5. Testicular descent. Reprinted with permission from Wilson (1979b).

the inguinal canal. The final phase is the movement of the testis from the peritoneal cavity into the processus vaginalis. The gubernaculum increases in size until the mass in the inguinal canal approaches that of the testis. As a result of abdominal pressure and degeneration of the proximal portion of the gubernaculum, the testis descends into the scrotum. The overall process appears to be gonadotropin dependent and mediated, in part, by androgen (Rajfer and Walsh, 1977).

2. *Female Development*

Development of the genital tract of the female is characterized by disappearance or failure of development of the wolffian ducts and by development of the mullerian ducts into the fallopian tubes and uterus (Fig. 3). The fallopian tubes are derived from the cranial portion of the mullerian ducts. Caudally, the paired mullerian ducts approach each other at the midline and fuse. This fused portion of the mullerian ducts develops into the uterus (Fig. 6). Development of the vagina begins with the formation of a solid mass of cells (the uterovaginal plate) between the caudal portions of the mullerian ducts and the urogenital sinus (Fig. 6) (O'Rahilly, 1977). The relative contributions of the mullerian and wolffian ducts and of the urogenital sinus to the development of the uterovaginal plate is not known. Participation of all these tissues is believed to be essential for complete vaginal development (Bulmer, 1957; Bok and Drews, 1983). The cells of the uterovaginal plate proliferate and elongate, and the vaginal plate eventually canalizes to form the vagina.

In contrast to the male in which the phallic and pelvic portions of the urogenital sinus are enclosed by fusion of the genital swellings, most of the urogenital sinus of the female remains exposed on the surface as a cleft into which the vagina and urethra open. The urogenital tubercle in the female undergoes limited growth and development to form the clitoris.

D. Breast Development

The breasts develop along "mammary lines," bilateral epidermal thickenings that extend from the forelimbs to the hindlimbs on the ventral side of the embryo. In the human the mammary lines shorten and condense into a single pair of buds, the only pair of mammary glands to develop. These mammary buds undergo little change until the fifth month of gestation when secondary epithelial buds appear and

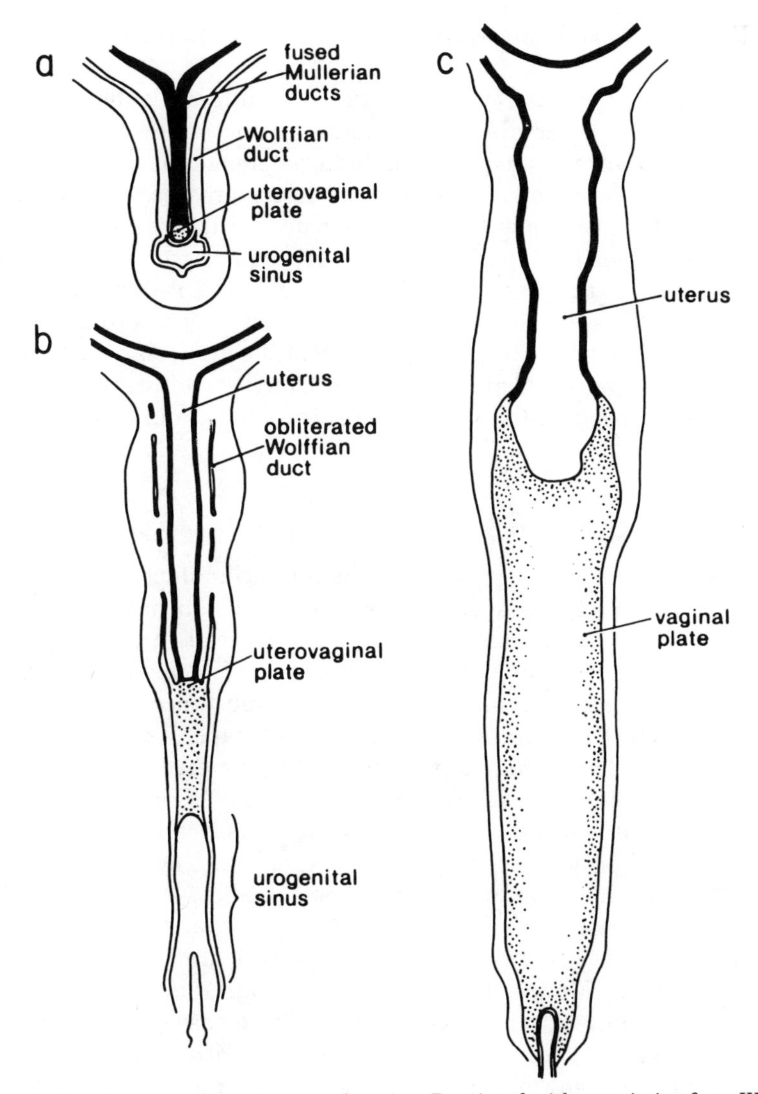

FIG. 6. Development of the uterus and vagina. Reprinted with permission from Wilson (1979b).

nipples develop. In species such as the mouse and rat the mammary buds of the male regress and disappear under the influence of androgens (Raynaud, 1947; Goldman *et al.*, 1976). Such dimorphism does not occur in humans, and the development of the breast in boys and girls is identical up to the time of puberty (Pfaltz, 1949).

IV. Hormonal Regulation of Male Phenotypic Development

The finding that castration of sexually indifferent rabbit embryos invariably leads to female development of embryos of either sex (Fig. 1), (Jost, 1953) established that the induced phenotype in mammals is male and that secretions from the fetal testes are necessary for male development. Development of the female urogenital tract occurs in the absence of gonads and apparently does not require secretions from the fetal ovaries. Furthermore, Jost deduced that two substances from the fetal testes are essential for male development: a nonsteroid hormone that acts ipsilaterally to cause regression of the mullerian duct (mullerian-inhibiting substance) and an androgenic steroid responsible for virilization of the wolffian duct, urogenital sinus, and urogenital tubercle.

A. Mullerian-Inhibiting Substance

In the male embryo regression of the mullerian duct begins shortly after formation of the spermatogenic cords (Blanchard and Josso, 1974), prior to the development of the Leydig cells and the onset of testosterone secretion by the testis. This process is mediated by a peptide hormone termed mullerian-inhibiting substance (mullerian regression factor). Mullerian-inhibiting substance, a glycoprotein formed by the Sertoli cells of the spermatogenic cords and tubules of the fetal and newborn testis (Donahoe *et al.*, 1977a; Picard *et al.*, 1978; Price, 1979; Tran and Josso, 1982), probably acts locally rather than as a circulating hormone to suppress mullerian duct development (van Niekerk, 1974; however, see Hutson and Donahoe, 1983).

Mullerian-inhibiting substance has been purified (for a review see Donahoe *et al.*, 1982); it is a large (140,000 Da), dimeric protein (Budzik *et al.*, 1983). Monoclonal antibodies to mullerian-inhibiting substance block mullerian regression in *in vitro* bioassays (Vigier *et al.*, 1982a; Mudgett-Hunter *et al.*, 1982), and a sensitive radioimmunoassay for mullerian-inhibiting substance has been developed (Vigier *et al.*, 1982b).

Even though they are not primarily responsible for mullerian duct regression, androgens and estrogens influence the process. For example, rat mullerian duct regression in organ culture is enhanced by testosterone, although testosterone itself is inactive (Ikawa *et al.*, 1982; Fallat *et al.*, 1984). Interestingly, neither dihydrotestosterone nor estradiol affects mullerian duct regression in this system. In other systems estrogens interfere with mullerian duct regression (McLachlan, 1977; Teng and Teng, 1979; Hutson *et al.*, 1982; Suzuki *et al.*, 1982; Kobayashi, 1984). Thus, although mullerian-inhibiting substance is required for mullerian duct regression, steroid hormones appear to influence its action.

The concept that mullerian duct regression in male development is an active process is supported by study of the persistent mullerian duct syndrome in the human (Sloan and Walsh, 1976; Brook, 1981). In this disorder, genetic and phenotypic males have fallopian tubes and a uterus (in addition to normal wolffian duct-derived structures) as the result of either an autosomal or X-linked gene defect. The pathogenesis of the disorder is uncertain but is probably either a failure of production of mullerian-inhibiting substance by the fetal testis or a failure of the tissue to respond to the hormone.

Persistence of mullerian ducts is usually accompanied by failure of the testes to descend (Josso *et al.*, 1983). Furthermore, mullerian-inhibiting activity is lower in testicular biopsies from newborn boys with cryptorchidism than from normal newborns (Donahoe *et al.*, 1977b). These findings suggest that mullerian-inhibiting substance may be crucial in the movement of the testis into the scrotum, possibly by influencing the anchoring cranially of the testis to the peritoneal fold.

B. Androgen

The second developmental hormone of the fetal testis was identified by Jost as an androgenic steroid. Testosterone is the principal steroid hormone formed by the testis in postnatal life and is also the androgen formed by the testes of rabbit and human embryos during male phenotypic development (Lipsett and Tullner, 1965; Wilson and Siiteri, 1973; Siiteri and Wilson, 1974). Testosterone formation by the testes begins shortly after the onset of differentiation of the spermatogenic cords and concomitant with the histological differentiation of the Leydig cells (Catt *et al.*, 1975; Gondos, 1980).

Testosterone is believed to perform two functions in male development. First, it probably exerts a local paracrine function within the testis to promote maturation of the spermatogonia. Second, it is essential in the endocrine control of development of the male phenotype.

In some species endocrine differentiation of the fetal ovary, as evidenced by the appearance of the capacity to synthesize estrogen (aromatase activity), develops simultaneously with the ability of the fetal testis to synthesize testosterone (Milewich *et al.*, 1977; George and Wilson, 1978a). The physiological significance of fetal ovarian endocrine function has not been established. It is not essential for the normal female phenotype, which can develop without the fetal gonads (Jost, 1953). Estrogen synthesis may also be important for ovarian development (Gondos *et al.*, 1983).

The critical action of testosterone for development of the male urogenital tract was deduced from three types of embryologic and endocrinologic evidence. First, the fact that testosterone synthesis immediately precedes the initiation of virilization of the urogenital tract in a variety of species suggested a cause and effect relationship between the two events (Lipsett and Tullner, 1965; Attal, 1969; Wilson and Siiteri, 1973; Siiteri and Wilson, 1974; Rigaudiere, 1979). Second, the administration of androgens to female embryos at the appropriate time induces male development of the internal and external genitalia (Schultz and Wilson, 1974). Third, administration of pharmacologic agents that inhibit the synthesis or action of androgens in embryogenesis impairs male development (Neumann *et al.*, 1970; Goldman, 1971).

In the human, five separate single gene defects in androgen synthesis have been identified as causes of inadequate testosterone synthesis and incomplete virilization of the male embryo (Wilson and Goldstein, 1975; Griffin and Wilson, 1978). Severely affected males may develop as phenotypic women with complete failure of virilization of the wolffian ducts, urogenital sinus, and external genitalia. At the other extreme, mildly affected men appear normal except for developmental abnormalities such as hypospadias. The fact that these individuals lack fallopian tubes and uterus indicates the regression of the mullerian ducts takes place normally during embryogenesis and that mullerian regression is not primarily dependent on testosterone biosynthesis and action.

1. *Regulation of Testosterone Synthesis in the Fetal Testis*

The regulation of testosterone synthesis during early sexual differentiation is incompletely understood. In fetal rabbits, which we have used as a model to investigate endocrine differentiation of the gonads, enzymatic differentiation of fetal ovaries and testes is apparent by day 18 of gestation and is manifested by an increase in the rate of 3β-hydroxysteroid dehydrogenase activity in the fetal testis and by an increase in aromatase activity in the fetal ovary (Milewich *et al.*, 1977). Activities of all other enzymes in the pathway of steroid hormone synthesis are similar in the ovaries and testes at this time (Fig. 7) (George *et al.*, 1979). Thus, in the rabbit, changes in the rates of only a few enzymatic reactions in the gonads at a critical time in embryonic development engender profound consequences for sexual differentia-

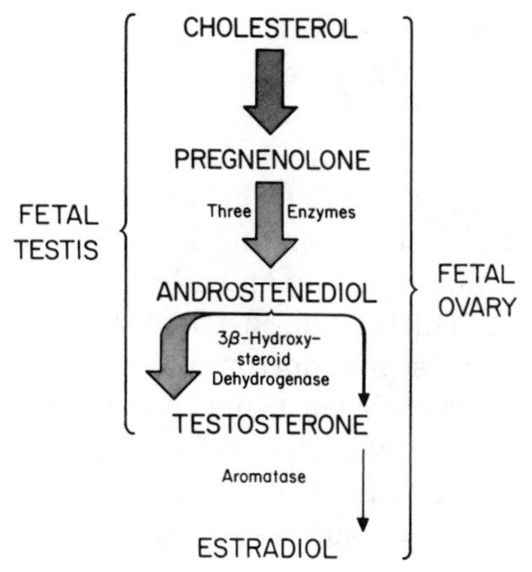

FIG. 7. Enzymatic differentiation of fetal rabbit ovaries and testes on day 18 of gestation. Reprinted with permission from Wilson *et al.* (1981a).

tion. Furthermore, this enzymatic differentiation appears to be an autonomous function of the gonads since it occurs at the appropriate time in the absence of gonadotropin stimulation in cultured fetal gonads exposed only to semisynthetic media (George and Wilson, 1980a).

Whether the actual rate of testosterone production in the rabbit fetal testis is regulated by fetal and/or placental gonadotropins at the onset of testosterone synthesis is not clear. On the one hand, receptors for luteinizing hormone (LH) are found in fetal rabbit testes at the time of initial testosterone synthesis (Catt *et al.*, 1975); moreover, these LH receptors are functional since human chorionic gonadotropin produces an increase in testicular cyclic AMP formation (George *et al.*, 1978a) and cholesterol side-chain cleavage activity (George *et al.*, 1979). On the other hand, the basal rate of cholesterol side-chain cleavage in fetal rabbit testes without gonadotropin stimulation is sufficient to provide enough steroid substrate to support testosterone synthesis at a maximum rate during the initial period of male phenotypic development. Later in embryogenesis when sexual differentiation is far advanced, testosterone synthesis is enhanced by gonadotropin treatment (George *et al.*, 1979). As a consequence, we believe that in rabbits the onset of testosterone synthesis and the resulting differentiation of the male urogenital tract are independent of gonadotropin control.

It is not known whether a similar situation exists in embryonic sexual differentiation in humans or in other animal species. LH receptors are found in human fetal testes as early as the twelfth week of gestation (Huhtaniemi *et al.*, 1977; Molsberry *et al.*, 1982), and human fetal testes respond to human chorionic gonadotropin stimulation with increased testosterone synthesis at this time (Huhtaniemi *et al.*, 1977). However, it is not known whether testosterone synthesis in human fetal testes (and consequently androgen-dependent virilization of male fetuses) is gonadotropin dependent between weeks 8 and 11 when the major portion of male phenotypic differentiation takes place. Such differentiation may be largely independent of pituitary and/or placental control in all species. During the last two-thirds of human gestation, testosterone synthesis is gonadotropin dependent, analogous to the situation in the rabbit embryo. Consequently those aspects of male sexual development that take place during the latter phases of gestation—growth of the penis and descent of the testes—are probably gonadotropin dependent in all species (Rajfer and Walsh, 1977).

2. *Testosterone Action in the Embryo*

The current concept of the mechanism of androgen action within target cells is schematically depicted in Fig. 8. Testosterone, the androgen secreted by the testis and the major androgen in plasma, enters target tissues by a passive diffusion process. Inside the cell testosterone may or may not be converted to 5α-dihydrotestosterone depending on the presence or absence of the 5α-reductase enzyme. Testosterone or 5α-dihydrotestosterone binds to a specific high-affinity receptor protein. After the hormone binds to its receptor the hormone–receptor complex undergoes an incompletely understood process termed *transformation* through which it acquires the capacity to bind to anionic substances such as DNA. It is not known whether hormone–receptor complexes form in the nucleus, the cytoplasm, or both, but in the nu-

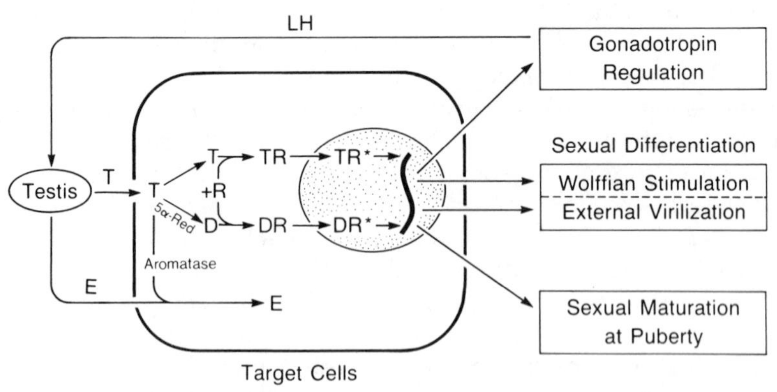

FIG. 8. Androgen action. LH, Luteinizing hormone; T, testosterone; D, 5α-dihydrotestosterone; E, estradiol; R, receptor; TR*, transformed receptor.

cleus the transformed hormone–receptor complexes interact with acceptor sites on the chromosomes. The nature of the acceptor sites within the nucleus (i.e., whether protein or DNA and their number) is not clear, but the overall result of the interaction of the hormone–receptor complexes with chromatin is to increase transcription of tissue-specific structural genes, with the subsequent appearance of new messenger RNAs and new proteins in the cytoplasm of the cell. Studies in other steroid hormone systems make it likely that the androgen–receptor complex binds to DNA at specific regulatory sites near the structural genes under regulatory control by the hormones (Pfahl, 1982; Dean *et al.*, 1984).

Much evidence (see below) indicates that testosterone–receptor complexes mediate fetal wolffian duct virilization and that 5α-dihydrotestosterone–receptor complexes mediate differentiation of the male external genitalia. In some tissues (e.g., hypothalamus) testosterone can be aromatized to estradiol, and androgen action is paradoxically mediated by an estrogen. Inappropriate increases in estrogen formation (aromatase) in gonadal or extragonadal tissue can change the ratio of androgen to estrogen and cause feminization.

a. Role of Testosterone and 5α-Dihydrotestosterone. Separate roles for testosterone in mediating virilization of the wolffian ducts and for 5α-dihydrotestosterone in mediating development of the external genitalia of the male were postulated on the basis of studies of androgen metabolism in embryos (Siiteri and Wilson, 1973; Wilson, 1971; Wilson and Lasnitzki, 1971). In rat, rabbit, guinea pig, and human embryos 5α-reductase activity is maximal in the anlagen of the prostate and external genitalia prior to virilization; the enzyme is virtually undetectable in the wolffian duct derivatives until after virilization is advanced (Fig. 9). Therefore, it was proposed that testosterone mediates virilization of the wolffian ducts whereas 5α-dihydrotestosterone is responsible for differentiation of the male urethra, prostate, and external genitalia (Wilson and Lasnitzki, 1971). This deduction received substantiation from studies of patients with a rare autosomal recessive form of abnormal sexual development due to deficiency of the 5α-reductase enzyme that catalyzes the conversion of testosterone to 5α-dihydrotestosterone (Walsh *et al.*, 1974; Peterson *et al.*, 1977; Fisher *et al.*, 1978). Affected persons are 46,XY males with predominately female external genitalia in association with bilateral testes and normally virilized wolffian duct structures (epididymis, vas deferens, seminal vesicle, and ejaculatory duct) that terminate in a pseudovagina (Fig. 10). At the time of expected puberty testosterone production increases into the male range, and the external genitalia

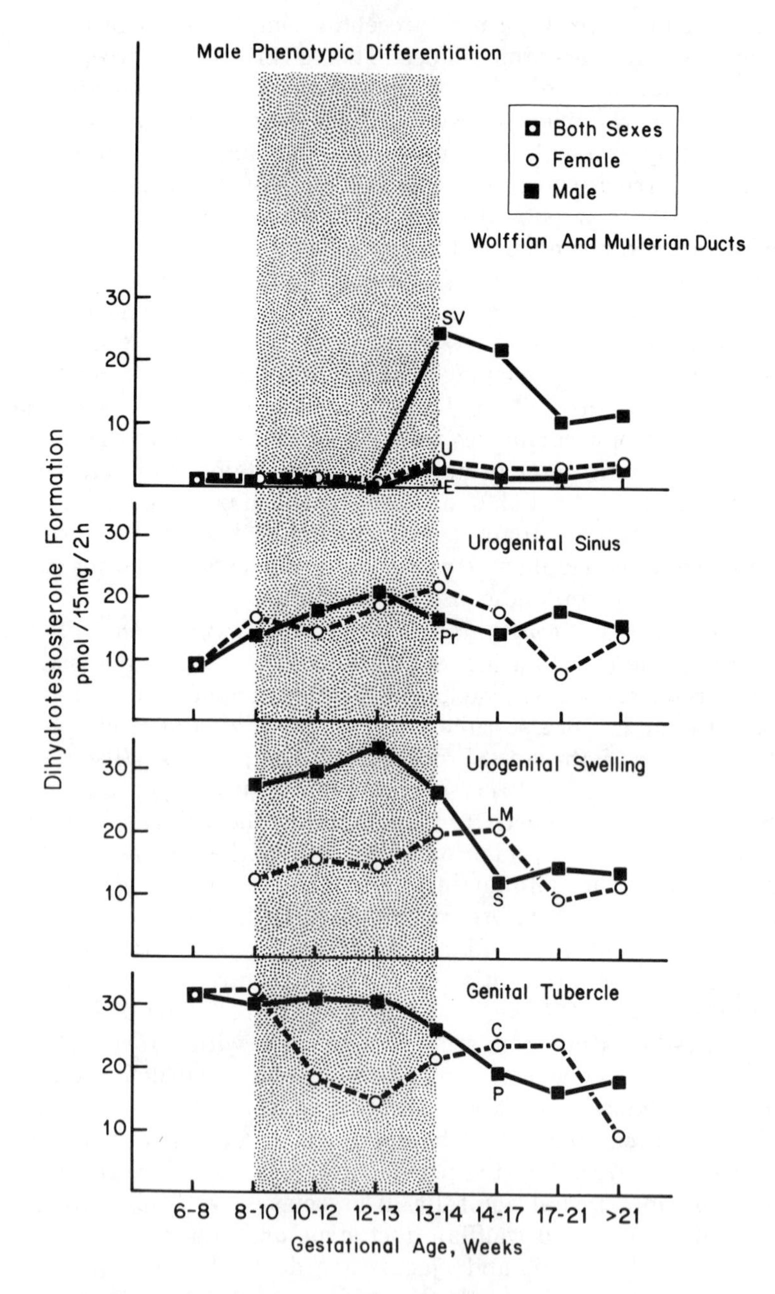

FIG. 9. Developmental study of 5α-reductase activity in urogenital tracts of human fetuses. Adapted with permission from Siiteri and Wilson (1974).

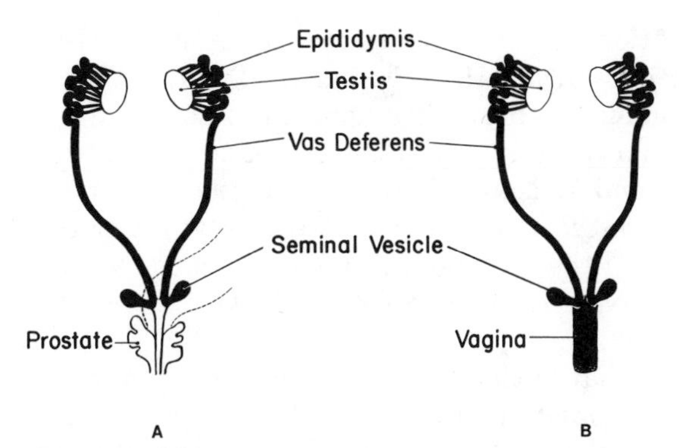

FIG. 10. Schematic diagram of the internal genitalia of normal males (A) and patients with 5α-reductase deficiency (B). Reprinted with permission from Wilson *et al.* (1981b).

may virilize to a limited extent. Axillary and pubic hair develop normally without gynecomastia.

Studies of 5α-reductase in fibroblasts cultured from genital skin of patients from different families with 5α-reductase deficiency have revealed that substantial genetic heterogeneity exists among affected families (Fig. 11). Sixteen families with defects in 5α-dihydrotestos-

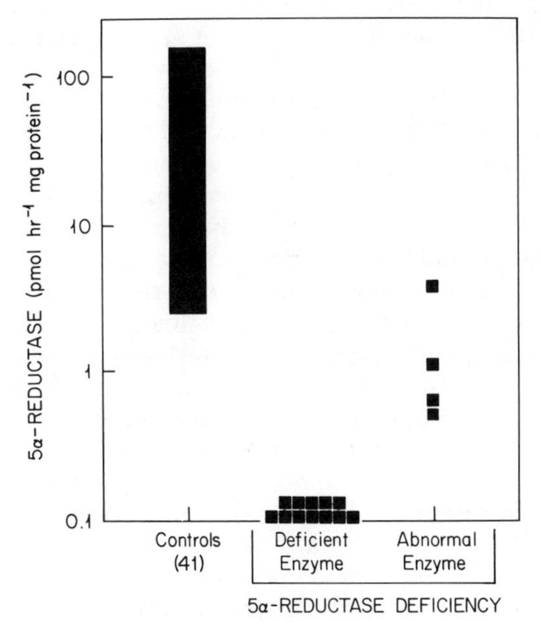

FIG. 11. Characteristics of 5α-reductase deficiency in 16 families.

terone formation have been characterized in detail (Imperato-McGinley *et al.,* 1974; Wilson, 1975; Fisher *et al.,* 1978; Wilson *et al.,* 1983). The most common abnormality appears to be a marked deficiency in the amount of a catalytically active 5α-reductase enzyme (Moore *et al.,* 1975; Moore and Wilson, 1976). Some patients show a less profound depression of *in vitro* enzyme activity. In the latter group structural abnormalities of the enzyme that affect cofactor (NADPH) and/or steroid binding have been described (Leshin *et al.,* 1978; Imperato-McGinley *et al.,* 1980).

Since no animal model for 5α-reductase defects (and decreased 5α-dihydrotestosterone formation) has yet been discovered, detailed endocrinological studies to directly characterize the importance of testosterone and 5α-dihydrotestosterone in differentiation of the male phenotype have been difficult. However, potent inhibitors of the 5α-reductase enzyme have been developed (Liang and Heiss, 1981; Brooks *et al.,* 1981, 1982; Leshin and Wilson, 1982). The administration of these inhibitors to pregnant rats during the period of embryonic sexual differentiation has reproduced many of the characteristics of the 5α-reductase deficiency phenotype in the male offspring. Virilization of the external genitalia is impaired, whereas no effect on the male differentiation of wolffian duct-derived structures is apparent (Brooks *et al.,* 1982; Imperato-McGinley *et al.,* 1985; George, unpublished observations). Since there appears to be nothing unique about the androgen receptor system of the wolffian duct derivatives that allows these structures to respond to testosterone preferentially (George and Noble, 1984), it has been difficult to understand why two androgens are necessary for complete male phenotypic development. It is possible that secretion of high concentrations of testosterone directly from the testis into the lumen of the wolffian duct might cause virilization of wolffian duct structures (epididymis, vas deferens, seminal vesicle) in normal individuals as well as those with impaired formation of 5α-dihydrotestosterone. Two types of evidence support this theory. First, active immunization of pregnant rabbits against testosterone reduces circulating androgen and causes pseudohermaphroditism in male offspring similar to the phenotype described for human males with 5α-reductase deficiency (Bidlingmaier *et al.,* 1977; Veyssière *et al.,* 1980), suggesting that androgens that are not exposed to antibody (lumenal androgens) may remain effective. Second, a heritable trait in the rat causes unilateral hypoplasia of the testis in 47% of males (Ikadai *et al.,* 1985). Hypoplasia of the testis is accompanied by ipsilateral aplasia of the epididymis and vas deferens despite the fact that prostate development and virilization of the external genitalia are normal, presumably mediated by androgens secreted by the normal testis. This mutation is consistent with a noncirculating factor from the testis (testosterone?) causing virilization of the adjacent wolffian duct.

A still-perplexing aspect of 5α-reductase deficiency is the partial virilization that occurs in some patients at the time of expected puberty (Peterson *et al.*, 1977; Price *et al.*, 1984). Late virilization in these patients may be due to the combination of higher levels of plasma testosterone at puberty than during embryogenesis and the presence of some residual 5α-reductase activity in all patients with this defect who have been characterized to date. Indeed, the small amounts of 5α-dihydrotestosterone formed in such patients are probably sufficient to effect partial virilization.

b. Role of the Androgen Receptor. A specific, high-affinity receptor protein mediates the postnatal actions of androgen in all androgen-dependent tissues. Studies in animals and humans of single-gene mutations causing resistance to androgen action and failure of male development of varying severity indicate that androgens act to virilize the male fetus by mechanisms fundamentally the same as those in the adult. Direct characterization of the androgen receptor of the urogenital tract of the rabbit embryo is in keeping with this concept (George and Noble, 1984).

The first disorder of the androgen receptor to be characterized in molecular terms was the testicular feminization (*Tfm*) mutation in the mouse, an X-linked disorder in which affected males have testes and normal testosterone production but differentiate as phenotypic females (Lyon and Hawkes, 1970; Goldstein and Wilson, 1972). The mullerian-inhibiting function of the fetal testis is presumed to be normal since no mullerian duct derivatives (uterus or fallopian tubes) are present in affected males. The profound resistance to androgen causes failure of all androgen-mediated aspects of male development in the wolffian duct, urogenital sinus, and external genitalia. 5α-Dihydrotestosterone formation is normal, but functional cytoplasmic androgen receptors are not detectable (Gehring *et al.*, 1971; Bullock *et al.*, 1971; Verhoeven and Wilson, 1976) (Fig. 12). Consequently, the hormone cannot reach the nucleus of the cell and interact with the chromosomes.

Studies of subjects with the human counterpart of the *Tfm* mouse, namely, testicular feminization and its variants, have provided additional insight into the role of the androgen receptor in embryonic virilization (Wilson *et al.*, 1983). Primary amenorrhea is the symptom usually prompting the patient with testicular feminization to seek medical attention. The karyotype is 46,XY, but the general habitus is female. Axillary, facial, and public hair is absent or scanty. The external geni-

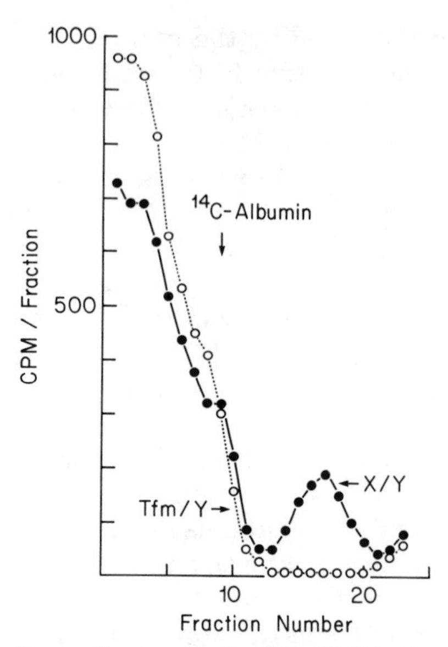

FIG. 12. Sucrose density gradient analysis of 5α-[^{3}H]dihydrotestosterone binding in kidney cytosol from normal (X/Y) and androgen-resistant (*Tfm*/Y) male mice. Adapted with permission from Verhoeven and Wilson (1976).

talia are unambiguously female, and the vagina is short and blind-ended. No internal genitalia are found except testes, located in the abdomen along the course of the inguinal canal, or in the labia majora. Female breast development at the time of expected puberty is due to increased estrogen synthesis by the testis (MacDonald *et al.*, 1979). A small percentage of patients with the phenotype of testicular feminization have axillary and pubic hair as well as a modest degree of virilization (Madden *et al.*, 1975). These patients are designated as having the "incomplete" form of testicular feminization. Reifenstein syndrome [most commonly characterized by a predominately male phenotype with the clinical findings of hypospadia, azoospermia, and gynecomastia (Wilson *et al.*, 1983)] and infertility in phenotypically normal men (Aiman *et al.*, 1979) complete the spectrum of disorders of the androgen receptor.

The molecular defect in many patients is similar to that in the *Tfm* mouse (i.e., no high-affinity androgen receptor can be detected; Keenan *et al.*, 1974; Griffin *et al.*, 1976). It is not known whether the loss of binding in these instances is due to total lack of the receptor protein or a protein defective in binding function. Other patients with testicular feminization have either a diminished amount of receptor or a qualitative abnormality of the receptor. Qualitative abnormalities of the androgen receptor were initially identified in studies documenting thermolability of androgen receptors in skin fibroblasts cultured from patients with phenotypic androgen resistance (Griffin, 1979). Subsequently, other mutations have been identified in which the cytosolic androgen receptor is unstable in molybdate-containing buffers (Griffin and Durrant, 1982). Studies of the process by which androgen–receptor complexes are "transformed" to the DNA-binding state have identified yet another subset of patients with qualitatively abnormal androgen receptors; the receptor abnormality becomes manifest under transforming conditions (Kovacs *et al.*, 1983, 1984). Qualitative abnormalities of the androgen receptor found in other laboratories include altered affinity of binding (Brown *et al.*, 1982), impaired nuclear retention (Eil, 1983), and impaired augmentation of receptor binding after prolonged incubation with ligand (Kaufman *et al.*, 1983). Since some patients with qualitatively abnormal receptor have androgen resistance as profound as that of patients showing no androgen binding it appears that such structural abnormalities can totally obliterate function. The normal gene coding for the androgen receptor and the mutant gene that causes absence of the receptor are X-linked (Meyer *et al.*, 1975; Migeon *et al.*, 1981); mutations causing qualitative abnormalities of the receptor are probably allelic mutations of the same gene (Elawady *et al.*, 1983).

Our laboratory has categorized the androgen receptor defects in genital skin fibroblasts grown from individuals from 71 families with androgen resistance (Fig. 13). Twenty-four were classified as complete

Phenotypic Spectrum: Female ⟶ Male

Type of Receptor Defect / Diagnostic Category	Complete Testicular Feminization	Incomplete Testicular Feminization	Reifenstein Syndrome	Infertile Male
Absent Binding	●●●●●●●●●●●●●●	●●●		
Qualitatively Abnormal	●●●●●●●●●	●●●●●●	●●●●●●●●●●●●	●●●●●●
Decreased Amount		●●	●●●●●	●●●●
Abnormality Unidentified	●	●●●●	●●●●	●

FIG. 13. Distribution of androgen receptor defects in 71 families with androgen resistance and phenotypes ranging from complete testicular feminization to the infertile male.

testicular feminization; in 14 of the 24 androgen binding was undetectable (absent binding), and in 9 the receptor was qualitatively abnormal (Griffin, 1979; Griffin and Durrant, 1982). In one of the individuals with the complete disorder no abnormality could be identified. Fifteen individuals phenotypically displaying incomplete testicular feminization were studied; three showed no detectable binding, six showed qualitative defects, two showed decreased amount of binding, and four had an abnormality not yet identified.

Partial androgen resistance (Reifenstein syndrome) constitutes a mixture of subtle qualitative and quantitative abnormalities of the receptor protein (Griffin *et al.*, 1976; Griffin, 1979; Griffin and Durrant, 1982). Partial (and variable) virilization here is probably mediated through residual androgen receptors. In approximately one-fifth of these patients an abnormality of the androgen receptor has yet to be discovered. The most subtle manifestation of a partial defect in the androgen receptor is infertility due to absence or profound deficiency of sperm in otherwise normal men (Aiman *et al.*, 1979). This latter disorder may be the most common phenotype associated with abnormalities of the androgen receptor (Aiman and Griffin, 1982).

In some patients androgen resistance is expressed with apparently normal androgen receptors that appropriately translocate to the nucleus. This was originally considered the consequence of defects in later phases of androgen action, so-called receptor-positive or postreceptor androgen resistance (Amrhein *et al.*, 1976). Individuals from 10 such families analyzed in our laboratory span a phenotypic spectrum from testicular feminization to the infertile male syndrome (Griffin *et al.*, 1985) (Fig. 13). As more sensitive techniques for characterizing qualitative abnormalities in the androgen receptor are developed, more and more of these cases, including the original family described by Amrhein *et al.* (1976), prove to represent subtle functional abnormalities of the androgen receptor.

c. Why Are Two Androgens Involved in Virilization? 5α-Dihydrotestosterone binds to the androgen receptor of most species with greater affinity than does testosterone (Maes *et al.*, 1979; Wilbert *et al.*, 1983; George and Noble, 1984; Kovacs *et al.*, 1984), and the 5α-dihydrotestosterone–receptor complex is more readily transformed to the DNA-binding state than is the testosterone–receptor complex (Kovacs *et al.*, 1983). These two features imply that 5α-dihydrotestosterone formation generally amplifies the androgenic signal. Furthermore, the characteristics of androgen receptors from fetal urogenital sinus and urogenital tubercle are similar, if not identical to those of adult prostate (George and Noble, 1984). Since a single androgen receptor appears to mediate the action of both androgens, a central, as yet unresolved question concerns the mechanisms whereby testosterone and 5α-dihydrotestosterone exert different actions during embryogenesis (see above). One possibility is that the two hormones act in exactly the same manner to promote virilization. By this schema, 5α-dihydrotestosterone, although amplifying the hormonal signal within most androgen target cells, is not absolutely required for androgen action, provided that the intracellular concentration of testosterone is sufficiently high and that sufficient time is available to allow registration of the weaker hormonal signal produced by testosterone. Alternatively, testosterone may promote virilization of the wolffian ducts indirectly, analogous to the involvement of erythropoietin in androgen-mediated control of erythopoiesis (Evens and Amerson, 1974).

d. The Critical Role of the Embryonic Mesenchyme in Androgen-Mediated Differentiation. The embryonic mesenchyme (stroma) of many tissues directs the phenotypic development of the epithelium, and steroid hormone receptors are found in the stroma of many tissues (reviewed by Cunha *et al.*, 1983). A compelling case for stromal–epithelial interactions in androgen action comes from studies of tissue recombinants in the development of the urogenital sinus. For example, co-grafting of mesenchyme from the urogenital sinus of embryonic mice with heterotypic integumental epithelium intraocularly in male animals yields epithelium characteristic of the glandular epithelium of the urogenital sinus (Cunha, 1972). Co-transplants with substitutes of mesenchyme from other embryonic sites are ineffective in causing glandular differentiation. Similar co-transplants utilizing mesenchyme from the urogenital sinus of androgen-resistant (*Tfm*/Y) mice with normal (+/Y) urogenital sinus epithelium exposed to androgen are also without effect. Reciprocal (*Tfm*/Y epithelium with +/Y mesenchyme) recombinants yield normal prostate development (Lasnitzki and Mizuno, 1980; Cunha and Chung, 1981).

Autoradiographic studies of androgen binding in the urogenital sinus of developing rats (Takeda *et al.*, 1985) provide additional support for the concept that the mesenchyme is the initial site of androgen action during morphogenesis of the male urogenital tract. At the time of prostatic bud formation androgen binding sites are located predominantly over the nuclei of mesenchymal cells that surround the developing buds. The urogenital sinus of female embryos also contains androgen binding sites in the nuclei of mesenchymal cells. In contrast, no sites were detected in the epithelia of fetal urogenital sinuses. By postnatal day 10, androgen binding is found in the epithelial cells of the prostate, and labeling in mesenchymal cells became less prominent. These results suggest that during morphogenesis of male urogenital tract androgen action is initiated through mesenchymal cells, whereas androgen responses of differentiated target tissues (such as the prostate) are mediated by interaction with the epithelial component.

A similar system is responsible for the androgen-mediated regression of the embryonic mammary bud in the mouse (Kratochwil and Schwartz, 1976; Drews and Drews, 1977). In this tissue, however, the response of the mesenchyme to androgen (the induction of androgen receptors) requires specific interaction of the mesenchyme with mammary epithelium (Heuberger *et al.,* 1982), suggesting that in some cases the epithelium may also take part in the differentiation process. There are also indications that epithelium of mesodermal origin when recombined with androgen-responsive mesenchyme responds differently than does epithelium of endoderm (Cunha *et al.,* 1983). Elucidating the nature of these mesenchymal–epithelial interactions is of critical importance in understanding androgen-mediated differentiative processes.

Despite evolving knowledge of hormonal control of differentiation in the urogenital tract and cellular sites of action, little is known about the specific gene products synthesized in response to hormones or how such products direct cellular organization during embryogenesis.

e. Virilization of the Female. Female embryos have the same androgen receptor system in the urogenital tract as do male embryos (George and Noble, 1984). For example, androgen receptors are as readily detectable in the urethra and vagina of the fetal female rabbit as they are in the prostatic urethra of the male (Fig. 14). In contrast, androgen binding is barely detectable in the urinary bladder of either sex. As a consequence, it is not surprising that exposure to androgens during the time of sexual differentiation causes virilization of female offspring (Schultz and Wilson, 1974). The anatomical consequences of such an experiment in rats are illustrated in Fig. 15. Figure 15A and B represent urogenital tracts dissected from female and male newborn rats born to mothers treated with oil (control) from day 14 through day 21 of gestation. Figure 15C depicts a urogenital tract from a newborn female exposed *in utero* to an inactive androgen analog (5β-dihydrotestosterone). Figure 15D depicts a urogenital tract from a female treated with 5α-dihydrotestosterone. This active androgen caused differentiation of the wolffian ducts in this female embryo into prominent epididymides, vasa deferentia, and seminal vesicles. Furthermore, the urogenital sinuses from female rats treated *in utero* with 5α-dihydrotestosterone contained prostatic buds with male-type ure-

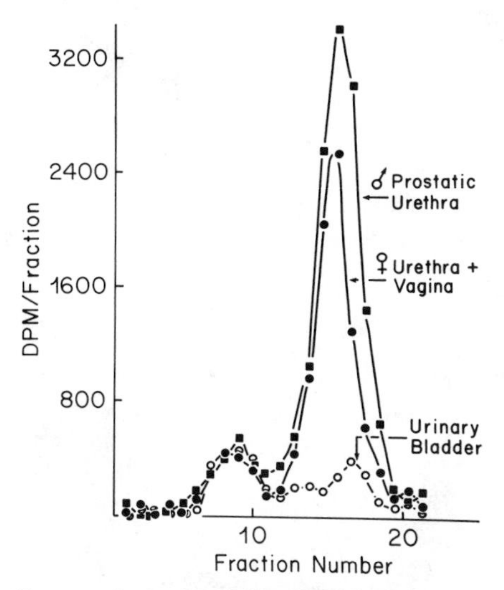

FIG. 14. Sucrose gradient analysis of 5 nM 5α-[^{3}H]dihydrotestosterone binding in cytosolic fractions of urogenital sinuses and bladder of fetal rabbits on day 28 of gestation.

thra and no vaginal development (George, unpublished observations). The fact that females are virilized when exposed to androgens suggests that differences in anatomical development between males and females depend on differences in the hormonal signals themselves and not on differences in the receptors for the hormones in target tissues.

The most common cause of virilization of human female embryos is congenital adrenal hyperplasia, an autosomal recessive mutation that produces a deficiency in steroid 21-hydroxylase enzyme activity (New *et al.,* 1983). Decreased synthesis of cortisol in the adrenal gland leads to a compensatory increase in ACTH secretion by the pituitary that, in turn, causes an increase in adrenal androgen secretion. The adrenal androgens then virilize the external genitalia of the female. The internal genitalia are, however, not virilized, and wolffian duct remnants are no more prominent in women with congenital adrenal hyperplasia than in controls. Therefore, it is likely that either the degeneration of the wolffian ducts precedes the onset of adrenal androgen sysnthesis or that the wolffian ducts are insensitive to the predominant androgens formed in affected females.

3. *Sex Hormones and Sexual Differentiation of the Brain*

In some animals gonadal steroids act in the central nervous system during fetal and/or postnatal life to influence sexual behavior and the

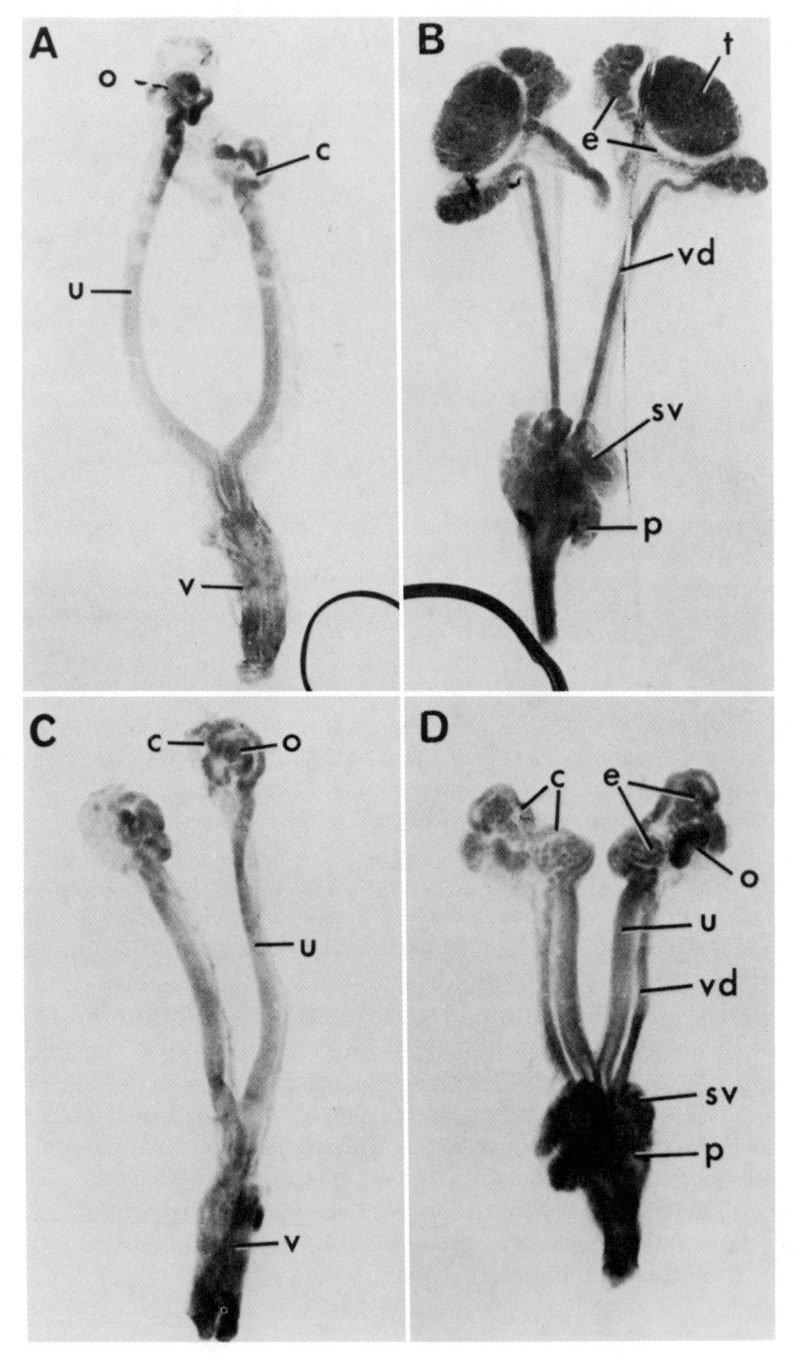

FIG. 15. Virilization of the female rat urogenital tract caused by 5α-dihydrotestosterone administration to the mother. (A, B) Female and male urogenital tracts, respectively, of newborn rats from a mother given oil from days 14–21 of gestation; (C) female

pattern of gonadotropin secretion by the hypothalamic–pituitary system. For example, the administration of testosterone for a short period to a newborn female rat can permanently imprint a tonic, "male-type" secretory pattern of gonadotropin and cause masculine sexual behavior (MacLuskey and Naftolin, 1981; McEwen, 1981). Likewise, gonadectomy of male rats at birth causes feminization of both neuroendocrine and sexual behavior components of the reproductive system (Harris, 1964). The facts that estrogens are more potent than androgens as inhibitors of ovulation in newborn female rats (Docke and Dorner, 1975; Doughty *et al.*, 1975) and that brain tissue forms estrogens from androgens in regions thought to control gonadotropin secretion and sexual behavior (Naftolin *et al.*, 1971; George and Ojeda, 1982; Roselli *et al.*, 1985) suggest that the defeminizing effect of androgens is paradoxically mediated by estrogen formed locally in specific areas of the brain. This concept is reinforced by experiments demonstrating that nonaromatizable androgens, such as 5α-dihydrotestosterone, are ineffective in suppressing reproductive cyclicity in female rats whereas androgens that can be aromatized to estrogens, such as testosterone, are effective in this regard (McDonald and Doughty, 1974; Arai, 1972). Hypothalamic estrogen receptors of neonatal male rats are partially occupied by estradiol derived from androgens (Westley and Salaman, 1976). Furthermore, nonsteroidal antiestrogens antagonize the defeminizing effect of androgens and estrogens on brain sexual differentiation (Doughty *et al.*, 1973; Lieberberg *et al.*, 1977).

Perhaps the strongest evidence that *in situ* conversion of androgens to estrogens is responsible for sexual differentiation of the brain is provided by the observation that administration of an inhibitor of aromatization (androst-1,4,6-triene-3,17-dione) to neonatal rats causes feminization of the sexual behavior of males and blocks the defeminizing effect of testosterone on lordosis behavior in females (McEwen *et al.*, 1977). Thus, in rats, at least, sexual dimorphism of both neuroendocrine function and behavior seems to be regulated directly by the conversion of androgenic steroids to estrogens in specific areas of the brain. This sexual dimorphism is another example of the importance of peripheral metabolism of testosterone (in this case to estrogen) in androgen action.

---

urogenital tract following administration of 16 mg 5β-dihydrotestosterone per day; (D) female urogenital tract following administration of 16 mg 5α-dihydrotestosterone per day; o, ovary; u, uterus; c, coils of oviduct; v, vagina; t, testis; e, epididymis; vd, vas deferens; sv, seminal vesicle; p, prostate. Reprinted with permission from Schultz and Wilson (1974).

The extent to which these findings in the rat can be applied to other species is unclear. Karsch *et al.* (1973) have demonstrated in the adult male rhesus monkey that the normal tonic pattern of gonadotropin secretion can be altered to the cyclic pattern characteristic of the female rhesus monkey by administration of ovarian steroids so as to mimic the pattern of secretion by the normal ovary. A similar phenomenon has been reported in men (Kulin and Reiter, 1976). In contrast to the rodent, however, regulation of gonadotropin secretion by gonadal steroids in humans or monkeys requires the continual presence or absence of the hormones in question, and gonadal hormones appear to have no permanent effects on the secretory pattern of gonadotropins analogous to that observed in the neonatal rodent. The role of gonadal hormones in the regulation of human sexual behavior is also unclear (Wilson, 1979a). While androgens clearly influence male sexual drive, a role for androgens or estrogens in controlling libido in women is not established. Furthermore, the complex phenomena loosely termed gender identity and gender role are difficult to study and poorly understood, but it is likely that androgens are important in development of male gender identity (Wilson, 1979a).

V. Possible Role of Hormones in Normal Female Development

A. Hormonal Control of Sexual Differentiation in Marsupials

In contrast to eutherian mammals in which sexual differentiation occurs *in utero,* marsupial young are born sexually indifferent. Development of the sexual phenotypes takes place in the pouch independent of the maternal milieu, and the pouch young are accessible for experimentation throughout development. Marsupials therefore represent an important model system for studying the hormonal factors controlling sexual differentiation. Pioneering work on the relationship between gonadal steroid hormones and phenotypic sex development was performed in the American opossum, *Didelphis virginiana* (Burns, 1939, 1945; Moore, 1941).

Burns (1945) studied the effects of the administration of androgen (testosterone propionate) or estrogen (estradiol dipropionate) on the development of the sexual phenotypes in newborn opossums. Testosterone administration caused a marked hypertrophy and male differentiation of the phallus in both male and female pouch young. In contrast, estrogen caused female-type development of the phallus and cloacal region in both sexes. Thus, estrogens are important in the development of the external genitalia of the female opossum.

The development of the pouch in female and the scrotum in male opossums occurs 10 days after birth, and it is believed that the two structures derive from common anlage (Bolliger, 1944). Pouch development is the earliest evidence of sexual dimorphism that can be identified grossly. Interestingly in all the pouch young that Burns treated with androgen or estrogen, some very soon after entering the pouch, the development of the pouch or scrotum was not influenced.

Thus, phenotypic differentiation in this marsupial appears to be an exception to Jost's formulation for sexual differentiation in eutherian mammals in that (1) estrogens may play a role in development of the female urogenital tract, and (2) some aspects of the sexual phenotype (scrotum and pouch development) appear to be independent of hormonal control. To provide additional insight into the control of phenotypic differentiation in this species, we have studied the synthesis and metabolism of gonadal steroids in pouch young of the American opossum (George *et al.*, 1985). The pattern of steroid hormone biosynthesis and metabolism in the opossum pouch young differs in at least two regards from that in embryos of eutherian mammals.

First, the ovaries and testes likely differentiate in the opossum before the pouch and scrotum (Fig. 16) and several weeks before onset of

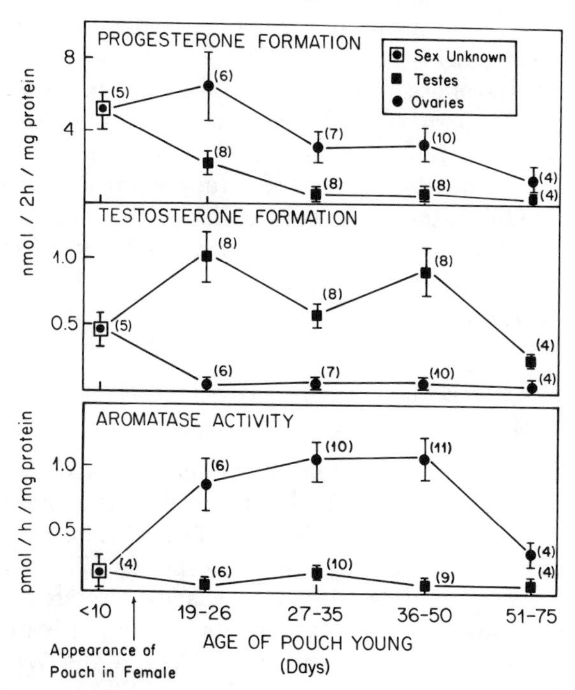

FIG. 16. Enzymatic differentiation of the ovary and testis of opossum (*Didelphis virginiana*) pouch young. Reprinted with permission from George *et al.* (1985).

virilization of the wolffian ducts and urogenital tubercle (Burns, 1939). In contrast, in rat, rabbit, guinea pig, mouse, and human embryos, virilization of the urogenital tract begins immediately after the onset of testosterone synthesis in the fetal testis (George and Wilson, 1984). This suggests that in the opossum the response mechanism to gonadal steroids (receptors, receptor transformation process, etc.) develops later than the formation of the hormones themselves, whereas in the eutherian mammal androgen receptors exist in target tissues prior to the onset of androgen biosynthesis. Furthermore, the fact that the ovary of the newborn opossum is capable of synthesizing substantial amounts of progesterone raises the possibility that ovarian hormones other than estrogen may influence female differentiation in this species.

Second, the pattern of 5α-reductase activity in peripheral tissues of opossum pouch young differs from that in other species. 5α-Reductase is high not only in urogenital sinus and tubercle but also in many tissues of the opossum pouch young as compared with rates in other mammalian species (George *et al.*, 1985). For example, activity is high in the early wolffian ducts of the opossum, whereas in most species the activity in wolffian ducts is low to undetectable prior to differentiation of the epididymis and seminal vesicle (Wilson and Lasnitzki, 1971; Siiteri and Wilson, 1974). It is not certain that these findings implicate 5α-dihydrotestosterone as the androgen responsible for virilization of the wolffian duct in marsupials. The apparent high content of 5α-reductase prior to differentiation might be coincidental and without significance prior to development of a functional androgen response mechanism. It is of interest, however, that in the adult male Australian phalanger, *Trichosurus vulpecula,* tissues derived from the wolffian ducts appear to be the major source of 5α-dihydrotestosterone synthesis (Cook *et al.*, 1978).

B. Possible Role of Estrogen in Embryonic Development of the Eutherian Mammal

No mutations are known that produce deficient estrogen synthesis or resistance to estrogen action. This contrasts with the androgen system in which single-gene mutations that interfere with hormone synthesis or action have been characterized in many species (Wilson *et al.*, 1983). In the rabbit, estrogen synthesis is temporarily activated in both male and female embryos at the time the blastocyst implants in the uterine wall between days 6 and 7 of gestation (George and Wilson, 1978b) (Fig. 17). Later in the embryogenesis of the rabbit, estrogen synthesis

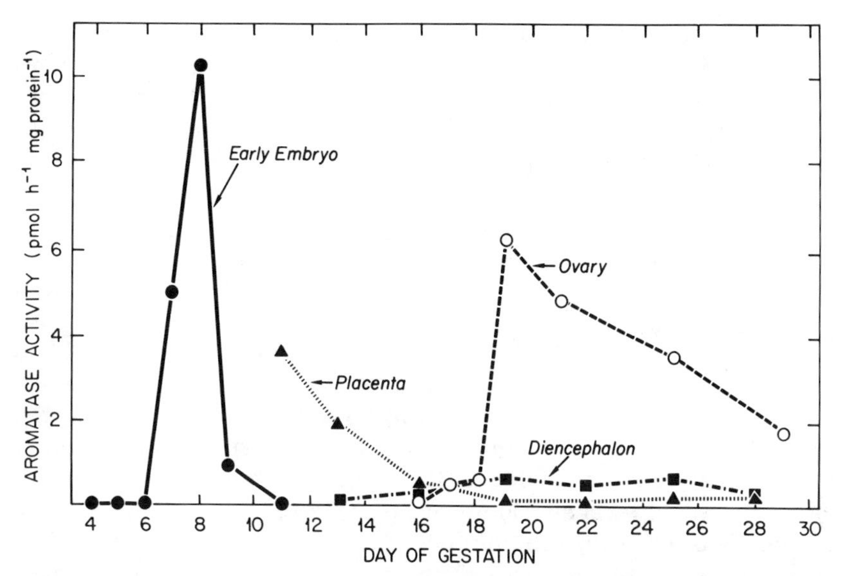

FIG. 17. Distribution of aromatase activity in the developing rabbit embryo. Composite of data in George *et al.* (1978b); George and Wilson (1978b); Milewich *et al.* (1977).

(aromatase activity) is activated in placenta (transiently), brain, and ovary, but specific activity of aromatase in these tissues is never as high as in the implanting blastocyst (Fig. 17). Estrogen action may be necessary for implantation and survival of the blastocyst (Dickmann and Dey, 1976; Dickmann *et al.,* 1977), suggesting that estrogen action is essential for life in eutherian mammals. If this is true, mutations that prevent either the synthesis or response to estrogens could be lethal at an early stage of development by preventing implantation of the blastocyst.

In many species estradiol synthesis is initiated in the ovary before definitive histological differentiation has occurred; it is possible that cellular organization of the ovary may be mediated in part by estrogens formed locally (Gondos *et al.,* 1983), analogous to the postulated role of testosterone in maturation of the spermatogenic cords of the testis. Whether estrogen affects phenotypic development of either sex is unknown. In the eutherian mammal, embryogenesis takes place in a "sea" of hormones (steroidal and nonsteroidal) derived from the placenta, the maternal circulation, and the fetal adrenal gland, the fetal testis, and possibly from the fetal ovary. It is not known whether any of these substances influence female phenotypic differentiation, because experimental agents that block estrogen synthesis or estrogen action interfere with placental function and cause abortion. Nevertheless, estrogens and progestogens may be involved in the growth and maturation of the urogenital tract of the female during the latter part of embryonic development, even if they are not required for their differentiation.

VI. Feminizing States in Males

A. Gynecomastia

In contrast to rodents, in which the mammary anlagen of the male are completely suppressed by androgens during embryogenesis (Kratochwil, 1971), there is no apparent sexual dimorphism of the human breast until puberty (Pfaltz, 1949) at which time a profound sexual dimorphism in breast development takes place. Estrogen is responsible for proliferation of the tubular duct network of the female breast (Lyon *et al.*, 1958) and is capable of causing a similar effect in males. Alveolar development at the ends of the ducts requires the synergistic action of progesterone, usually in an estrogen to progesterone ratio of 1 to 20–100. Even when breast tissue cannot be palpated in men, remnants of a duct system can be demonstrated histologically. Sexual dimorphism in human breast development is the consequence of the differences in estrogen secretion at puberty between the two sexes.

Men may become feminized (most often breast enlargement, termed *gynecomastia*) when estrogen action is increased relative to that of androgen in target tissues (Wilson *et al.*, 1980) by one of two mechanisms. The first is through decreased androgen production or action with or without compensatory enhancement in estrogen formation. This situation can result from mutations of the androgen receptor or from primary gonadal defects. Examples of the latter include testicular failure after bilateral mumps orchitis and late embryonic failure of testicular development (as in the syndrome of congenital anorchia). The second mechanism of feminization in males is attendant upon estrogen excess, e.g., secretion of estradiol by certain testicular tumors; drugs, as in diethylstilbestrol treatment of patients with carcinoma of the prostate; or accelerated extragonadal conversion of circulating androgens to estrogens. Estrogen formation by the latter mechanism can be enhanced through increased availability of androgen substrate for extraglandular estrogen synthesis, as in patients with cirrhosis of the liver or hyperthyroidism or through increased activity of the enzyme system that converts androgen to estrogen in nongonadal sites. This latter mechanism was first recognized as a cause of severe feminization in studies of an 8-year-old boy with profound gynecomastia (Hemsell *et al.*, 1977). In this patient the extent of extragonadal (and extrahepatic) conversion of androstenedione to estrone (aromatization) was 50 times normal, but the site of peripheral aromatization was never identified. Recently Berkovitz *et al.* (1985) have described a family in which five boys developed gynecomastia in association with increased peripheral aromatization. Of the mechanisms of feminization, enhanced estrogen formation in extragonadal tissues is the least understood, and valuable insight into the process has been gained from the study of the phenomenon in certain breeds of chickens.

B. The Henny Feathering Mutation of the Sebright Bantam Chicken

Normal male chickens (Fig. 18D) display long neck feathers and tail feathers that sometimes droop to the ground; in contrast, the normal hen has short neck feathers and short tail feathers that stand erect (Fig. 18B). Normal female feathering is determined by estrogen

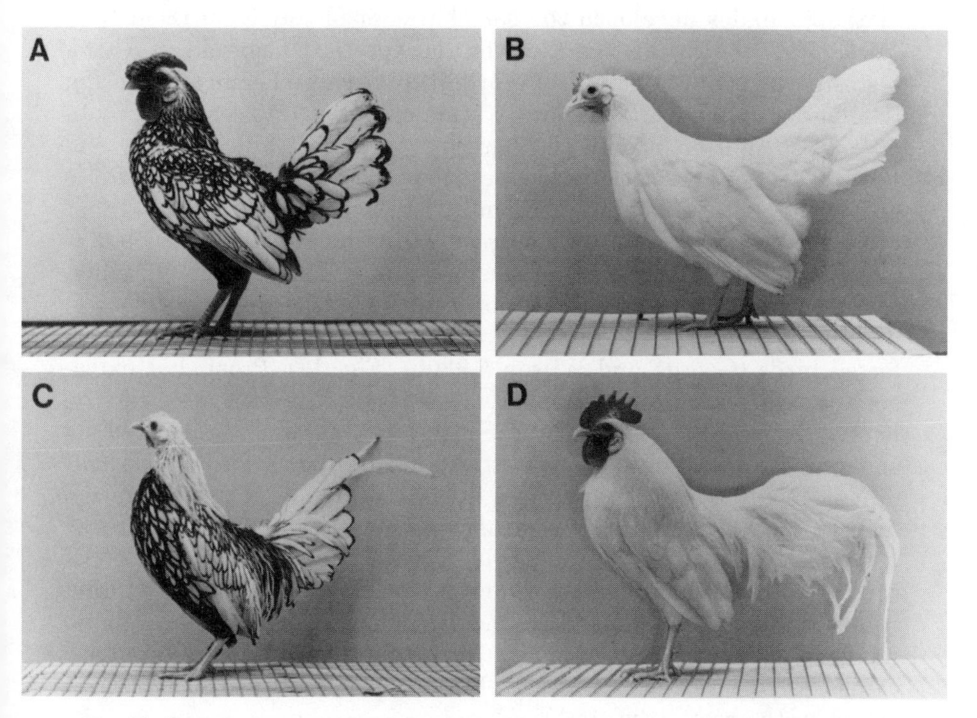

Fig. 18. Sexual phenotypes of Sebright bantam and Leghorn bantam chickens. (A) Sebright cock; (B) Leghorn hen; (C) castrated Sebright cock; (D) Leghorn cock.

formed in the ovary, whereas male feathering is not under hormonal control and is identical to the feathering pattern of castrated male or female chickens (Domm, 1939). The feathering pattern of the Sebright bantam male is distinctly female in character (Fig. 18A), and this trait is termed henny feathering (Tegetmeir, 1867).

1. *Endocrine Features*

The defect responsible for henny feathering causes testosterone to act aberrantly as an estrogen in the skin of affected birds. Three early lines of evidence helped clarify the abnormality responsible for henny feathering. First, castration of henny-feathered chickens of either sex caused henny feathering to revert to male-type plumage (Morgan, 1917) (Fig. 18C). Furthermore, transplantation of the testis from a Sebright cock to the Leghorn capon produced typical male feathering pattern and normal male comb development, suggesting that the testis of the Sebright produces normal male hormones (Roxas, 1926). Second, skin transplants from Sebright males to normal males maintained henny feathering; skin transplanted from normal males to henny-feathered males developed the sex character of the donor (Danforth, 1935, 1944), indicating that the defect is expressed in skin itself. Third, testosterone given to castrated Sebright cocks caused henny feathering (Gallagher *et al.,* 1933). Administration of estrogen to castrated cocks either Sebright or normal produced henny feathering (Deansley and Parkes, 1937). These studies suggest that the defect in the Sebright is due to the metabolism of androgen to estrogen in skin.

This hypothesis was proved correct on finding that the henny feathering trait reflects a mutation causing enhanced expression of aromatase activity (the enzyme complex that catalyzes the conversion of androgens to estrogens) in skin and other extragonadal tissues of affected birds (George and Wilson, 1980b) (Fig. 19). Proof that extragonadal conversion of androgens to estrogens is responsible for the henny feathering phenotype of Sebright cocks was established by showing that testosterone (a substrate for aromatization) but not 5α-dihydrotestosterone (an androgen that cannot undergo aromatization to estradiol) causes henny feathering in castrated Sebright cocks (George *et al.,* 1981). Interestingly, the comb and wattle of the Sebright, both of which express abnormal elevation of aromatase activity, appear to be unaffected by the mutation that causes a profound increase in circulating estrogen (George and Wilson, 1980b). Thus, excess estrogen does not adversely affect (or antagonize) androgen action in the comb (Fig. 18A).

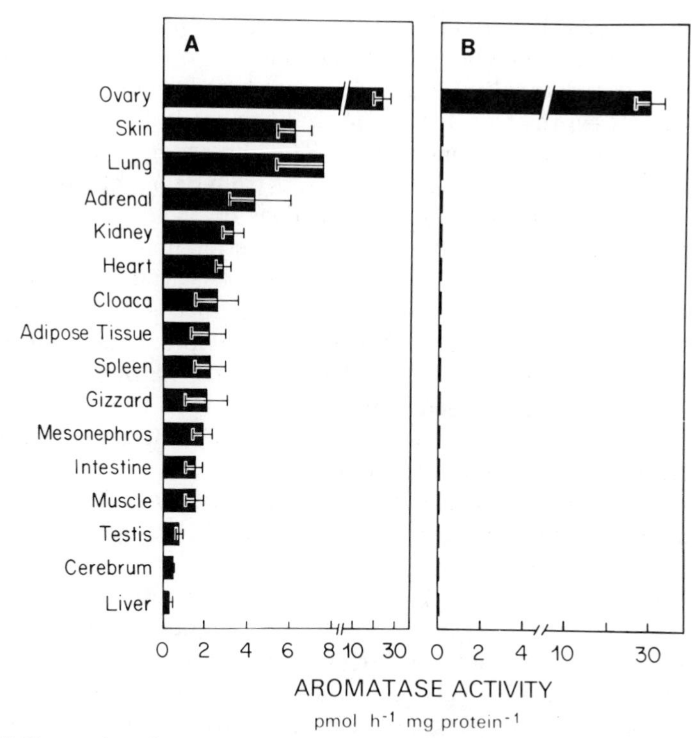

FIG. 19. Expression of aromatase activity in Sebright (A), but not control (B), nonovarian tissues. Adapted with permission from George and Wilson (1982).

2. *Genetic Defect*

Fibroblasts cultured from skin of chickens with the henny feathering trait also express increased aromatase activity (Leshin *et al.*, 1981a), and thus have been used to characterize the aromatase of the mutant birds in detail. Increased aromatase activity in the Sebright is due to an increase in the specific androgen-binding cytochrome P-450 oxidase component of the aromatase complex (Leshin *et al.*, 1981b). Since the aromatase enzyme is not normally expressed in skin fibroblasts from control chickens, direct comparison of normal and Sebright fibroblast enzymes has not been possible. As an alternative approach, we have compared properties of the aromatase enzyme in Sebright fibroblasts with those of the enzymes from control and Sebright ovaries. We have shown that the kinetic properties, substrate specificity, and pH optimum of membrane-bound aromatase from Sebright skin fibroblasts are the same as those of the ovarian enzymes from Sebright and control hens (Leshin *et al.*, 1983). Consequently, our working hypothesis is that Sebright bantam chickens synthesize an increased amount of a structurally normal "ovarian-type" aromatase in peripheral tissues (Leshin *et al.*, 1983) and that this mutation in the Sebright represents a regulatory abnormality. The abnormality in the Sebright is cis acting. Co-culture of skin fibroblasts from Sebright chickens with skin fibroblasts from normal chickens does not lead to suppression of aromatase activity in Sebright cells or induction of aromatase activity in normal cells (Leshin *et al.*, unpublished observations). Furthermore, the mutation that causes expression of aromatase activity in nonovarian tissues of the Sebright is inherited in a simple mendelian codominant manner (Somes *et al.*, 1984). Thus it seems unlikely that expression of the gene for increased aromatase activity in the Sebright is the result of either a diffusible activator or lack of a diffusible suppressor regulating the activity of both alleles of the gene.

The precise nature of this mutation is thus unclear. The mutation in the Sebright bantam chicken causes expression of a gene in virtually every tissue of affected birds that is normally expressed only in the ovary (Fig. 19) (George and Wilson, 1982). The rate of expression of this enzyme in peripheral tissues of the Sebright is increased several hundredfold above normal. Mutations that cause an increase in enzymatic activity are relatively uncommon, but the few that have been described fall into four categories. First, mutations can lead to compensatory increase in synthesis of a structurally normal enzyme in response to a primary defect in another protein; e.g., increased activity of β-hydroxy-β-methylglutaryl coenzyme reductase in familial hypercholesterolemia is due to lack of negative regulation of enzyme expression because of a defect in the cell-surface receptor for low-density lipoprotein (Goldstein and Brown, 1977). Second, mutations affecting the structure of the enzyme molecule can produce increased activity by any of several mechanisms. Rare structural mutations can cause an increase in catalytic activity per molecule (such as in one variant of increased plasma cholinesterase activity) (Neitlich, 1966). Alternatively, structural mutations that do not affect the catalytic properties of the enzyme can cause increased expression of the enzyme (as in a human variant of glucose-6-phosphate dehydrogenase) (Dern *et al.*, 1969). Finally, mutations can cause the appearance of unique isozymes that result in an increase in overall catalytic activity, presumably the result of gene duplication (Wilson and Taylor, 1982). In the latter three instances, the mutant proteins can be distinguished from the wild-type proteins by physicochemical techiques. The kinetic properties of the aromatase enzyme in Sebright skin fibroblasts, however, appear to be indistinguishable from those of the ovarian enzyme of either Sebright or control chickens (Leshin *et al.*, 1983). For this reason, as well as the fact that the magnitude of the increased expression of aromatase activity is so great, it seems unlikely that the increase in aromatase activity in peripheral tissues of the Sebright is due to a mutation of the structural gene(s) for the protein. Indeed, the ubiquitous expression of aromatase activity in the tissues of the Sebright, as well as the finding that the combination of 5-azacytidine (an inhibitor of DNA methylation) and sodium butyrate causes a severalfold induction of aromatase activity in fibroblasts cultured from a variety of Sebright but not control tissues (Leshin, 1985), suggest that the mutation may be due to a regulatory abnormality in the expression of this gene.

VII. Summary

It is now clear that Jost's formulation for sexual differentiation is fundamentally correct. Chromosomal sex determines gonadal sex, and gonadal sex in turn determines phenotypic sex. A minimum of 19 genes have been implicated in sexual differentiation in man (Wilson and Goldstein, 1975). Some of these are located on sex chromosomes, some on autosomes. Thus, the relatively simple mechanism that imposes male development on the indifferent embryo requires the participation of many genes common to both the male and female embryo. Much of our understanding of the process of sexual differentiation is due to the fact that, unlike many other congenital defects, abnormalities of sexual differentiation are not lethal, and even individuals with mild abnormalities of sexual development come to the attention of physicians and scientists and are systematically studied. Many of these abnormalities reflect single-gene defects, and detailed analyses of these disorders in man and animals have provided a great deal of insight into the endocrine, molecular, and genetic determinants that regulate sexual differentiation.

Determinants on the Y chromosome cause the indifferent gonad to develop into a testis. Two hormonal secretions from the fetal testis, mullerian-inhibiting substance and testosterone, then transform the indifferent urogenital tract into one characteristic of the male. Mullerian-inhibiting substance, secreted by the Sertoli cells, causes regression of the female (mullerian) duct system. Testosterone, secreted by the Leydig cells, is responsible for the remainder of male development including stabilization and differentiation of the wolffian ducts into the male accessory organs of reproduction as well as differentiation of the male external genitalia and prostate.

The role of hormones in female development is less clear. In the opossum ovarian hormones are probably involved in differentiation of the female urogenital tract and in pouch development as well. In the eutherian mammal it has not been possible to test whether hormones from the placenta, the maternal circulation, or the fetal ovary regulate female development.

A major portion of androgen action in the fetus and in postembryonic life is mediated by 5α-reduced metabolites of testosterone rather than by testosterone itself. Thus, a genetic deficiency in the 5α-reductase enzyme that catalyzes formation of 5α-dihydrotestosterone from testosterone impairs androgen action and can cause male pseudohermaphrditism. Although wolffian duct development is apparently normal in these individuals, other aspects of male development are defective.

Testosterone and 5α-dihydrotestosterone act via a common receptor to virilize male fetuses. Consequently, normal phenotypic sexual development is determined by the presence (in males) or the absence (in females) of specific hormonal signals at the critical time in embryonic development. At the time of sexual differentiation altered function of only a few gonadal enzymes in the steroid biosynthesis pathway profoundly affect the character of the hormones secreted and thus the sexual development of the fetus.

Testosterone, secreted by the fetal and adult testis, can be metabolized to a second active metabolite, estradiol. In some extragonadal tissues such as the hypothalamus the local formation of estradiol causes male differentiation. In most tissues the rate of estrogen formation from androgens is small, but an increase in circulating estrogen, either relative or absolute, can cause feminization in males. In man feminization is most often manifest as an increase in breast size (gynecomastia). In male birds estrogen excess is reflected in development of a female feathering pattern.

Although we now understand the hormonal and genetic factors responsible for mammalian sexual differentiation in considerable detail, many fundamental issues in the embryonic development of the urogenital tract remain poorly understood. What, for instance, is the mechanism by which the same hormonal signal is translated into different physiological effects in different tissues? What are the molecular and cellular changes that cause these diverse differentiative events? Ultimately, these fundamental issues of embryogenesis will have to be clarified before we can understand the entire program through which the myriad of genetic determinants and hormones interact to cause development of phenotypic sex.

ACKNOWLEDGMENT

The original work presented in this review was aided by Grant 5-R01-AM03892 from the National Institutes of Health.

REFERENCES

Aiman, J., and Griffin, J. E. (1982). The frequency of androgen receptor deficiency in infertile men. *J. Clin. Endocrinol. Metab.* **54,** 725–732.

Aiman, J., Griffin, J. E., Gazak, J. M., Wilson, J. D., and MacDonald, P. C. (1979). Androgen insensitivity as a cause of infertility in otherwise normal men. *N. Engl. J. Med.* **300,** 223–227.

Amrhein, J. A., Meyer, W. J., III, Jones, H. W., Jr., and Migeon, C. J. (1976). Androgen insensitivity in man: Evidence for genetic heterogeneity. *Proc. Natl. Acad. Sci. U.S.A.* **73,** 891–894.

Arai, Y. (1972). Effect of 5α-dihydrotestosterone on differentiation of masculine pattern of the brain in the rat. *Endocrinol. Jpn.* **19,** 389–393.

Attal, J. (1969). Levels of testosterone, androstenedione, estrone and estradiol-17β in the testes of fetal sheep. *Endocrinology* **85,** 280–289.

Bardin, C. W., Bullock, L. P., Sherins, R. J., Mowszowisz, I., and Blackburn, W. R. (1973). Androgen metabolism and mechanism of action in male pseudohermaphroditism: A study of testicular feminization. *Recent Prog. Horm. Res.* **29,** 65–105.

Baum, M. J., and Vreeburg, J. T. M. (1973). Copulation in castrated male rats following combined treatment with estradiol and dihydrotestosterone. *Science* **182,** 283–285.

Berkovitz, G. D., Guerami, A., Brown, T. R., MacDonald, P. C., and Migeon, C. J. (1985). Familial gynecomastia with increased extraglandular aromatization of plasma carbon 19-steroids. *J. Clin. Invest.* **75,** 1763–1769.

Beutler, B., Nagai, Y., Ohno, S., Klein, G., and Shapiro. I. M. (1978). The HLA-dependent expression of testis-organizing H-Y antigen by human male cells. *Cell* **13,** 509–513.

Bidlingmaier, F., Knorr, D., and Neumann, F. (1977). Inhibition of masculine differentiation in male offspring of rabbits actively immunized against testosterone before pregnancy. *Nature (London)* **266,** 647–648.

Blanchard, M. G., and Josso, N. (1974). Source of the anti-mullerian hormone synthesized by the fetal testis: Mullerian-inhibiting activity of the fetal bovine Sertoli cells in tissue culture. *Pediatr. Res.* **8,** 968–971.

Bok, G., and Drews, U. (1983). The role of the wolffian ducts in the formation of the sinus vagina; an organ culture study. *J. Embryol. Exp. Morphol.* **73,** 275–295.

Bolliger, A. (1944). An experiment on the complete transformation of the scrotum into a marsupial pouch in *Trichosurus vulpecula*. *Med. J. Aust.* **2,** 56–58.

Bouin, P., and Ancel, P. (1903). Sur la signification de la glande interstitielle du testicule embryonnaire. *C.R. Soc. Biol.* **55,** 1682–1684.

Brook, C. G. D. (1981). Persistent mullerian duct syndrome. *Pediatr. Adolesc. Endocrinol.* **8,** 100–104.

Brooks, J. R., Baptista, E. M., Berman, C., Ham, E. A., Hichens, M., Johnston, D. B. R., Primka, R. L., Rasmusson, G. H., Reynolds, G. F., Schmitt, S. M., and Arth, G. E. (1981). Response of rat ventral prostate to a new and novel 5α-reductase inhibitor. *Endocrinology* **109,** 830–836.

Brooks, J. R., Berman, C., Hichens, M., Primka, R. L., Reynolds, G. F., and Rasmusson, G. H. (1982). Biological activities of a new steroidal inhibitor of Δ^4-5α-reductase (41309). *Proc. Soc. Exp. Biol. Med.* **169,** 67–73.

Brown, T. R., Maes, M., Rothwell, S. W., and Migeon, C. J. (1982). Human complete androgen insensitivity with normal dihydrotestosterone receptor binding capacity in cultured genital skin fibroblasts. Evidence for a qualitative abnormality of the receptor. *J. Clin. Endocrinol. Metab.* **55,** 61–69.

Budzik, G. P., Powell, S. M., Kamagata, S., and Donahoe, P. K. (1983). Mullerian-inhibiting substance fractionation by dye affinity chromatography. *Cell* **34,** 307–314.

Bullock, L. P., Bardin, C. W., and Ohno, S. (1971). The androgen insensitive mouse: Absence of intranuclear androgen retention in the kidney. *Biochem. Biophys. Res. Commun.* **44,** 1537–1543.

Bulmer, D. (1957). The development of the human vagina. *J. Anat.* **91,** 490–509.

Burns, R. K. (1979). Sex differentiation during the early pouch stages of the opossum (*Didelphys virginiana*) and a comparison of the anatomical changes induced by male and female sex hormones. *J. Morphol.* **65,** 497–542.

Burns, R. K. (1945). The differentiation of the phallus in the opossum and its reactions to sex hormones. *Contrib. Embryol.* **31,** 149–162.

Catt, K. J., Dufau, M. L., Neaves, W. B., Walsh, P. C., and Wilson, J. D. (1975). LH-hCG receptors and testosterone content during differentiation of the testis in the rabbit embryo. *Endocrinology* **97,** 1157–1165.

Chemke, J., Carmichael, R., Stewart, J., Geer, R. H., and Robinson, A. (1970). Familial XY gonadal dysgenesis. *J. Med. Genet.* **7,** 105–111.

Cohen, M. M., and Shaw, M. W. (1965). Two XY siblings with gonadal dysgenesis and a female phenotype. *N. Engl. J. Med.* **272,** 1083–1088.

Cook, B., McDonald, I. R., and Gibson, W. R. (1978). Prostatic function in the brush-tailed possum. *J. Reprod. Fertil.* **53,** 369–375.

Cunha, G. R. (1972). Tissue interactions between epithelium and mesenchyme of uro-genital and integumental origin. *Anat. Rec.* **172,** 529–542.

Cunha, G. R., and Chung, L. W. K. (1981). Stromal-epithelial interactions. I. Induction of prostatic phenotype of urothelium of testicular feminized (Tfm/Y) mice. *J. Steroid Biochem.* **14,** 1317–1321.

Cunha, G. R., Chung, L. W. K., Shannon, J. M., Taguchi, O., and Fujii, H. (1983). Hormone-induced morphogenesis and growth: Role of mesenchymal–epithelial interactions. *Recent Prog. Horm. Res.* **39,** 559–595.

Danforth, C. H. (1935). Testicular hormones and Sebright plumage. *Proc. Soc. Exp. Biol. Med.* **32,** 1474–1476.

Danforth, C. H. (1944). Relation of the follicular hormone to feather form and pattern in the fowl. *Yale J. Biol. Med.* **17,** 13–18.

Dean, D. C., Gope, R., Knoll, B. J., Riser, M. E., and O'Malley, B. W. (1984). A similar 5'-flanking region is required for estrogen and progesterone induction of ovalbumin gene expression. *J. Biol. Chem.* **259,** 9967–9970.

Deansley, R., and Parkes, A. S. (1937). Multiple activities of androgenic compounds. *Q. J. Exp. Physiol.* **26,** 393–402.

Dern, R. J., McCurdy, P. R., and Yoshida, A. (1969). A new structural variant of glucose-6-phosphate dehydrogenase with a high production rate (G6PD Hektoen). *J. Lab. Clin. Med.* **73,** 283–290.

Dickmann, Z., and Dey, S. K. (1976). A new concept: Control of early pregnancy by steroid hormones originating in the preimplantation embryo. *Vitam. Horm.* **34,** 215–242.

Dickmann, Z., Gupta, J. S., and Dey, S. K. (1977). Does "blastocyst estrogen" initiate implantation? *Science* **195,** 687–688.

Docke, F., and Dorner, G. (1975). Anovulation in adult female rats after neonatal intracerebral implantation of oestrogen. *Endokrinologie* **65,** 375–377.

Domm, L. V. (1939). Modifications in sex and secondary sexual characters in birds. *In* "Sex and Internal Secretions" (E. Allew, C. H. Danforth, and E. A. Doisy, eds.), pp. 227–327. Williams & Wilkins, Baltimore.

Donahoe, P. K., Ito, Y., Price, J. M., and Herndon, W. H., III. (1977a). Mullerian inhibiting substance activity in bovine fetal, newborn and prepubertal testes. *Biol. Rep.* **16,** 238–243.

Donahoe, P. K., Ho, Y., Morikawa, Y., and Hendren, W. H. (1977b). Mullerian inhibiting substance in human testes after birth. *J. Pedriatr. Surg.* **12,** 323–330.

Donahoe, P. K., Budzik, G. P., Trelstad, R., Mudgett-Hunter, M., Fuller, A., Jr., Hutson, J. M., Ikawa, H., Hayashi, A., and MacLaughlin, D. (1982). Mullerian-inhibiting substance: An update. *Recent Prog. Horm. Res.* **38,** 279–326.

Doughty, C., Booth, J. E., McDonald, P. G., and Parrot, R. F. (1973). Inhibition by the antioestrogen MER-25 of defeminization induced by the synthetic oestrogen RU-2858. *Endocrinology* **67,** 459–460.

Doughty, C., Booth, J. E., McDonald, P. G., and Parrot, R. F. (1975). Effect of oestradiol-17β, oestradiol benzoate and the synthetic oestrogen RU2858 on sexual differentiation in the neonatal female rat. *J. Endocrinol.* **67,** 419–424.

Drews, U., and Drews, U. (1977). Regression of mouse mammary gland anlagen in recombinants of Tfm and wild-type tissues: Testosterone acts via the mesenchyme. *Cell* **10,** 401–404.

Eichwald, E. J., and Silmser, C. R. (1955). Untitled communication. *Transplant. Bull.* **2,** 148–149.

Eil, C. (1983). Familial incomplete male pseudohermaphroditism associated with impaired nuclear androgen retention. *J. Clin. Invest.* **71,** 850–858.

Elawady, M. K., Allman, D. R., Griffin, J. E., and Wilson, J. D. (1983). Expression of a mutant androgen receptor in cloned fibroblasts derived from a heterozygous carrier for the syndrome of testicular feminization. *Am. J. Hum. Genet.* **35,** 376–384.

Espiner, E. A., Veale, A. M. O., Sands, V. E., and Fitzgerald, P. H. (1970). Familial syndrome of streak gonads and normal male karyotype in five phenotypic females. *N. Engl. J. Med.* **203,** 6–11.

Evens, R. P., and Amerson, A. B. (1974). Androgens and erythropoiesis. *J. Clin. Pharmacol.* **14,** 94–101.

Faiman, C., Winter, J. S. D., and Reyes, F. I. (1981). Endocrinology of the fetal testis. *In* "The Testis," Comprehensive Endocrinology Series (H. Burger and D. deKretser, eds.), pp. 81–105. Raven, New York.

Fallat, M. E., Hutson, J. M., Budzik, D. P., and Donahoe, P. K. (1984). Androgen stimulation of nucleotide pyrophosphatase during mullerian duct regression. *Endocrinology* **114,** 1592–1598.

Ferguson-Smith, M. A. (1961). Chromosomes and human disease. *Prog. Med. Genet.* **1,** 292–334.

Fisher, L. K., Kogut, M. D., Moore, R. J., Goebelsmann, U., Weitzman, J. J., Isaacs, H., Jr., Griffin, J. E., and Wilson, J. D. (1978). Clinical, endocrinological, and enzymatic characterization of two patients with 5α-reductase deficiency. Evidence that a single enzyme is responsible for the 5α-reduction of cortisol and testosterone. *J. Clin. Endocrinol.* **47,** 653–664.

Ford, C. E., Jones, K. W., Polani, P. E., de Almeida, J. C., and Briggs, J. H. (1959). A sex chromosome anomaly in a case of gonadal dysgenesis (Turner's syndrome). *Lancet* **1,** 711–713.

Fujimoto, T., Miyayama, Y., and Fuyuta, M. (1977). The origin, migration and fine morphology of human primordial germ cells. *Anat. Rec.* **188,** 315–330.

Gallagher, T. F., Domm, L. V., and Koch, F. C. (1933). The problem of hen-feathering in Sebright cocks. *J. Biol. Chem.* **100,** 47 (Abstr.).

Gardner, R. L., Lyon, M. F., Evans, E. P., and Burtenshaw, M. D. (1985). Clonal analysis of X-chromosome inactivation and the origin of the germ line in the mouse embryo. *J. Embryol. Exp. Morphol.* **88,** 349–363.

Gasser, D. L., and Silvers, W. K. (1972). Genetics and immunology of sex-linked antigens. *Adv. Immunol.* **15,** 215–247.

Gehring, U., Tomkins, G. M., and Ohno, S. (1971). Effect of the androgen-insensitivity mutation on a cytoplasmic receptor for dihydrotestosterone. *Nature (London) New Biol.* **232,** 106–107.

George, F. W., and Noble, J. F. (1984). Androgen receptors are similar in fetal and adult rabbits. *Endocrinology* **115,** 1451–1458.

George, F. W., and Ojeda, S. R. (1982). Changes in aromatase activity in the rat brain during embryonic, neonatal, and infantile development. *Endocrinology* **111,** 522–529.

George, F. W., and Wilson, J. D. (1978a). Conversion of androgen to estrogen by the human fetal ovary. *J. Clin. Endocrinol. Metab.* **47,** 550–555.

George, F. W., and Wilson, J. D. (1978b). Estrogen formation in the early rabbit embryo. *Science* **199,** 200–202.

George, F. W., and Wilson, J. D. (1980a). Endocrine differentiation of the fetal rabbit ovary in culture. *Nature (London)* **283,** 861–863.

George, F. W., and Wilson, J. D. (1980b). Pathogenesis of the henny feathering trait in the Sebright bantam chicken. Increased conversion of androgen to estrogen in skin. *J. Clin. Invest.* **66,** 57–65.

George, F. W., and Wilson, J. D. (1982). Developmental pattern of increased aromatase activity in the Sebright bantam chicken. *Endocrinology* **110,** 1203–1207.

George, F. W., and Wilson, J. D. (1984). Sexual differentiation. *In* "Fetal Physiology and Medicine: The Basis of Perinatology" (R. W. Beard and P. W. Nathanielsz, eds.), Chap. 2, pp. 57–79. Dekker, New York.

George, F. W., Catt, K. J., Neaves, W. B., and Wilson, J. D. (1978a). Studies on the regulation of testosterone synthesis in the rabbit fetal testis. *Endocrinology* **102,** 106–107.

George, F. W., Tobleman, W. T., Milewich, L., and Wilson, J. D. (1978b). Aromatase activity in the developing rabbit brain. *Endocrinology* **102,** 86–91.

George, F. W., Simpson, E. R., Milewich, L., and Wilson, J. D. (1979). Studies on the regulation of steroid hormone biosynthesis in fetal rabbit gonads. *Endocrinology* **105,** 1100–1106.

George, F. W., Noble, J. F., and Wilson, J. D. (1981). Female feathering in Sebright cocks is due to conversion of testosterone to estradiol in skin. *Science* **213,** 557–559.

George, F. W., Hodgins, M. B., and Wilson, J. D. (1985). The synthesis and metabolism of gonadal steroids in pouch young of the opossum, *Didelphis virginiana. Endocrinology* **116,** 1145–1150.

Gier, H. T., and Marion, G. B. (1969). Development of the mammalian testis and genital ducts. *Biol. Reprod.* **1,** 1–23.

Gillman, J. (1948). The development of the gonads in man, with a consideration of the role of fetal endocrines and the histogenesis of ovarian tumors. *Carnegie Contrib. Embryol.* **32,** 83–131.

Goldman, A. S. (1971). Production of hypospadias in the rat by selective inhibition of fetal testicular 17a-hydroxylase and $C_{17\text{-}20}$-lyase. *Endocrinology* **88,** 527–531.

Goldman, A. S., Shapiro, B. H., and Neuman, F. (1976). Role of testosterone and its metabolites in the differentiation of the mammary gland in rats. *Endocrinology* **99,** 1490–1495.

Goldstein, J. L., and Brown, M. S. (1977). The low density lipoprotein pathway and its relation to atherosclerosis. *Annu. Rev. Biochem.* **46,** 897–930.

Goldstein, J. L., and Wilson, J. D. (1972). Studies on the pathogenesis of the pseudohermaphroditism in the mouse with testicular feminization. *J. Clin. Invest.* **51,** 1647–1658.

Gondos, B. (1980). Development and differentiation of the testis and male reproductive tract. *In* "Testicular Development, Structure, and Function" (A. Steinberger and E. Steinberger, eds.), pp. 3–20. Raven, New York.

Gondos, B., George, F. W., and Wilson, J. D. (1983). Granulosa cell differentiation and estrogen synthesis in the fetal rabbit ovary. *Biol. Reprod.* **29,** 791–798.

Griffin, J. E. (1979). Testicular feminization associated with a thermolabile androgen receptor in cultured human fibroblasts. *J. Clin. Invest.* **64,** 1624–1631.

Griffin, J. E., and Durrant, J. L. (1982). Qualitative receptor defects in families with androgen resistance: Failure of stabilization of the fibroblast cytosol androgen receptor. *J. Clin. Endocrinol. Metab.* **55,** 465–474.

Griffin, J. E., and Wilson, J. D. (1978). Hereditary male pseudohermaphroditism. *Clin. Obstet. Gynaecol.* **5,** 457–479.

Griffin, J. E., and Wilson, J. D. (1980). The syndromes of androgen resistance. *N. Engl. J. Med.* **203,** 198–209.

Griffin, J. E., Punyashthiti, K., and Wilson, J. D. (1976). Dihydrotestosterone binding by cultured human fibroblasts. Comparison of cells from control subjects and from patients with hereditary male pseudohermaphroditism due to androgen resistance. *J. Clin. Invest.* **57,** 1342–1351.

Griffin, J. E., Kovacs, W. J., and Wilson, J. D. (1985). Characteristics of androgen resistance. *In* "Regulation of Androgen Action" (N. Bruchovsky, A. Chapdelaine, and F. Neumann, eds.), The Proceedings of an International Symposium, pp. 127–131. Congressdruck R. Brückner, Berlin.

Harris, G. W. (1964). Sex hormones, brain development and brain function. *Endocrinology* **75,** 627–648.

Hemsell, D. L., Edman, C. D., Marks, J. F., Siiteri, P. K., and MacDonald, P. C. (1977). Massive extraglandular aromatization of plasma androstenedione resulting in feminization of a prepubertal boy. *J. Clin. Invest.* **60,** 455–464.

Heuberger, B., Fritzka, I., Wasner, G., and Kratochwil, K. (1982). Induction of androgen receptor formation by epithelium–mesenchyme interaction in embryonic mouse mammary gland. *Proc. Natl. Acad. Sci. U.S.A.* **79,** 2957–2961.

Huhtaniemi, I. T., Korenbrat, C. C., and Jaffe, R. B. (1977). hCG binding and stimulation of testosterone biosynthesis in the human fetal testis. *J. Clin. Endocrinol. Metab.* **44,** 963–967.

Hutson, J. M., and Donahoe, P. K. (1983). Is mullerian-inhibiting substance a circulating hormone in the chick–quail chimera? *Endocrinology* **113,** 1470–1475.

Hutson, J. M., Ikawa, H., and Donahoe, P. K. (1982). Estrogen inhibition of mullerian inhibiting substance in the chick embryo. *J. Pediatr. Surg.* **17,** 953–959.

Ikadai, H., Sakuma, Y., Suzuki, K., and Imamichi, T. (1985). Congenital abnormalities of the male genital organs in the newly established TW rat strain. *Cong. Anom.* **25,** 65–71.

Ikawa, H., Hutson, J. M., Budzik, D. P., MacLaughlin, D. T., and Donahoe, P. K. (1982). Steroid enhancement of mullerian duct regression. *J. Pediatr. Surg.* **17,** 453–458.

Imperato-McGinley, J., Guerrero, L., Gautier, T., and Peterson, R. E. (1974). Steroid 5α-reductase deficiency in man: An inherited form of male pseudohermaphroditism. *Science* **186,** 1213–1215.

Imperato-McGinley, J., Peterson, R. E., Leshin, M., Griffin, J. E., Cooper, G., Draghi, S., Berenyi, M., and Wilson, J. D. (1980). Steroid 5α-reductase deficiency in a 65 year old pseudohermaphrodite: The natural history, ultrastructure of the testis and evidence for inherited enzyme heterogeneity. *J. Clin. Endocrinol. Metab.* **50,** 15–22.

Imperato-McGinley, J., Binienda, Z., Arthur, A., Mininberg, D. T., Vaughan, D., Jr., and Quimby, F. W. (1985). The development of a male pseudohermaphroditic rat using an inhibitor of the enzyme 5α-reductase. *Endocrinology* **116,** 807–812.

Jones, H. W., Jr., Rary, J. M., Rock, J. A., and Cummings, D. (1979). The role of H-Y antigen in human sexual development. *Johns Hopkins Med. J.* **145,** 33–43.

Josso, N., de Grouchy, J., Frézal, J., and Lamy, M. (1963). Le syndrome de Turner familial, étude de deux familles avec caryotypes XO et XX. *Ann. Pediatr. Paris* **10,** 163–167.

Josso, N., Fekete, C., Cachin, O., Nezelof, C., and Rappaport, R. (1983). Persistence of mullerian ducts in male pseudohermaphroditism, and its relationship to cryptorchidism. *Clin. Endocrinol.* **19,** 247–258.

Jost, A. (1953). Problems in fetal endocrinology: The gonadal and hypophyseal hormones. *Recent Prog. Horm. Res.* **8,** 379–418.

Jost, A. (1961). The role of fetal hormones in prenatal development. *Harvey Lect.* **55,** 201–226.

Jost, A. (1972). A new look at the mechanisms controlling sexual differentiation in mammals. *Johns Hopkins Med. J.* **130,** 38–53.

Karsch, F. J., Dierschke, D. J., and Knobil, E. (1973). Sexual differentiation of pituitary function: Apparent differences between primates and rodents. *Science* **179,** 484–486.

Kaufman, M., Pinsky, L., Hollander, R., and Bailey, J. D. (1983). Regulation of the androgen receptor in normal and androgen resistant genital skin fibroblasts. *J. Steroid Biochem.* **18,** 383–390.

Keenan, B. S., Meyer, W. J., III, Hadjian, A. J., Jones, H. W., and Migeon, C. J. (1974). Syndrome of androgen insensitivity in man: Absence of 5α-dihydrotestosterone binding protein in skin fibroblasts. *J. Clin. Endocrinol. Metab.* **38,** 1143–1146.

Kelch, R. P., Jenner, M. R., Weinstein, R., Kaplan, S. L., and Grumbach, M. M. (1972). Estradiol and testosterone secretion by human, simian, and canine testes, in males with hypogonadism and in male pseudohermaphrodites with feminizing testes syndrome. *J. Clin. Invest.* **51,** 824–830.

Kellokumpo-Lehtinen, P., Santti, R., and Pelliniemi, L. J. (1980). Correlation of early cytodifferentiation of the human fetal prostate and Leydig cells. *Anat. Rec.* **196,** 263–273.

Kobayashi, S. (1984). Induction of mullerian duct derivatives in testicular feminized (Tfm) mice by prenatal exposure to diethylstilbestrol. *Anat. Embryol.* **169,** 35–39.

Kovacs, W. J., Griffin, J. E., and Wilson, J. D. (1983). Transformation of human androgen receptors to the deoxyribonucleic acid-binding state. *Endocrinology* **113,** 1574–1581.

Kovacs, W. J., Griffin, J. E., Weaver, D. D., Carlson, B. R., and Wilson, J. D. (1984). A mutation that causes lability of the androgen receptor under conditions that normally promote transformation to the DNA-binding state. *J. Clin. Invest.* **73,** 1095–1104.

Kratochwil, K. (1971). *In vitro* analysis of the hormonal basis for the sexual dimorphism in the embryonic development of the mouse mammary gland. *Embryol. Exp. Morphol.* **25,** 141–153.

Kratochwil, K., and Schwartz, P. (1976). Tissue interaction in androgen response of embryonic mammary rudiment of mouse: Identification of target tissue for testosterone. *Proc. Natl. Acad. Sci. U.S.A.* **73,** 4041–4044.

Kulin, H. E., and Reiter, E. O. (1976). Gonadotropin and testosterone measurements after estrogen administration to adult men, prepubertal and pubertal boys, and men with hypogonadotropism: Evidence for maturation of positive feedback in the male. *Pediatr. Res.* **10,** 46–51.

Larsson, K., Sodersten, P., and Beyer, C. (1973). Induction of male sexual behavior by estradiol-benzoate in combination with dihydrotestosterone. *J. Endocrinol.* **57,** 563–564.

Lasnitzki, I., and Mizuno, T. (1980). Prostatic induction: Interaction of epithelium and mesenchyme from normal wild-type and androgen insensitive mice with testicular feminization. *J. Endocrinol.* **85,** 423–428.

Leshin, M. (1985). 5-Azacytidine and sodium butyrate induce expression of aromatase in fibroblasts from chickens carrying the henny-feathering trait but not from wild-type chickens. *Proc. Natl. Acad. Sci. U.S.A.* **82,** 3005–3009.

Leshin, M., and Wilson, J. D. (1982). Inhibition of steroid 5α-reductase from human skin fibroblasts by 17β-*N,N*-diethylcarbamoyl-4-methyl-4-aza-5α-androstan-3-one. *J. Steroid Biochem.* **17,** 245–250.

Leshin, M., Griffin, J. E., and Wilson, J. D. (1978). Hereditary male pseudohermaphroditism associated with an unstable form of 5α-reductase. *J. Clin. Invest.* **62,** 685–691.

Leshin, M., Baron, J., George, F. W., and Wilson, J. D. (1981a). Increased estrogen formation and aromatase activity in fibroblasts cultured from the skin of chickens with the henny feathering trait. *J. Biol. Chem.* **256,** 4341–4344.

Leshin, M., George, F. W., and Wilson, J. D. (1981b). Increased estrogen synthesis in the Sebright bantam is due to a mutation that causes increased aromatase activity. *Trans. Assoc. Am. Phys.* **94,** 97–105.

Leshin, M., Noble, J. F., George, F. W., and Wilson, J. D. (1983). Characterization of the increased estrogen synthesis in skin fibroblasts from the Sebright bantam. *J. Steroid Biochem.* **18,** 33–39.

Liang, T., and Heiss, C. E. (1981). Inhibition of 5α-reductase, receptor binding, and nuclear uptake of androgens in the prostate by a 4-methyl-4-aza-steroid. *J. Biol. Chem.* **256,** 7998–8005.

Lieberburg, I., Wallach, G., and McEwen, B. S. (1977). The effects of an inhibitor of aromatization (1,4,6-androstatriene-3,17-dione) and an antiestrogen (C-1628) on *in vivo* formed testosterone metabolites recovered from neonatal rat brain tissues and purified cell nuclei. Implications for sexual differentiation of the rat brain. *Brain Res.* **128,** 176.

Lillie, F. R. (1916). The theory of the free-martin. *Science* **43,** 611–613.

Lipsett, M. B., and Tullner, W. W. (1965). Testosterone synthesis by the fetal rabbit gonad. *Endocrinology* **77,** 273–277.

Lowsley, O. S. (1912). The development of the human prostate with reference to the development of other structures of the neck of the urinary bladder. *Am. J. Anat.* **13,** 299–349.

Lyon, M. F., and Hawkes, S. G. (1970). X-Linked gene for testicular feminization in the mouse. *Nature (London)* **227,** 1217–1219.

Lyon, W. R., Li, C. H., and Johnson, R. F. (1958). The hormonal control of mammary growth and lactation. *Recent Prog. Horm. Res.* **14,** 219–248.

MacDonald, P. C., Madden, J. D., Brenner, P. F., Wilson, J. D., and Siiteri, P. K. (1979). Origin of estrogen in normal men and in women with testicular feminization. *J. Clin. Endocrinol. Metab.* **49,** 905–916.

McDonald, P. G., and Doughty, C. (1974). . Effect of neonatal administration of different androgens in the female rat: Correlation between aromatization and the induction of sterilization. *J. Endocrinol.* **61,** 95–103.

McEwen, B. (1981). Neural gonadal steroid actions. *Science* **211,** 1303–1311.

McEwen, B. S., Lieberburg, I., Chaptal, C., and Krey, L. C. (1977). Aromatization: Important for sexual differentiation of the neonatal rat brain. *Horm. Behav.* **9,** 249–263.

McLachlan, J. A. (1977). Prenatal exposure to diethylstilbestrol in mice: Toxicological studies. *J. Toxicol. Environ. Health* **2,** 527–537.

MacLuskey, N. J., and Naftolin, F. (1981). Sexual differentiation of the central nervous system. *Science* **211,** 1294–1303.

Madden, J. D., Walsh, P. C., MacDonald, P. C., and Wilson, J. D. (1975). Clinical and endocrinological characterization of a patient with the syndrome of incomplete testicular feminization. *J. Clin. Endocrinol. Metab.* **40,** 751–760.

Maes, M., Sultan, C., Zerhouni, N., Rothwell, S. W., and Migeon, C. J. (1979). Role of testosterone binding to the androgen receptor in male sexual differentiation of patients with 5α-reductase deficiency. *J. Steroid Biochem.* **11,** 1385–1390.

Magre, S., and Jost, A. (1984). Dissociation between testicular organogenesis and endocrine cytodifferentiation of Sertoli cells. *Proc. Natl. Acad. Sci. U.S.A.* **81,** 7831–7834.

Marcus, R., and Korenman, S. G. (1976). Estrogens and the human male. *Annu. Rev. Med.* **27,** 357–370.

Meyer, W. J., III, Migeon, B. R., and Migeon, C. J. (1975). Locus on human X chromosome for dihydrotestosterone receptor and androgen insensitivity. *Proc. Natl, Acad. Sci. U.S.A.* **72,** 1469–1472.

Migeon, B. R., Brown, T. R., Axelman, J., and Migeon, C. J. (1981). Studies of the locus for androgen receptor: Localization on the human X chromosome and evidence for homology with the *Tfm* locus in the mouse. *Proc. Natl. Acad. Sci. U.S.A.* **78,** 6339–6343.

Milewich, L., George, F. W., and Wilson, J. D. (1977). Estrogen formation by the ovary of the rabbit embryo. *Endocrinology* **100,** 187–196.

Mintz, B., and Russell, E. S. (1957). Gene-induced embryological modification of primordial germ cells in the mouse. *J. Exp. Zool.* **134,** 207–230.

Molsberry, R. L., Carr, B. R., Mendelson, C. R., and Simpson, E. R. (1982). Human chorionic gonadotropin binding to human fetal testes as a function of gestation age. *J. Clin. Endocrinol. Metab.* **55,** 791–794.

Moore, C. R. (1941). On the role of sex hormones in sex differentiation in the opossum (*Didelphys virginiana*). *Physiol. Zool.* **14,** 1–45.

Moore, R. J., and Wilson, J. D. (1976). Steroid 5α-reductase in cultured human fibroblasts: Biochemical and genetic evidence for two enzyme activities. *J. Biol. Chem.* **251,** 5895–5900.

Moore, R. J., Griffin, J. E., and Wilson, J. D. (1975). Diminished 5α-reductase activity in extracts of fibroblasts cultured from patients with familial incomplete male pseudohermaphroditism, type 2. *J. Biol. Chem.* **250,** 7168–7172.

Morgan, T. H. (1917). Demonstration of the effects of castration on Seabright cockerals. *Proc. Soc. Exp. Biol. Med.* **15,** 3–4.

Mudgett-Hunter, M., Budzik, G. P., Sullivan, M., and Donahoe, P. K. (1982). Monoclonal antibody to mullerian inhibiting substance. *J. Immunol.* **128,** 1327–1333.

Müller, U., Aschmoneit, I., Zenzes, M. T., and Wolf, U. (1978). Binding studies of H-Y antigen in rat tissues: Indications for a gonad specific receptor. *Hum. Genet.* **43,** 151–157.

Müller, U., Wolf, U., Siebers, J.-W., and Gunter, E. (1979). Evidence for a gonad-specific receptor for H-Y antigen: Binding of exogenous H-Y antigen to gonadal cells is independent of β_2-microgbloulin. *Cell* **17,** 331–335.

Naftolin, F., Ryan, K. J., and Petro, Z. (1971). Aromatization of androstenedione by the diencephalon. *J. Clin. Endocrinol. Metab.* **33,** 368–370.

Neitlich, H. W. (1966). Increased plasma cholinesterase activity on succinylcholine resistance: A genetic variant. *J. Clin. Invest.* **45,** 380–387.

Neumann, F., von Berswordt-Wallrabe, R., Elger, W., Steinbeck, H., Hahn, J. D., and Kramer, M. (1970). Aspects of androgen-dependent events as studied by antiandrogens. *Recent Prog. Horm. Res.* **26,** 337–405.

New, M. I., Dupont, B., Grunback, K., and Levine, L. S. (1983). Congenital adrenal hyperplasia and related conditions. *In* "The Metabolic Basis of Inherited Disease" (J. B. Stanbury, J. B. Wyngaarden, D. S. Fredrickson, J. L. Goldstein, and M. S. Brown, eds.), 5th Ed., pp. 973–1000. McGraw-Hill, New York.

Ohno, S. (1978). The role of H-Y antigen in primary sex determination. *J. Am. Med. Assoc.* **239,** 217–220.

Ohno, S. (1979). "Major Sex-Determining Genes." Springer-Verlag, New York.

Ohno, S., Nagai, Y., and Ciccarese, S. (1978). Testicular cells lysostripped of H-Y antigen organize ovarian follicle-like aggregates. *Cytogenet. Cell Genet.* **20,** 351–364.

O'Rahilly, R. (1977). The development of the vagina in the human. *In* "Morphogenesis and Malformation of the Genital System" (R. J. Blandua and D. Bergsma, eds.), *Birth Defects Orig. Art. Ser.* **13,** 123–136.

Patsavoudi, E., Magre, S., Castanier, M., Schooler, R., and Jost, A. (1985). Dissociation between testicular morphogenesis and functional differentiation of Leydig cells. *J. Endocrinol.* **105,** 235–238.

Peterson, R. E., Imperato-McGinley, J., Gautier, T., and Sturla, E. (1977). Male pseudohermaphroditism due to steroid 5α-reductase deficiency. *Am. J. Med.* **62,** 170–191.

Pfahl, M. (1982). Specific binding of the glucocorticoid-receptor complex to the mouse mammary tumor proviral promotor region. *Cell* **31,** 475–482.

Pfaltz, C. R. (1949). Das embryonale und postnatale Verhalten der männlichen BrustDruese beim Menschen. II. Das Mammarorgan im Kindes-, Jünglings-, Mannes- und Greisenalter. *Acta Anat.* **8,** 293–328.

Picard, J. Y., Tran, D., and Josso, N. (1978). Biosynthesis of labelled anti-müllerian hormone by fetal testes: Evidence for the glycoprotein nature of the hormone and for its disulfide-bonded structure. *Mol. Cell. Endocrinol.* **12,** 17–30.

Price, J. M. (1979). The secretion of mullerian inhibiting substance by cultured isolated Sertoli cells of the neonatal calf. *Am. J. Anat.* **156,** 147–157.

Price, P., Wass, J. A. H., Griffin, J. E., Leshin, M., Savage, M. O., Large, D. M., Bu'Lock, D. E., Anderson, D. C., Wilson, J. D., and Besser, G. M. (1984). High dose androgen therapy in male pseudohermaphroditism due to 5α-reductase deficiency and disorders of the androgen receptor. *J. Clin. Invest.* **74,** 1496–1508.

Rajfer, J., and Walsh, P. C. (1977). Hormonal regulation of testicular descent: Experimental and clinical observations. *J. Urol.* **118,** 985–990.

Raynaud, A. (1947). Effet des injections d'hormones sexuelles à la souris gravide, sur le développement des ébauches de la glande mammaire des embryons. I. Action des substances androgenes. *Ann. Endocrinol.* **8,** 248–253.

Rigaudiere, N. (1979). The androgens in the guinea-pig foetus throughout the embryonic development. *Acta Endocrinol.* **92,** 174–186.

Roselli, C. E., Horton, L. E., and Resko, J. A. (1985). Distribution and regulation of aromatase activity in the rat hypothalamus and limbic system. *Endocrinology* **117,** 2471–2477.

Roxas, H. A. (1926). Gonad cross-transplantation in the Sebright and Leghorn fowls. *Endocrinology* **4,** 381–385.

Russell, W. L., Russell, L. B., and Gower, J. S. (1959). Exceptional inheritance of a sex-linked gene in the mouse explained on the basis that the X/O sex-chromosome constitution is female. *Proc. Natl. Acad. Sci. U.S.A.* **45,** 554–560.

Schultz, F. M., and Wilson, J. D. (1974). Virilization of the wolffian duct in the rat fetus by various androgens. *Endocrinology* **94,** 979–986.

Siiteri, P. K., and Wilson, J. D. (1974). Testosterone formation and metabolism during male sexual differentiation in the human embryo. *J. Clin. Endocrinol. Metab.* **38,** 113–125.

Silvers, W. K., and Wachtel, S. S. (1977). H-Y antigen: Behavior and function. *Science* **195,** 956–960.

Silvers, W. K., Gasser, D. L., and Eicher, E. M. (1982). H-Y antigen, serologically detectable male antigen and sex determination. *Cell* **28,** 439–440.

Simpson, J. L., Christakos, A. C., Horwith, M., and Silverman, F. S. (1971). Gonadal dysgenesis in individuals with apparently normal chromosomal complements: Tabulation of cases and compilation of genetic data. *Birth Defects Orig. Art. Ser.* **7,** 215–228.

Simpson, J. L., Blagowidow, N., and Martin, A. O. (1981). XY gonadal dysgenesis. Genetic heterogeneity based upon clinical observations. H-Y antigen status and segregation analysis. *Hum. Genet.* **58,** 91–97.

Sloan, W. R., and Walsh, P. C. (1976). Familial persistent müllerian duct syndrome. *J. Urol.* **115,** 459–461.

Somes, R. G., Jr., George, F. W., Baron, J., Noble, J. F., and Wilson, J. D. (1984). Inheritance of the henny-feathering trait of the Sebright bantam chicken. *J. Hered.* **75,** 99–102.

Stern, C. (1961). The genetics of sex determination in man. *Int. Congr. Genet.* **2,** 1121–1127.

Sternberg, W. H., Barclay, D. L., and Skoepfer, H. W. (1968). Familial XY gonadal dysgenesis. *N. Engl. J. Med.* **278,** 695–700.

Suzuki, Y., Ishii, H., Furuya, H., and Arai, Y. (1982). Developmental changes of the hypogastric ganglion associated with the differentiation of the reproductive tracts in the mouse. *Neurosci. Lett.* **32,** 271–276.

Takeda, H., Mizuno, T., and Lasnitzki, I. (1985). Autoradiographic studies of androgen-binding sites in the rat urogenital sinus and postnatal prostate. *J. Endocrinol.* **104,** 87–92.

Tegetmeir, W. B. (1867). "The Poultry Book." Routledge & Kegan Paul, London.

Teng, C. S., and Teng, C. T. (1979). Prenatal effect of the estrogenic hormone on embryonic genital organ differentiation. *In* "Ontogeny of Receptors and Reproductive Hormone Action" (T. H. Hamilton, J. H. Clark, and N. A. Sadler, eds.), pp. 421–440. Raven, New York.

Tran, D., and Josso, N. (1982). Localization of antimullerian hormone in the rough endoplasmic reticulum of the developing bovine Sertoli cell using immunocytochemistry with a monoclonal antibody. *Endocrinology* **111,** 1562–1567.

Van Niekerk, W. A. (1974). "True Hermaphroditism. Clinical Morphologic and Cytogenetic Aspects." Harper, New York.

Verhoeven, G., and Wilson, J. D. (1976). Cytosol androgen binding in submandibular gland and kidney of the normal mouse and the mouse with testicular feminization. *Endocrinology* **99,** 79–92.

Veyssière, G., Corre, M., Berger, M., Jean-Faucher, Ch., de Turikheim, M., and Jean, Cl. (1980). Androgines circulants et organogenèse sexuelle mali chez le foetus delapin. Etude après immunisation active delarnère contre la testostérone. *Arch. Anat. Microsc. Morphol. Exp.* **69,** 17–28.

Vigier, B., Picard, J.-Y., and Josso, N. (1982a). A monoclonal antibody against bovine anti-mullerian hormone. *Endocrinology* **110,** 131–137.

Vigier, B., Legali, L., Picard, J.-Y., and Josso, N. (1982b). A sensitive radioimmunoassay for bovine anti-müllerian hormone, allowing its detection in male and freemartin fetal serum. *Endocrinology* **111,** 1409–1411.

Wachtel, S. S. (1983). "H-Y Antigen and the Biology of Sex Determination." Gruen & Stratton, New York.

Walsh, P. C., Madden, J. D., Harrod, M. J., Goldstein, J. L., MacDonald, P. C., and Wilson, J. D. (1974). Familial incomplete male pseudohermaphroditism, type 2. Decreased dihydrotestosterone formation in pseudovaginal perineoscrotal hypospadias. *N. Engl. J. Med.* **291,** 944–949.

Weinstein, R. L., Kelch, R. P., Jenner, M. R., Kaplan, S. L., and Grumbach, M. M. (1974). Secretion of unconjugated androgens and estrogens by the normal and abnormal human testis before and after human chorionic gonadotropin. *J. Clin. Invest.* **53,** 1–6.

Welshons, W. J., and Russell, L. B. (1959). The Y-chromosome as the bearer of male determining factors in the mouse. *Proc. Natl. Acad. Sci. U.S.A.* **45,** 560–566.

Westley, B. R., and Salaman, D. F. (1976). Role of oestrogen receptor in androgen-induced sexual differentiation of the brain. *Nature (London)* **262,** 407–408.

Wilbert, D. M., Griffin, J. E., and Wilson, J. D. (1983). Characterization of the cytosol androgen receptor of the human prostate. *J. Clin. Endocrinol. Metab.* **56,** 113–120.

Wilson, C. M., and Taylor, B. A. (1982). Genetic regulation of mouse submaxillary gland renin. *J. Biol. Chem.* **257,** 217–233.

Wilson, J. D. (1971). Testosterone metabolism in skin. *Symp. Dtsch. Ges. Endokrinol.* **17,** 11–18.

Wilson, J. D. (1975). Metabolism of testicular androgens. *In* "Handbook of Physiology" (R. O. Greep and E. B. Astwood, eds.), Sect. 7: Endocrinology, Vol. V, Male Reproductive System, Chap. 25, pp. 491–508. American Physiological Society, Washington, D.C.

Wilson, J. D. (1979a). Sex hormones and sexual behavior. *N. Engl. J. Med.* **300,** 1269–1270.

Wilson, J. D. (1979b). Embryology of the genital tract. *In* "Urology" (J. H. Harrison, R. F. Gittes, A. D. Perlmutter, T. A. Stamey, and P. C. Walsh, eds.), 4th Ed., Vol. 2, Chap. 41, pp. 1469–1483. Saunders, Philadephia.

Wilson, J. D., and Goldstein, J. L. (1975). Classification of hereditary disorders of sexual development. *Birth Defects Orig. Art. Ser.* **11,** 1–16.

Wilson, J. D., and Lasnitzki, I. (1971). Dihydrotestosterone formation in fetal tissues of the rabbit and rat. *Endocrinology* **89,** 659–668.

Wilson, J. D., and Siiteri, P. K. (1973). Developmental pattern of testosterone synthesis in the fetal gonad of the rabbit. *Endocrinology* **92,** 1182–1191.

Wilson, J. D., Aiman, J., and MacDonald, P. C. (1980). The pathogenesis of gynecomastia. *Adv. Intern. Med.* **25,** 1–32.

Wilson, J. D., Griffin, J. E., Leshin, M., and MacDonald, P. C. (1983). The androgen resistance syndromes: 5α-Reductase deficiency, testicular feminization, and related disorders. *In* "The Metabolic Basis of Inherited Disease" (J. B. Stanbury, J. B. Wyngaarden, D. S. Fredrickson, J. L. Goldstein, and M. S. Brown, eds.), pp. 1001–1026. McGraw-Hill, New York.

Wilson, J. D., Griffin, J. E., George, F. W., and Leshin, M. (1984). Androgen action and the mechanisms of hormone resistance. *In* "Medicine, Science, and Society: Symposium Celebrating the Harvard Medical School Bicentennial" (K. Isselbacher, ed.), Chap 26, pp. 463–481. Wiley, New York.

Wolf, U. (1981). Genetic aspects of H-Y antigen. *Hum. Genet.* **58,** 25–28.

Wolfe, J., and Goodfellow, P. N. (1985). The elusive testis determining factor. *Trends Genet.* **1,** 3–4.

Zenzes, M. T., Wolf, U., Gunter, E., and Engel, W. (1978). Studies on the function of H-Y antigen: Dissociation and reorganization experiments on rat gonadal tissue. *Cytogenet. Cell Genet.* **20,** 365–372.

The Hormonal Regulation of Prolactin Gene Expression: An Examination of Mechanisms Controlling Prolactin Synthesis and the Possible Relationship of Estrogen to These Mechanisms

JAMES D. SHULL[1] AND JACK GORSKI

Department of Biochemistry,
University of Wisconsin,
Madison, Wisconsin 53706

I. Introduction

Prolactin (Prl) is a polypeptide hormone produced in the anterior pituitary gland of most vertebrates by a specialized population of cells termed lactotrophs or mammotrophs. In the rat, Prl is synthesized as a prehormone (Maurer *et al.*, 1976; Evans and Rosenfeld, 1976) containing a leader peptide of 29 amino acids at its amino-terminus (Maurer *et al.*, 1977); this leader peptide is removed prior to its secretion into the systemic circulation. At its target tissues, Prl interacts with a specific receptor present on the cytoplasmic membrane (Kelly *et al.*, 1984; Rillema, 1980) and mediates a wide variety of physiological processes involved in growth, development, and reproduction (Nicoll, 1980); Prl functions in the regulation of electrolyte balance (Horrobin, 1980), gonadotropin secretion, and gonad function in female (Smith, 1980) as well as male (Bartke, 1980) mammals.

A large body of data shows that Prl production, usually assayed by measuring circulating Prl levels or the release of Prl from pituitary explants or cultured pituitary cells, is controlled by a number of circulating hormones and hypothalamic factors. As our knowledge expands, it becomes clear that Prl production represents a composite of rates of Prl synthesis and degradation by lactotrophs and the rate of its release into the systemic circulation, all of which appear to be independently regulated. Although it is difficult to discuss these parameters separately, an attempt has been made to focus this review on the regulation of Prl synthesis, and more specifically the possible interrelationships between estrogen and other regulatory factors. In Section II we present data on the molecular structure of the Prl gene domain. Section III

[1] Present address: McArdle Laboratory for Cancer Research, University of Wisconsin, Madison, Wisconsin 53706.

details the effects of estrogen on Prl synthesis and emphasizes our recent studies on the regulation of Prl gene transcription. In Section IV the regulation of Prl gene expression by factors other than estrogen is briefly discussed. Finally, Section V illustrates a number of possible mechanisms whereby estrogen might modulate this regulation by other factors. The regulation of Prl secretion has been the topic of a number of recent reviews (Clemens and Shaar, 1980; Leong *et al.*, 1983; Gunnet and Freeman, 1983).

II. Molecular Nature of the Prolactin Gene

A. Prolactin Gene Structure

Prolactin, growth hormone, and chorionic somatomammotropin (placental lactogen) are related protein hormones coded from structurally similar genes which appear to have evolved from a common precursor (Miller and Eberhardt, 1983). In an attempt to elucidate the molecular mechanisms controlling synthesis of these hormones, several groups have examined the structure of these genes in a number of species. The rat Prl gene, extending from the transcription initiation site at its 5′ end to the polyadenylic acid [poly(A)] addition site at its 3′ end, spans approximately 10 kilobases (kb) of DNA and consists of 5 exons separated by 4 large introns (Chien and Thompson, 1980; Gubbins *et al.*, 1980; Maurer *et al.*, 1981). The human Prl gene, described recently, shows a very similar structure (Truong *et al.*, 1984). The fourth intron and flanking regions of the rat Prl gene contain repetitive-sequence DNA (Cooke and Baxter, 1982; Weber *et al.*, 1985). In addition a polymorphic, Alu-like element has been localized approximately 7.6 kb upstream of the first exon and is found in 0–2 copies per genome in outbred Holtzman rats, but is not observed at this locus in the inbred Fischer 344 strain (Schuler *et al.*, 1983). The biological functions of these repetitive DNA elements are not known.

B. Prolactin Gene Chromatin Structure

Transcriptionally active genes exist in an "open" chromatin structure which is more sensitive to nicking during a limited nuclease digestion than is the "closed" chromatin structure of nontranscribed genes (Weintraub and Groudine, 1976). In an estrogen-induced pituitary tumor consisting mainly of lactotrophs (Phelps and Hymer, 1983), the rat Prl gene and its flanking regions exist in a DNase-sensitive chromatin structure, whereas in liver it exists in a closed conformation characteristic of a nonexpressed gene (Durrin *et al.*, 1984). Two sites hypersensitive to DNase digestion have been localized near the 5′ end of the rat Prl gene in chromatin prepared from these tumors and may represent regulatory domains (Durrin *et al.*, 1984). Furthermore, in these pituitary tumors, the Prl gene is not methylated at a number of cytosine residues relative to the methylated state of these sites in Prl DNA prepared from liver (Durrin *et al.*, 1984). In these experiments, methylation was assayed through the use of isoschizomeric restriction enzymes which recognize identical sequences but differ in their abilities to cleave sequences that are methylated. These data on nuclease-sensitive chromatin structure, DNase-hypersensitive sites, and cytosine residue methylation are illustrated in Fig. 1.

In GH_3 cells, a clonal pituitary tumor cell line, the Prl gene exists in a chromatin structure with intermediate sensitivity to digestion by micrococcal nuclease (Levy-Wilson, 1983). Furthermore, there was no detectable change in sensitivity to digestion with chromatin prepared from cultures expressing high versus low levels of Prl mRNA. In another strain of pituitary tumor cells (GH_1) capable of expressing the Prl gene, it has been shown that the three *Msp*I/*Hpa*II sites present within the Prl gene are methylated (Stanley and Samuels, 1984). It remains to be determined whether these differences in cytosine residue methylation among these *in vivo* and *in vitro* systems are biologically relevant or are simply a reflection of our ability to examine only a small percentage of total cytosine residues.

C. Prolactin RNA Structure

Putative Prl transcripts ranging in size from 1.0 kb for the mature Prl mRNA to 7.0 kb (Maurer *et al.*, 1980), 10.0 kb (Maurer, 1982a), and

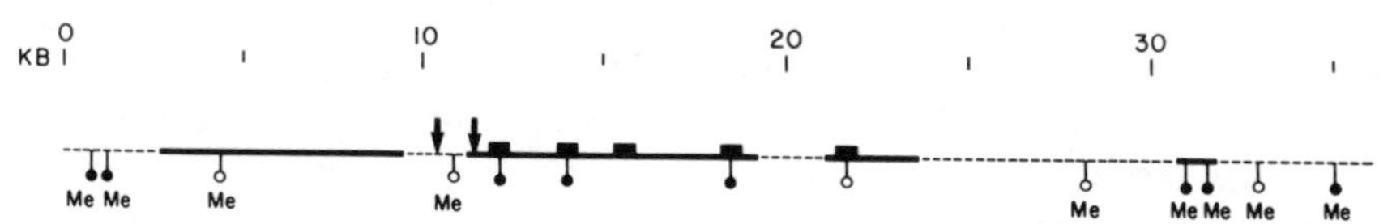

Fig. 1. Summary of the methylation pattern, location of repetitive DNA sequences, and DNase I-hypersensitive sites associated with the prolactin gene domain in rat pituitary tumors. Translated regions of the Prl gene are represented by filled boxes. Unique DNA sequences within and around the Prl gene are represented by the solid line; regions of DNA containing repetitive sequences are represented by the dotted line. *Msp*I/*Hpa*II and *Hha*I restriction sites are shown as solid and open circles, respectively. Me, Sites which are methylated in pituitary tumors or control pituitaries of rats. The two heavy arrows 5′ to the first exon indicate the location of the hypersensitive sites observed in pituitary tumors. Data from Durrin *et al.* (1984).

approximately 14.0 kb (Hoffman *et al.*, 1981; Potter *et al.*, 1981; White and Bancroft, 1983) have been reported. These transcripts were detected by resolving, by gel electrophoresis, nuclear RNA molecules according to size, transferring the separated RNAs to nitrocellulose or DBM paper, and probing for RNAs that exhibit sequence homology to radiolabeled Prl cDNA. The discrepancy between the size of the largest transcripts (14 kb) and the reported size of the Prl gene (10 kb) may possibly be due to inaccuracies in estimating the size of the large transcripts or to multiple poly(A) addition sites or transcription initiation sites being utilized during Prl gene transcription. The relative levels of these putative Prl RNAs increase in response to estrogen (Maurer, 1982a), thyrotropin-releasing hormone (Potter *et al.*, 1981; Biswas *et al.*, 1982), calcium (White and Bancroft, 1983), epidermal growth factor (Murdoch *et al.*, 1983), and vasoactive intestinal peptide (Carillo *et al.*, 1985) and decrease in response to ergocryptine, a dopamine agonist (Maurer, 1981). These observations suggest that the expression of the Prl gene is regulated either at the level of transcription or during processing of the primary Prl gene transcript to mature Prl mRNA.

III. Regulation of Prolactin Synthesis by Estrogen

A. Model of Estrogen Action in Regulating Gene Expression

Until recently it was held that estrogens and other steroid hormones interact specifically with receptors in the cytoplasm of target cells and that the hormone–receptor complex is by some unknown mechanism translocated into the nucleus where it functions in regulating the expression of specific genes (Gorski and Gannon, 1976). This model of steroid hormone action has been revised (Gorski *et al.*, 1984; and Fig. 2) in light of evidence which suggests that the estrogen receptor resides permanently in the nucleus (Welshons *et al.*, 1984; King and Greene, 1984). We still lack specific knowledge of the molecular mechanisms whereby the steroid hormone–receptor complex regulates gene expression. However, recent reports indicating that the glucocorticoid receptor complex interacts specifically with the murine mammary tumor virus genome (Payvar *et al.*, 1983), an element whose transcription is stimulated by glucocorticoids (Ringold *et al.*, 1977), suggest the possibility that steroid hormones may regulate gene expression at the transcriptional level through an interaction of the hormone–receptor complex with specific regulatory domains of controlled genes. More

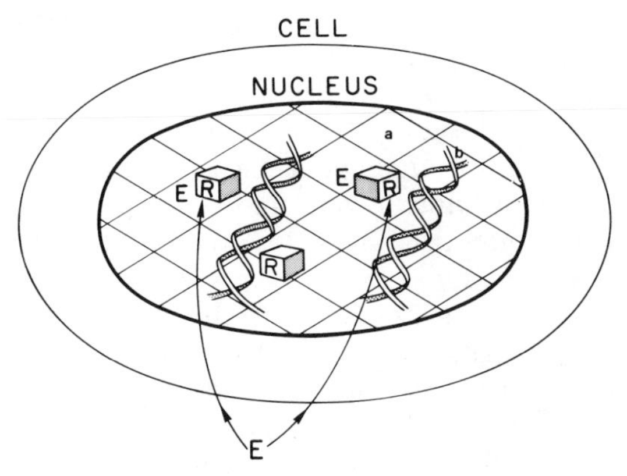

FIG. 2. "New" model of estrogen receptor. R, Receptor; E, estrogen; a, nuclear matrix or scaffold; b, DNA. Reproduced from Gorski *et al.* (1984).

recently, Maurer has shown that the estrogen receptor binds selectively to a region 1.2–2.0 kb upstream of the rat prolactin gene (Maurer, 1985). As we will discuss, estrogen stimulates the transcription of the rat prolactin gene. It should be noted, however, that the relative affinities of steroid receptors for these "specific" regulatory domains are approximately 10-fold greater than their affinities for nonspecific DNA sequences. In comparison, the relative affinity of the *lac* repressor for the *lac* operator exceeds by three or four orders of magnitude its affinity for nonoperator DNA (Lin and Riggs, 1972). A similarly large difference in relative binding affinity has recently been demonstrated for the interaction of a specific nuclear factor with the nuclease-hypersensitive region of the chicken adult β-globin gene (Emerson *et al.*, 1985).

B. Estrogen Stimulates the Synthesis of Prolactin by the Rat Anterior Pituitary

It has been known for many years that estrogen is a positive regulator of Prl production. During the estrous cycle of the rat, the major surge in circulating Prl occurs on the afternoon and evening of proestrus, only a few hours after the peak in circulating estrogen (Butcher *et al.*, 1974). Furthermore, an anti-estrogen antiserum administered to cycling rats at diestrus blocked this Prl surge (Neill *et al.*, 1971). Based on these reports, it was conceivable that this estrogen effect could be mediated either at the level of Prl synthesis or secretion.

Analysis of pituitary proteins by starch gel electrophoresis (Baker *et al.*, 1963) showed that pituitaries from intact female rats contain more Prl than pituitaries from ovariectomized rats and that estrogen administration increases the amount of Prl in pituitaries from these ovariectomized animals. MacLeod *et al.* (1969) demonstrated that estrogen, administered *in vivo* in a single pharmacological dose, stimulated the incorporation of [^{3}H]leucine, by cultured whole pituitaries removed 5 or 9 days after estrogen treatment, into the pituitary proteins which migrated with a Prl standard on polyacrylamide gels. This estrogen effect was observed in intact males, castrated males, and intact female rats (MacLeod *et al.*, 1969). Similar results were reported by Yamamoto *et al.* (1975), who used similar techniques in examining the effect of 8 daily injections (50 μg) of 17β-estradiol on Prl synthesis in ovariectomized female rats. These authors also observed that a single 10-μg injection of 17β-estradiol increased Prl synthesis in ovariectomized rats within 12 hours of treatment (Yamamoto *et al.*, 1975). These results were confirmed by Maurer and Gorski (1977) who demonstrated that daily injections of 17β-estradiol (10 μg) stimulated synthesis of Prl in pituitaries of male and ovariectomized female rats. Significant increases in Prl synthesis were observed 24 hours after the first injection and peak levels of Prl synthesis were achieved after 2–3 injections in ovariectomized female and 7 injections in male rats (Maurer and Gorski, 1977). These studies provided conclusive evidence that estrogen stimulates Prl synthesis by the anterior pituitary gland, but did not identify the target site(s) of the estrogen or the mechanisms involved in this stimulation.

C. The Effects of Estrogen on Prolactin Synthesis Are Pretranslational

Stone *et al.* (1977) found that Prl mRNA activity, assayed by translation of pituitary RNA in a cell-free system coupled with immunoprecipitation of the labeled Prl, was increased in male rats within 24 hours of a single injection of 17β-estradiol (10 μg). Further increases were observed upon successive daily injections to a total of 7 injections. In ovariectomized retired breeders, 4 daily injections of 17β-estradiol (10 μg) increased Prl mRNA activity approximately fivefold, an increase considerably greater than observed in male rats treated in the same manner. This result was likely due to the fact that lactotrophs represent a larger proportion of the pituitary cell population in female rats as compared to male rats (Hymer *et al.*, 1974; Neill and Frawley, 1983). No increase in Prl mRNA activity was observed in intact retired breeder females in response to this estrogen treatment, possibly because Prl mRNA activity was already at its maximum level in intact females (Stone *et al.*, 1977). In the same study, it was reported that Prl mRNA activity in the male rat pituitary decreased by approximately 50% within 72 hours of the last of 4 daily injections of 17β-estradiol (10 μg). This observation suggested that Prl mRNA is quite stable with a half-life in excess of 48 hours.

Through the use of DNA complementary to Prl mRNA (cDNA) synthesized *in vitro,* Ryan *et al.* (1979) demonstrated that 17β-estradiol (3–6 daily injections of 10 μg) increases Prl mRNA levels in the pituitaries of male or immature female rats. In this study the levels of Prl mRNA reached after treatment closely paralleled the levels of Prl synthesized by whole pituitaries incubated *in vitro.* 17β-Estradiol (14 daily injections of 10 μg) also increased the amount of Prl mRNA in the pituitaries of ovariectomized female rats (Maurer, 1980a). These reports suggested that estrogen stimulates Prl synthesis by acting at a pretranslational level.

Seo *et al.* (1979a) reported that a single injection of 17β-estradiol (80 μg/100 g body weight) into male rats caused a significant increase in Prl mRNA within 12 hours of treatment. However, there was no parallel increase in Prl synthesized by cultured whole pituitaries from these animals. Animals treated with estradiol valerate (400 μg/100 g) gave similar results. In animals chronically stimulated by estrogen for 4 weeks and subsequently withdrawn from estrogen treatment for 13 days, a single injection of estradiol valerate produced a more rapid increase in Prl mRNA and Prl synthesis. This observation was likely due to an estrogen-induced increase in the number of lactotrophs in the chronically stimulated animals, although the level of Prl synthesis still lagged behind that of Prl mRNA (Seo *et al.*, 1979a). The investigators therefore hypothesized that estrogen may stimulate Prl synthesis by acting at pretranslational as well as translational levels.

D. Estrogen Acts, at Least in Part, Directly on the Cells of the Anterior Pituitary

The studies discussed up to this point clearly indicated that estrogen stimulates Prl synthesis *in vivo* and that this increased level of Prl synthesis is due at least in part, and perhaps totally, to an increase in the level of Prl mRNA. However, these studies did not indicate whether the estrogen effects are mediated directly at the pituitary level, or indirectly through another estrogen target tissue. Physiological concentrations of 17β-estradiol were shown to stimulate Prl synthesis in primary cultures of anterior pituitary cells (Lieberman *et al.*, 1978). In these experiments, cultured cells treated for 7 days with 17β-estradiol synthesized Prl at a rate fivefold higher than control cells. These data were supported by Vician *et al.* (1979) who showed that 17β-estradiol-treated (5×10^{-9} *M*) ovine pituitary cells synthesized Prl at twice the rate of control cells and that this elevated level of Prl synthesis was paralleled by increased amounts of Prl mRNA. Furthermore, significantly increased Prl synthesis and Prl mRNA were observed as early as 24 hours after adding 17β-estradiol to the cultures (Vician *et al.*, 1979). These *in vitro* studies clearly showed that estrogen acts in stimulating Prl synthesis at least partially through a direct action on the pituitary.

Chronic estrogen treatment (pellets of 2 mg 17β-estradiol implanted subcutaneously for at least 1 week) stimulated Prl synthesis and increased Prl mRNA in thyroidectomized male rats (Seo *et al.*, 1979b). Increased Prl synthesis in response to chronic 17β-estradiol treatment was also observed in pituitaries transplanted under the kidney capsule, away from direct contact with the hypothalamus (Wiklund *et al.*, 1981). These *in vivo* studies indicated that neither the thyroid nor direct contact with the hypothalamus are required for induction of Prl synthesis in response to chronic estrogen treatment.

A more recent study showed that Prl synthesis and Prl mRNA increase 2.7- and 3.2-fold, respectively, in anterior pituitary cells cultured for 5 days with 17β-estradiol (10^{-8} *M*) while the number of lactotrophs, as measured by immunocytochemical staining, increased by only 30% (Lieberman *et al.*, 1982). This observation, along with the data of Vician *et al.* (1979) showing significantly increased Prl synthesis and Prl mRNA within 24 hours of estrogen treatment, suggested that the stimulatory effects of estrogen on Prl synthesis are not simply due to an estrogen-induced increase in the number of Prl synthesizing cells in the cultured cell population.

E. Estrogen Regulates the Expression of the Rat Prolactin Gene at the Level of Transcription

1. *Estrogen Stimulates Prolactin Gene Transcription by a Mechanism Independent of Pituitary Protein Synthesis*

a. An Examination in Vivo. We have recently investigated the effects of estrogen on transcription of the rat Prl and growth hormone (GH) genes. In these studies, the rates of Prl and GH gene transcription were measured by quantitating the amount of radiolabeled uridine triphosphate (UTP) incorporated with time into Prl- and GH-specific messenger RNA sequences by nuclei isolated from anterior pituitary glands after hormone treatment (Fig. 3). These nuclei synthesized RNA for at least 60 minutes when isolated and incubated as described (Shull and Gorski, 1984). RNA polymerases I, II, and III were active in 20–25%, 65–70%, and 5–10% of this RNA synthesis, respectively, as indicated by the concentration-dependent inhibition of polymerases II and III by the fungal toxin α-amanitin (Shull and Gorski, 1984). The inhibition of nuclear RNA synthesis by actinomycin D indicated that this RNA was synthesized from a DNA template (Shull and Gorski, 1984). Nuclei isolated from estrogen-treated rats (10 μg, ip) synthesized RNA at a rate significantly greater than nuclei from control animals; nuclear RNA synthesis was stimulated approximately 30% at 3 and 6 hours after injection of 17β-estradiol (Table I).

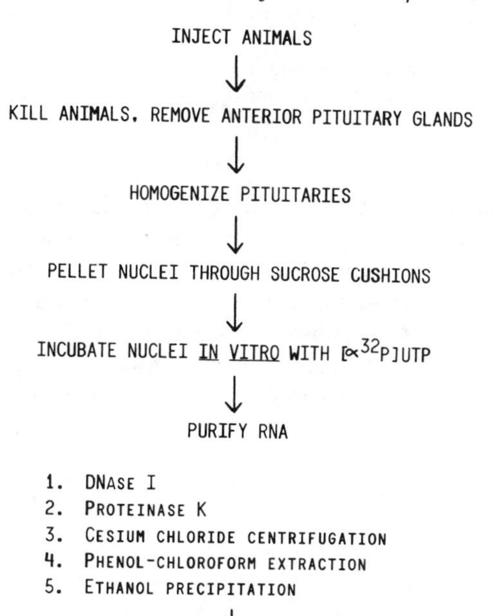

Fig. 3. A summary of procedures used in studying hormonal effects on prolactin gene transcription. See Shull and Gorski (1984, 1985) for more detailed procedures.

TABLE I
STIMULATORY EFFECT OF 17β-ESTRADIOL ON TOTAL RNA SYNTHESIS BY ISOLATED PITUITARY NUCLEI[a]

Treatment group	Picomole UMP incorporated per microgram DNA[b]	-Fold stimulation[c]	p value[d]
Control	0.40 ± 0.02	1.00 ± 0.09	
30 minutes	0.42 ± 0.02	1.05 ± 0.09	0.294
3 hours	0.51 ± 0.03	1.28 ± 0.11	0.014
6 hours	0.51 ± 0.01	1.28 ± 0.08	0.007
24 hours	0.42 ± 0.01	1.04 ± 0.06	0.321

[a] At the indicated times after hormone treatment, pituitary nuclei were isolated and total RNA synthesis was measured as described (Shull and Gorski, 1984).

[b] Each value represents the mean and standard error of the mean (n = 3).

[c] The ratio of each treatment group relative to the control value and a calculated standard error is represented.

[d] Student's p value.

A single injection of 17β-estradiol (10 μg, ip) into male rats significantly stimulated the transcription of the Prl gene (Fig. 4). Prolactin gene transcription was increased as early as 30 minutes after estrogen treatment and remained elevated for at least 48 hours (Fig. 4). Maurer, using similar procedures, observed similar stimulatory effects of estrogen on Prl gene transcription in ovariectomized female rats (Maurer, 1982a). Although we observed some variability in the time to peak Prl gene transcription (6–24 hours) and the magnitude of the peak response (1.5- to 5.0-fold), we consistently observed rapid (within minutes) and prolonged (48–72 hours) stimulation of Prl gene transcription by 17β-estradiol (Shull and Gorski, 1982, 1983, 1984, 1985).

In contrast to the stimulatory effects of 17β-estradiol on Prl gene transcription, this estrogen did not significantly affect the transcription of the GH gene (Table II). The level of GH gene transcription in untreated male rats was usually 40–60% of that observed for the Prl gene.

In this nuclear transcription system, the Prl and GH RNAs were asymmetrically transcribed from a DNA template by RNA polymerase II (Shull and Gorski, 1984). The fungal toxin α-amanitin at a concentration of 1.0 μg/ml (a concentration known to inhibit RNA polymerase II selectively) inhibited Prl gene transcription by greater than 95% in nuclei prepared from both control and estrogen-treated animals (Fig.

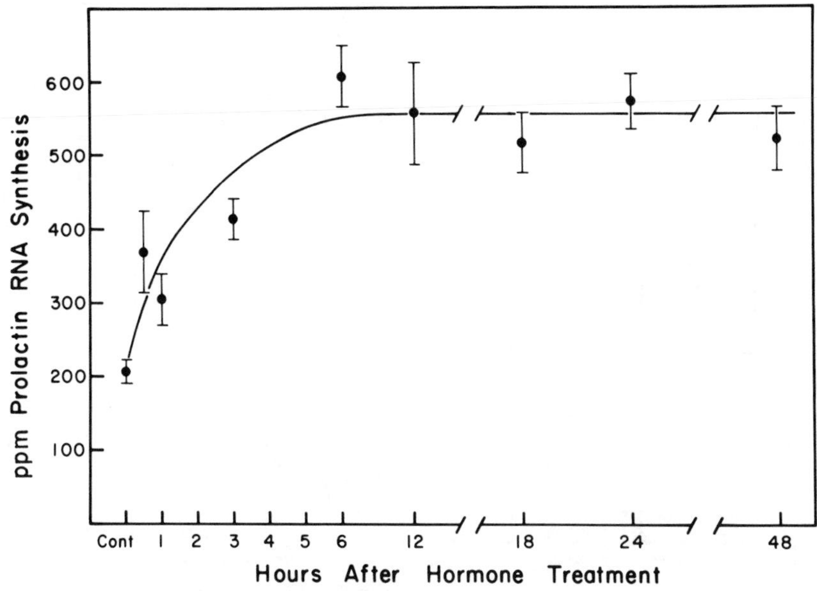

FIG. 4. Stimulatory effect of 17β-estradiol on prolactin gene transcription. At the indicated times prior to sacrifice, male rats were injected ip with 10 μg of estradiol in sesame oil. Anterior pituitary nuclei were then prepared and prolactin gene transcription was assayed as described in Shull and Gorski (1984).

5A and B). Actinomycin D at 10 μg/ml inhibited both Prl gene transcription and total RNA synthesis by approximately 50% (Shull and Gorski, 1984). Therefore, the rate of Prl gene transcription when expressed relative to total RNA synthesis (i.e., levels given in parts per million of total RNA) was not affected in nuclei from either control

TABLE II
GROWTH HORMONE GENE TRANSCRIPTION IS NOT REGULATED BY 17β-ESTRADIOL[a]

Treatment group	Growth hormone RNA synthesis (ppm)
Control	101 ± 34
30 minutes	140 ± 24
6 hours	138 ± 61
12 hours	141 ± 25
24 hours	118 ± 22

[a] Growth hormone transcription was assayed as described in legend to Fig. 3 and Shull and Gorski (1984).

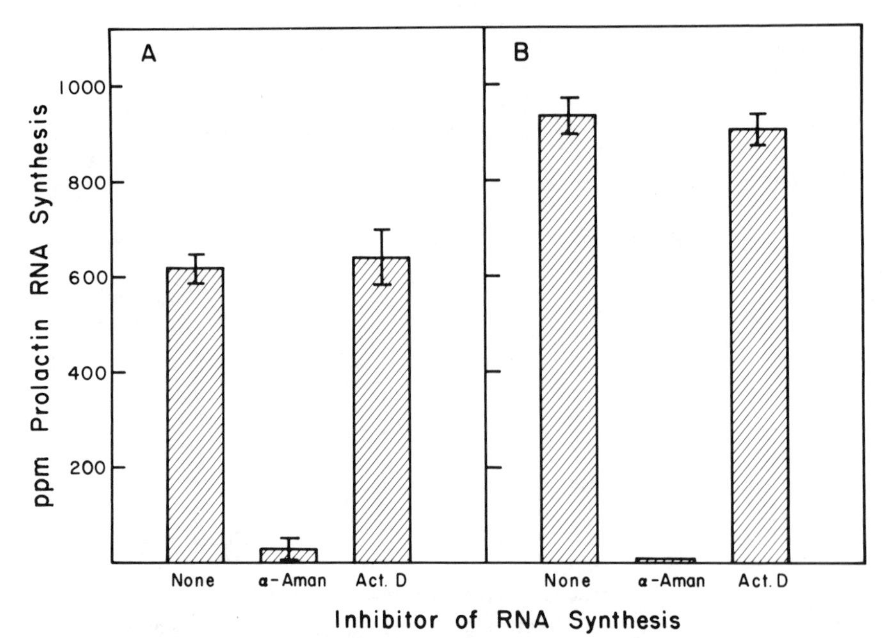

FIG. 5. Effects of transcriptional inhibitors on prolactin RNA synthesis by isolated pituitary nuclei. Anterior pituitary nuclei were isolated 24 hours after injection of the sesame oil vehicle (A) or 10 μg of 17β-estradiol (B) and were incubated under normal conditions or in the presence of α-amanitin (1 μg/ml) or actinomycin D (10 μg/ml). See Shull and Gorski (1984) for details.

animals (Fig. 5A) or animals treated with 17β-estradiol (Fig. 5B). The inhibitors equally affected GH RNA synthesis by nuclei from control or estrogen-treated animals (Shull and Gorski, 1984). The asymmetry of Prl RNA synthesis by isolated nuclei incubated under our conditions was determined with single-stranded Prl DNAs as hybridization probes (J. D. Shull and J. Gorski, unpublished data).

Maurer has reported that during the initial hour after injection of 17β-estradiol (20 μg, ip) into ovariectomized female rats the increase in the level of Prl gene transcription paralleled an increase in the level of estrogen receptors located in the nucleus (Maurer, 1982a). We have shown that although this relationship between the rate of Prl gene transcription and numbers of nuclear-form estrogen receptors (occupied or transformed receptors) may hold during the initial hour following 17β-estradiol injection, at later time points such a relationship no longer held (Shull and Gorski, 1984). Figure 6A illustrates that the amount of nuclear-form estrogen receptor peaked approximately 1 hour after injection and returned virtually to baseline between 6 and

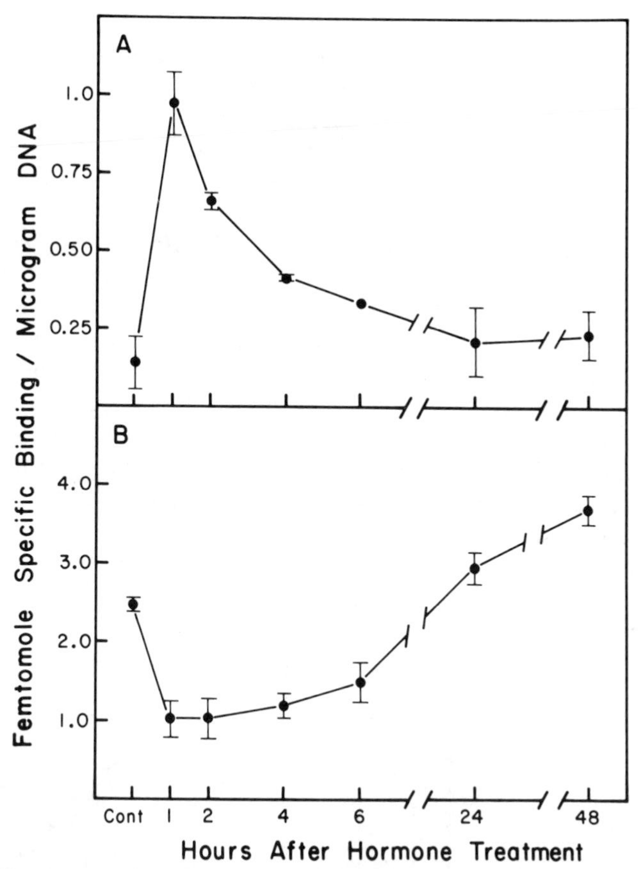

FIG. 6. Time course of estrogen receptor transformation following an injection of 17β-estradiol. The levels of transformed nuclear receptors (A) and nontransformed cytosolic receptors (B) were assayed at the indicated times following a single injection of 17β-estradiol (10 μg in sesame oil, ip). See Shull and Gorski (1984) for experimental details.

24 hours after injection. In contrast, an equivalent injection of 17β-estradiol stimulated Prl gene transcription for 48–72 hours (Fig. 4). In explanation of these data we suggested that 17β-estradiol might regulate Prl gene transcription through a stable mechanism involving the modification of chromatin proteins or DNA sequences within or surrounding the Prl gene, by inducing a change in the level of a second regulator of Prl gene transcription, by altering the responsiveness of the anterior pituitary to a second regulator, or through a combination of these mechanisms (Shull and Gorski, 1984). Data to be presented illustrate that estrogen regulates the transcription of the Prl gene *in vivo* through both direct and indirect mechanisms.

If the proposed mechanism of estrogen action is correct (Fig. 2), then the induction of transcription of estrogen-regulated genes should not require the synthesis of any intermediary proteins. We have investigated the effects of inhibitors of protein synthesis on the induction of Prl gene transcription by 17β-estradiol. Three hours after injection of 17β-estradiol or its sesame oil vehicle, cycloheximide was without effect; Prl gene transcription was stimulated approximately twofold in either cycloheximide- or saline-pretreated animals (Fig. 7). Similar results were obtained 8 hours after 17β-estradiol injection in cycloheximide-pretreated (Fig. 8B) or saline-pretreated animals (Fig. 8A). In these experiments, cycloheximide administration caused an approximate 80% inhibition of protein synthesis by the anterior pituitary glands of animals treated with either sesame oil or 17β-estradiol (Fig. 9). These data suggest that the induction of Prl gene transcription by 17β-estradiol is through a mechanism which does not require the synthesis of an intermediary protein or proteins by the anterior pituitary gland. We cannot, however, exclude the possibility that under conditions of an 80% inhibition of pituitary protein synthesis a required

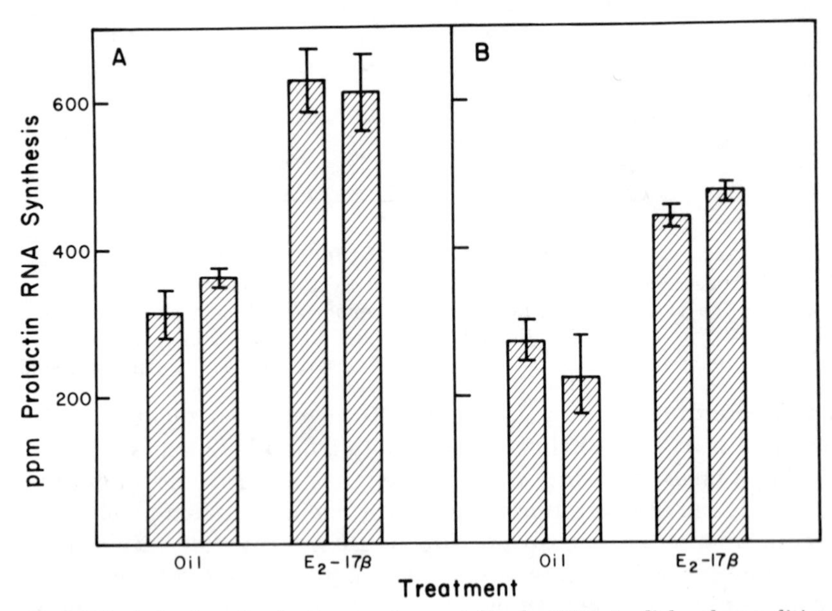

FIG. 7. The induction of prolactin gene transcription by 17β-estradiol under conditions of inhibited pituitary protein synthesis; examined at 3 hours. Sterile saline (A) or cycloheximide (B) was injected 10 minutes prior to 17β-estradiol (10 μg, ip) or its sesame oil vehicle. The animals were sacrificed 3 hours after hormone treatment and Prl gene transcription was assayed as described in Shull and Gorski (1984).

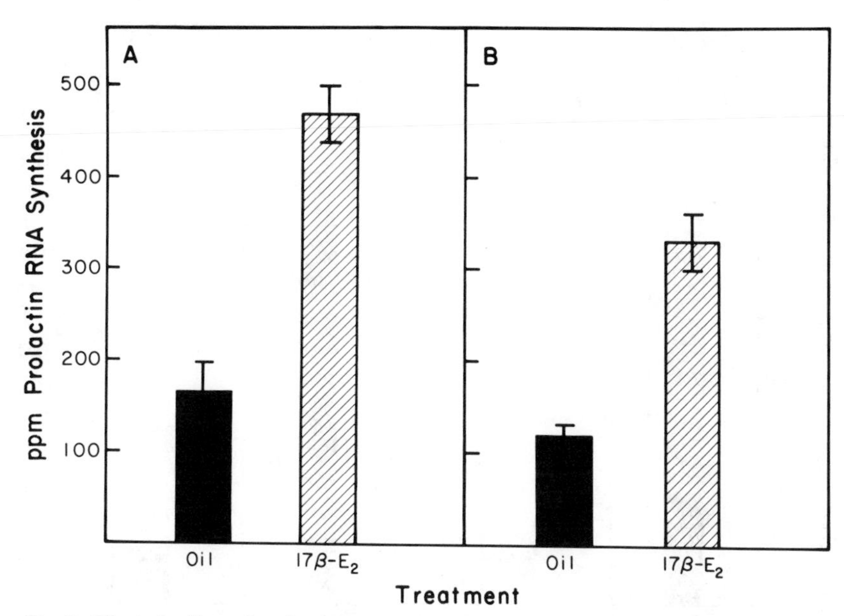

FIG. 8. The induction of prolactin gene transcription by 17β-estradiol under conditions of inhibited pituitary protein synthesis; examined at 8 hours. Sterile saline (A) or cycloheximide (B) was injected and animals were treated as described in Shull and Gorski (1984) and Fig. 9B.

protein (or proteins) might have been synthesized in a reduced but sufficient level to allow the full induction of Prl gene transcription by 17β-estradiol.

b. An Examination in Cultured Anterior Pituitary Cells. Estrogen has been shown to stimulate Prl synthesis in primary cultures of rat anterior pituitary cells (Lieberman *et al.*, 1978, 1982). However, significant increases in the rate of Prl synthesis were not generally observed until after 2–3 days of estrogen treatment (Lieberman *et al.*, 1978, 1982). Therefore, it is difficult to ensure that the number of lactotrophs in the cultured cell population remains constant throughout the culture period (Lieberman *et al.*, 1982). *In vivo,* estrogen increases Prl synthesis at least in part by stimulating the transcription of the Prl gene (Maurer, 1982a; Shull and Gorski, 1982, 1983, 1984, 1985) through a mechanism independent of pituitary protein synthesis (Shull and Gorski, 1984; Figs. 7–9 this review). *In vivo,* however, it is possible to inhibit pituitary protein synthesis by only approximately 80–90% without prematurely killing the experimental animals (J. D. Shull and J. Gorski, unpublished observations). We have, therefore, investigated the effects of 17β-estradiol on the transcription of the Prl

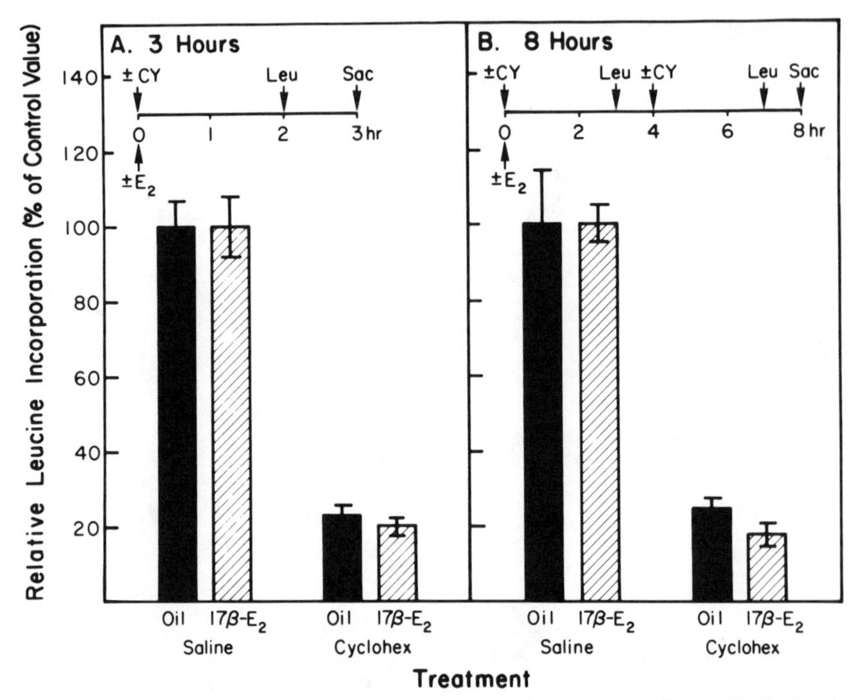

FIG. 9. Inhibitory effects of cycloheximide on pituitary protein synthesis. (A) Cycloheximide (or its saline vehicle) was injected 10 minutes prior to 17β-estradiol (or its oil vehicle). Two hours after hormone injection, [^{3}H]leucine was injected. (B) Cycloheximide (or its saline vehicle) was injected 10 minutes prior to 17β-estradiol (or its oil vehicle) and again 4 hours later. [^{3}H]Leucine was injected 3 and 7 hours following hormone treatment. At the indicated times, the animals were sacrificed and leucine incorporation into pituitary protein was measured as described in Shull and Gorski (1984).

gene in cultured pituitary cells. The time course of induction of Prl gene transcription by this estrogen has been examined as well as the ability of this estrogen to induce Prl gene transcription under conditions of grossly inhibited protein synthesis.

In these experiments the cells were prepared for culture by the procedure of Vale *et al.* (1972). Dispersed cells were plated at a density of 3.5×10^6 cells per 100-mm dish in Dulbecco's modified Eagle's medium (DMEM) supplemented with HEPES (25 m*M*), insulin (10μg/ml), horse serum (15%, v/v), fetal calf serum (2.5%, v/v), gentamycin (50 μg/ml), and penicillin (100 U/ml). To remove endogenous steroids, the sera were stripped three to four times with acid-washed, dextran-coated charcoal prior to use. After 3 days of culture the medium was removed and replaced with 10 ml of fresh medium, 17β-estradiol was added to a concentration of 10^{-9} *M*, and incubation at 37°C was continued as indicated. The medium was then removed, the cells were rinsed and homogenized, and nuclei were isolated for Prl gene transcription as described (Fig. 3).

Nuclei prepared from anterior pituitary cells derived from 6-week-old male rats and treated for 24 hours with 17β-estradiol beginning on day 3 of culture synthesized Prl RNA in amounts significantly greater

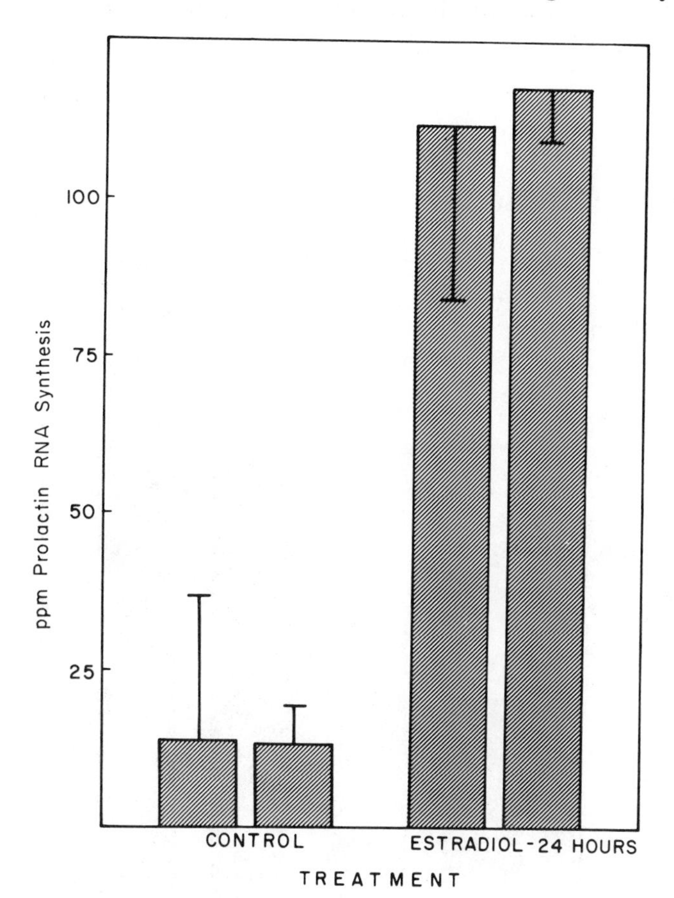

FIG. 10. The stimulatory effects of estradiol on prolactin gene transcription in primary cultures of pituitary cells prepared from male rats. On day 3 of culture, the medium was changed and estradiol was added to a final concentration of 10^{-9} *M*. Control cultures received an equivalent volume of the DMEM–ethanol vehicle. The cells were harvested 24 hours later, nuclei were prepared, and prolactin gene transcription was assayed as described in the text and Shull and Gorski (1984). Each bar represents the level (mean ± the standard error of the mean; $n = 3$) of prolactin RNA synthesized by nuclei isolated from cells harvested from six 100-mm culture dishes. Data are from Shull *et al.* (1984a).

($p < 0.001$) than nuclei prepared from control cultures (Fig. 10). In this experiment, estradiol stimulated prolactin gene transcription 6.5-fold over control. We next examined Prl gene transcription after 1, 6, and 24 hours of estradiol treatment *in vitro*. In duplicate groups of control cultures, the amounts of Prl gene transcription were 45.6 ± 9.6 and 21.1 ± 23.5 ppm (Fig. 11). In cultures treated with estradiol for 1 hour the amounts were 82.7 ± 15.5 and 10.9 ± 20.0 ppm. We consistently observed large variability in the rate of Prl gene transcription follow-

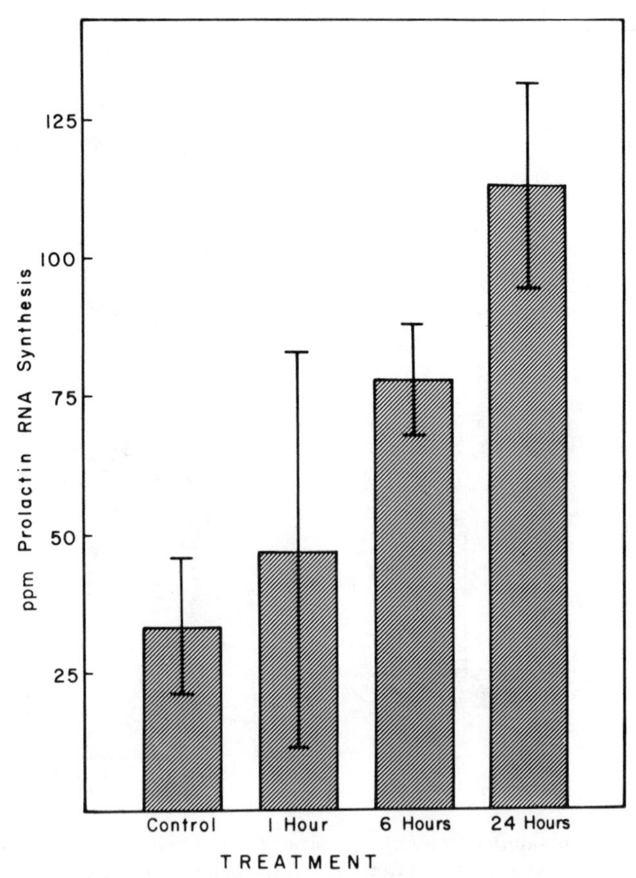

FIG. 11. Time course of estradiol-stimulated prolactin gene transcription in primary cultures of pituitary cells prepared from male rats. The culture protocol was described in Fig. 10. Estradiol or its vehicle was added to the cultures at the indicated times prior to harvest. Each bar represents the level (mean ± range) of prolactin RNA synthesized by duplicate preparations of nuclei. Each preparation was from cells harvested from six 100-mm culture dishes and the RNA purified from each of these preparations of nuclei was assayed in triplicate. Data are from Shull *et al.* (1984a).

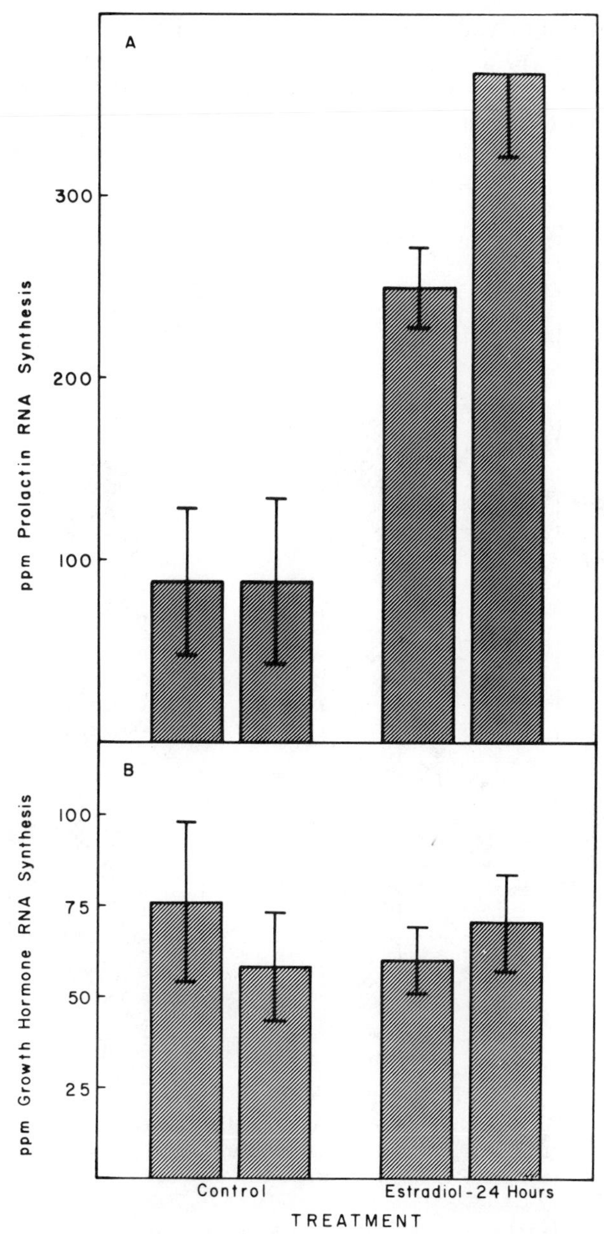

FIG. 12. The contrasting effects of estradiol on the transcription of the prolactin and growth hormone genes in primary cultures of pituitary cells prepared from female rats. Procedures were as described in Fig. 10. (A) Estradiol effects on prolactin gene transcription; (B) estradiol effects on growth hormone gene transcription. Data are from Shull *et al.* (1984a).

ing 1–2 hours of estradiol treatment (J. D. Shull and J. Gorski, unpublished observation). In duplicate sets of cultures treated with estradiol for 6 hours, the Prl gene was transcribed at 88.1 ± 23.5 and 67.7 ± 10.0 ppm. This represents a significant ($p = 0.015$), 2.3-fold induction of Prl gene transcription over control. By 24 hours of estrogen treatment, the

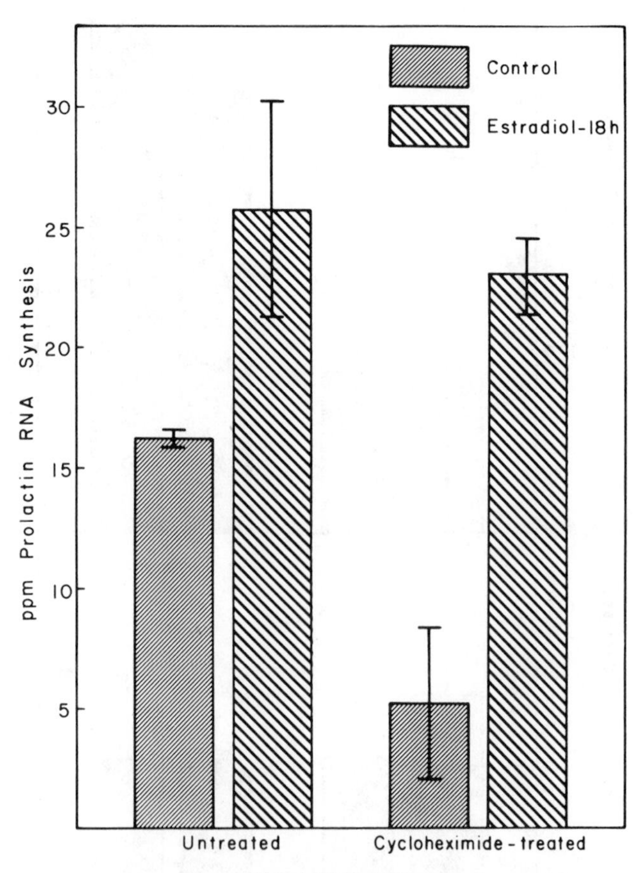

FIG. 13. Estradiol stimulates the transcription of the prolactin gene in cycloheximide-treated cultures of pituitary cells prepared from male rats. On day 3 of culture, the medium was changed and cycloheximide was added to a concentration of 10^{-5} *M*. Parallel cultures received the DMEM vehicle. Estradiol (or its vehicle) was added to 10^{-9} *M* 30 minutes following cycloheximide. The cells were harvested 18 hours later, nuclei were prepared, and prolactin gene transcription was assayed as described in Fig. 10. Each bar represents the level (mean ± range) of prolactin RNA synthesized by duplicate preparations of nuclei. Each preparation was from cells harvested from six 100-mm culture dishes and the RNA purified from each of these preparations of nuclei was assayed in triplicate. Data are from Shull *et al.* (1984a).

transcription of the Prl gene was significantly stimulated 3.4-fold ($p = 0.005$); the amounts of transcription in duplicate sets of cultures were 131.5 ± 28.7 and 94.7 ± 27.7 ppm (Fig. 11).

Estradiol also stimulated the transcription of the Prl gene in primary cell cultures prepared from the anterior pituitaries of female retired breeders (Fig. 12A); a significant ($p = 0.032$), 3.5-fold induction of Prl gene transcription was observed. In contrast, estradiol had no effect on the transcription of the closely related GH gene (Fig. 12B). These data indicate that the stimulatory effects of estradiol on Prl gene transcription are specific.

Estradiol stimulated the transcription of the Prl gene in cultured pituitary cells treated with an inhibitor of protein synthesis. In pituitary cells derived from male rats and cultured for 3 days, an 18-hour treatment with estradiol caused a 1.6 ± 0.3-fold stimulation of Prl gene transcription (Fig. 13). A 4.6 ± 2.8-fold stimulation of Prl gene transcription was observed in response to estradiol in cultures containing cycloheximide at a concentration of 10^{-5} *M* (Fig. 13). Cycloheximide inhibited by greater than 95% the rate of incorporation of [^{3}H]leucine into trichloroacetic acid-precipitable material (Fig. 14). The inhibitory actions of cycloheximide were for the most part reversible as [^{3}H]leucine incorporation returned virtually to control rates upon removal of the inhibitor (Fig. 14). In cultures derived from female retired breeders and pretreated with cycloheximide, the transcription of the Prl gene was stimulated 2.4 ± 0.2-fold upon 8 hours of estradiol treatment, while a 1.9 ± 0.5-fold stimulation by estradiol was observed in untreated cultures (Fig. 15). Protein synthesis was inhibited by greater than 95% by cycloheximide treatment in estrogen-treated or control cultures (Fig. 16).

The data presented clearly indicate that 17β-estradiol stimulates the transcription of the rat Prl gene through a mechanism independent of pituitary protein synthesis. These data in conjunction with those illustrating that 17β-estradiol stimulates Prl gene transcription *in vivo* within minutes of its injection are compatible with and lend indirect support to the hypothesis that estrogen acts in regulating gene expression through an interaction of the estrogen–receptor complex with control regions of regulated genes. As the unoccupied estrogen receptor appears to reside permanently in the nucleus of target cells (Welshons *et al.*, 1984; King and Greene, 1984; Gorski *et al.*, 1984), it is possible that this receptor is normally in close association with specific domains of regulated genes and that estrogen binding is the requisite signal for transcriptional enhancement. If this is the case, one would expect that the level of stimulated transcription would decline as the steroid dissociates from its receptor. A single injection of 17β-estradiol

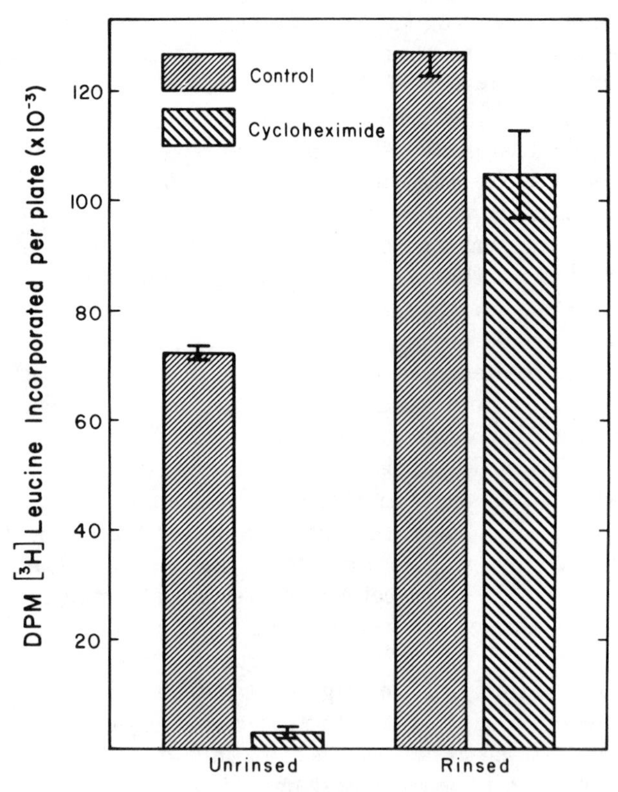

FIG. 14. The reversible inhibition of pituitary cell protein synthesis by cycloheximide. On day 3 of culture, the medium was changed and cycloheximide (or its DMEM vehicle) was added to the medium to a concentration of 10^{-5} *M*. Following 17 hours of incubation, [^{3}H]leucine was added to one group of cultures (unrinsed) to a concentration of 10 μCi/ml. From a second group of plates the medium was removed, the plates were rinsed with 5 ml DMEM, and fresh DMEM containing [^{3}H]leucine at 10 μCi/ml was readded. Following an additional hour of incubation, the cells from both groups were harvested and the incorporation of [^{3}H]leucine into acid-precipitable material was assayed. Data are from Shull *et al.* (1984a).

stimulated Prl gene transcription *in vivo* for 48–72 hours (Fig. 4), whereas the amount of occupied, nuclear-form receptor returned to baseline within 24 hours of injection (Fig. 6). Furthermore, circulating estradiol was undetectable within 24 hours after a single injection (10 μg, ip) of this estrogen (J. D. Shull and J. Gorski, unpublished observation). Upon initial inspection, these data suggest that the above-mentioned model of estrogen action is too simplistic. In the next section, however, we will show that the time course of stimulation of Prl gene

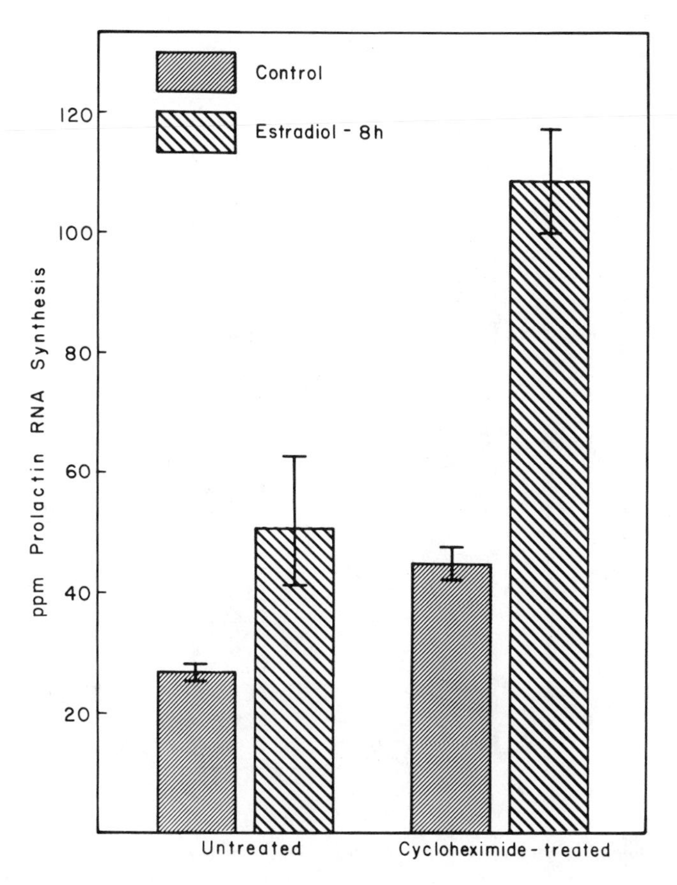

FIG. 15. Estradiol stimulates the transcription of the prolactin gene in cycloheximide-treated cultures of pituitary cells prepared from female rats. Procedures were as described in Fig. 13 except the length of estrogen treatment was 8 hours. Data are from Shull *et al.* (1984a).

transcription by 17β-estradiol (Fig. 4) is actually a composite of direct and indirect stimulatory effects of this estrogen.

Prolactin gene transcription in cultured pituitary cells was stimulated by 17β-estradiol at all time points examined between 6 and 24 hours after addition of estrogen to the cultures (Figs. 10–13, 15). These pituitary cells have little capacity for metabolizing estrogen, and the level of estrogen in the culture medium remains relatively constant. Therefore, it is not surprising that Prl gene transcription was stimulated at these time points. This difference in estrogen clearance between these *in vivo* and *in vitro* systems is extremely important and

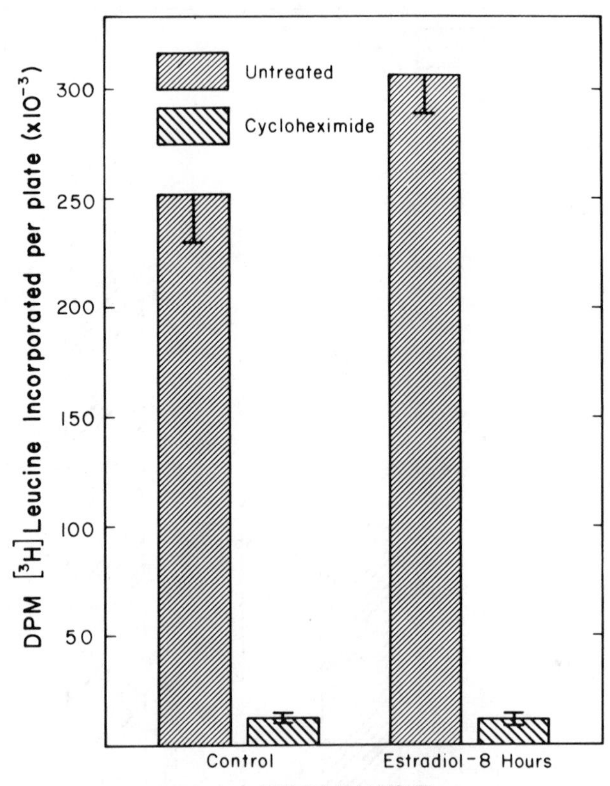

FIG. 16. The inhibitory effects of cycloheximide on protein synthesis in control and estradiol-treated pituitary cells. On day 3 of culture, the medium was changed and cycloheximide was added to a concentration of 10^{-5} *M*. Parallel cultures received the DMEM vehicle. Estradiol (or its vehicle) was added to 10^{-9} *M* 30 minutes following cycloheximide. After 5 hours of incubation, [^{3}H]leucine was added to a concentration of 10 μCi/ml. The cells were incubated for an additional 3 hours. The cells were harvested and the incorporation of [^{3}H]leucine into acid-precipitable material was assayed. Data are from Shull *et al.* (1984a).

should always be considered when one attempts to confirm through *in vitro* experimentation observations made *in vivo* and vice versa.

Estrogen stimulates the proliferation of GH_4C_1 cells, a clonal pituitary tumor cell line (Amara and Dannies, 1983), induces *in vivo* the formation of pituitary tumors which are composed almost entirely of lactotrophs (Phelps and Hymer, 1983), and may stimulte slightly the proliferation of lactotrophs in primary cultures of anterior pituitary cells (Lieberman *et al.,* 1982). Therefore the question has been raised whether the stimulatory effects of estrogen on Prl synthesis by cultured cells may be simply due to lactotroph proliferation. The data illustrating that 17β-estradiol stimulates the transcription of the Prl gene in as few as 6 hours after its addition to cultured cells (Fig. 11) and that cycloheximide does not interfere with this stimulation (Figs. 13 and 15) clearly indicate that lactotroph proliferation is not a prerequisite for the induction of this response by 17β-estradiol.

2. *Estrogen Regulates the Transcription of the Rat Prolactin Gene in Vivo through at Least Two Independent Mechanisms*

A short-acting estrogen stimulates early estrogenic responses such as water imbibition and the synthesis of the "induced protein" by the rat uterus, but not delayed responses such as uterine DNA synthesis. One such estrogen, 16α-estradiol, induced the transformation of the uterine estrogen receptor from its cytosolic form to its nuclear form; however, the level of nuclear-form receptor rapidly diminished toward baseline with a half-life of approximately 30 minutes, in contrast to a half-life of approximately 2 hours for nuclear-form receptor associated with 17β-estradiol (Kassis and Gorski, 1981). If properly administered through multiple injections, 16α-estradiol is equipotent with 17β-estradiol in its ability to stimulate DNA synthesis in the rat uterus (Stack, 1983). We have used the short-acting estrogens 16α-estradiol and estriol in our *in vivo* studies in an attempt to define further the mechanisms through which estrogen stimulates the transcription of the rat Prl gene.

16α-Estradiol stimulated the transcription of the rat Prl gene in a biphasic manner (Fig. 17). The initial phase of stimulated Prl gene transcription was detectable within 30 minutes of 16α-estradiol injection, peaked within approximately 1 hour (1.9 $\pm$ 0.4-fold stimulation) and was completed within 3 hours (1.1 $\pm$ 0.1-fold stimulation). The second phase of stimulated Prl gene transcription was observed within 6 hours of 16α-estradiol injection and continued for 24–48 hours. During this second phase, the transcription of the Prl gene was stimulated approximately 1.5-fold (Fig. 17).

The stimulatory effects of 16α-estradiol on the transcription of the rat Prl gene appeared to be specific because this estrogen did not affect the level of GH gene transcription (Fig. 18). The biphasic stimulation of Prl gene transcription by 16α-estradiol was apparent; transcription was significantly stimulated when examined 1 hour (2.9-fold; $p < 0.001$) and 6 hours (1.9-fold; $p < 0.01$) but not 3 hours ($p > 0.05$) following injection, while the transcription of the GH gene was unaffected over the entire 6-hour time course (Fig. 18).

Estriol also stimulated the transcription of the Prl gene in a biphasic

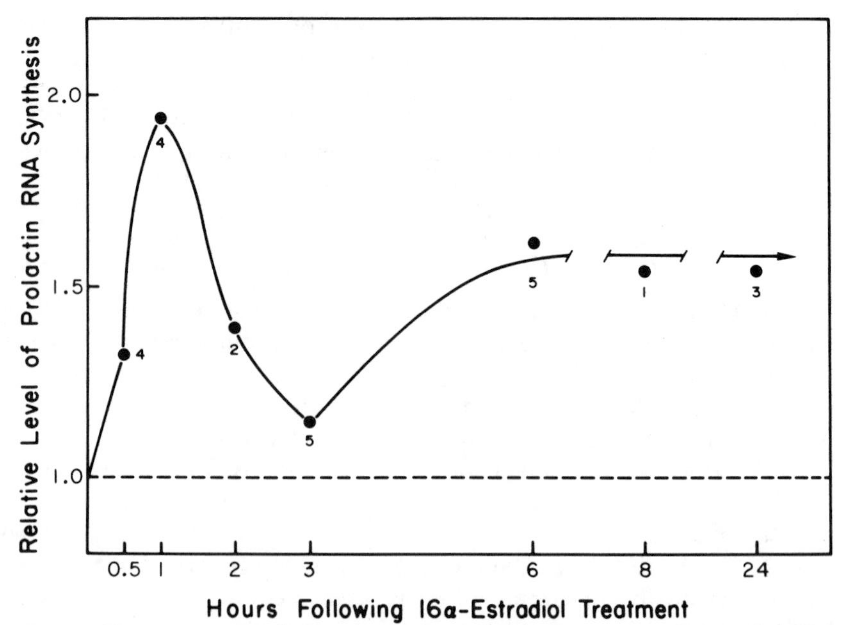

FIG. 17. Time course of prolactin gene transcription in response to 16α-estradiol. Male rats received a single injection of 16α-estradiol (10 μg, ip) at the indicated times prior to sacrifice. Nuclei were then isolated from the anterior pituitary glands and the level of prolactin gene transcription was determined as described in Shull and Gorski (1985). Each data point represents the level of prolactin gene transcription (relative to control levels) observed at the indicated time following treatment. The averaged results of several experiments are presented. As all time points were not examined in each of these experiments, the number of experiments in which each time point was examined is presented. The standard errors of these averaged values were less than 10% at all time points, except the 1-hour point where it was 21%.

manner (Fig. 19), but the initial phase extended into the second phase and the phases were distinguishable only in degree of stimulation. The first phase of stimulated Prl gene transcription was observed within 1 hour of treatment and continued for at least 3 hours. The second phase was observed by at least 6 hours following estriol injection and continued through at least 24 hours (Fig. 19).

The data presented in Table III directly contrast the stimulatory effects of 17β-estradiol, 16α-estradiol, and estriol on the transcription of the Prl gene. 17β-Estradiol and 16α-estradiol each stimulated Prl gene transcription when tested at 30 minutes or 6 hours after injection. However, 3 hours after injection of 17β-estradiol, 16α-estradiol, or estriol, transcription was stimulated by 17β-estradiol and estriol but not by 16α-estradiol (Table III).

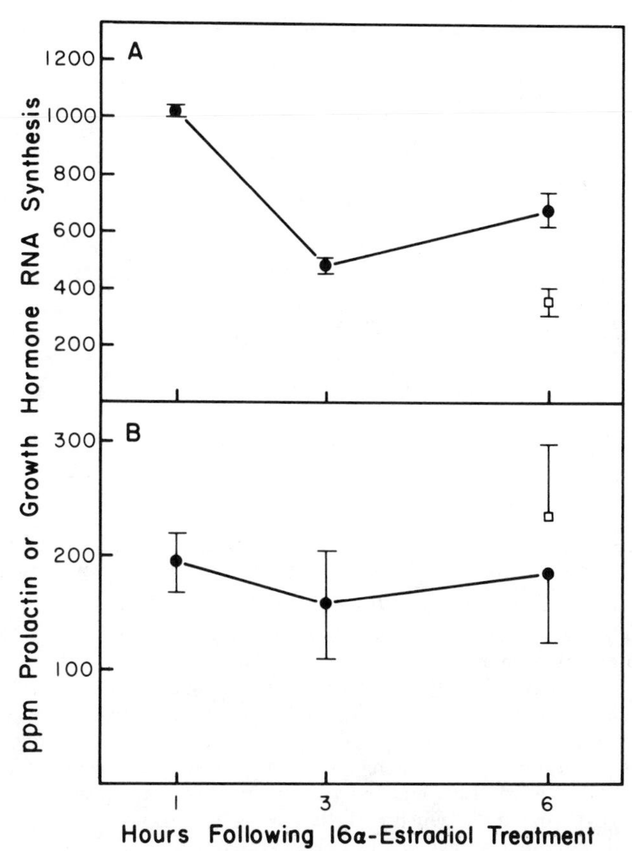

FIG. 18. Time course of prolactin and growth hormone gene transcription in response to 16α-estradiol. Procedures are as described in Shull and Gorski (1985). Each data point represents the mean (± standard error of the mean; $n = 3$) for the assay of RNA purified from a single *in vitro* transcription reaction which included nuclei isolated from 8–10 anterior pituitary glands. (A) Prolactin gene transcription: (●) 16α-estradiol (10 μg, ip); (□) sesame oil. (B) Growth hormone gene transcription; symbols as in (A).

A single injection of 16α-estradiol (10 μg, ip) caused a transitory increase in the nuclear form of the pituitary estrogen receptor and a parallel decrease in the cytosol form of this receptor (Fig. 20). The amount of nuclear-form receptor peaked within 1 hour of 16α-estradiol injection and returned virtually to the control value within 4 hours (Fig. 20A). The cytosol-form receptor decreased from 87% of total receptor in control animals to 65% within 1 hour of 16α-estradiol injection and to control amounts within 4 hours (Fig. 20B). Within the same experiment, the amount of nuclear-form receptor remained elevated, and the cytosol-form receptor diminished, for at least 6 hours after an

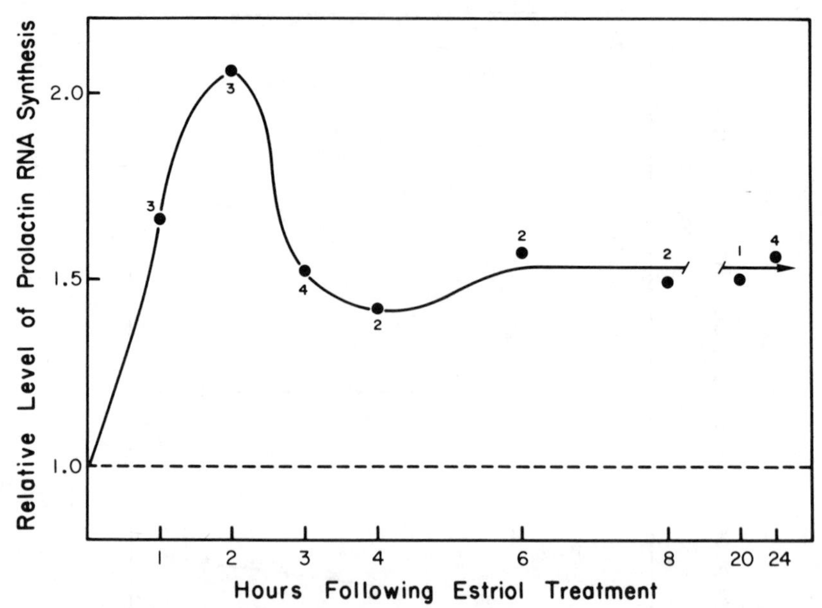

FIG. 19. Time course of prolactin gene transcription in response to estriol. Male rats received a single injection of estriol (10 μg, ip) at the indicated times prior to sacrifice. Nuclei were then isolated from the anterior pituitary glands and the level of prolactin gene transcription was determined as described in Shull and Gorski (1985). Each data point represents the level of prolactin gene transcription (relative to control levels) observed at the indicated times following treatment. The averaged results of five experiments are presented. As all time points were not examined in each of these experiments, the number of experiments in which each time point was examined is presented. The standard errors of these averaged values were less than 10% at all time points, except the 8- and 24-hour points where they were less than 15%.

equivalent injection of 17β-estradiol (Fig. 20A and B). The total amount of pituitary estrogen receptor remained constant throughout the 6 hours after an injection of 16α-estradiol while 17β-estradiol caused an approximate 25% loss of total receptor within 6 hours (Fig. 20C). This loss of estrogen receptor upon treatment with 17β-estradiol has been termed *receptor processing* and has been discussed in a recent review (Kassis and Gorski, 1983). A 24-hour response of pituitary nuclear-form and cytosol-form receptors to 17β-estradiol is illustrated in Fig. 6.

We have examined the effects of inhibitors of pituitary protein synthesis on the induction of the two phases of stimulated Prl gene transcription by 16α-estradiol. Within 1 hour after injection of 16α-estradiol, 17β-estradiol, or estriol, the transcription of the Prl gene was enhanced approximately twofold in animals pretreated with cyclohexi-

TABLE III
THE STIMULATION OF PROLACTIN GENE TRANSCRIPTION BY 17β-ESTRADIOL, 16α-ESTRADIOL, AND ESTRIOL[a]

Hours following treatment	Prolactin gene transcription (ppm) after injection with			
	Sesame oil	17β-E_2	16α-E_2	E_3
Experiment 1				
0.5 hour	228.9[b] ± 7.6 (1.0)	310.6 ± 6.6 (1.4)	355.8 ± 12.4 (1.6)	N.D.
3.0 hours	240.4 ± 9.2 (1.0)	379.1 ± 4.4 (1.6)	282.2 ± 44.3 (1.2)	N.D.
6.0 hours	245.1 ± 17.6 (1.0)	385.1 ± 12.6 (1.6)	461.9 ± 24.6 (1.9)	N.D.
Experiment 2				
3.0 hours	106.9 ± 7.0 (1.0)	178.9 ±7.0 (1.7)	103.4 ± 12.4 (1.0)	192.8 ± 24.2 (1.8)

[a] At the indicated times prior to sacrifice, male rats were injected with either 17β-estradiol (17β-E_2), 16α-estradiol (16α-E_2), estriol (E_3) (all 10 μg, ip), or the sesame oil vehicle. Nuclei were then isolated from the anterior pituitary glands (8–10 per group) and the level of Prl gene transcription was determined as described (Shull and Gorski, 1985).

[b] Three values for each data point are given. The first represents the mean ($n = 3$), and the second represents the standard error of the mean. Relative levels of Prl gene transcription are given in parentheses. N.D., Not determined.

mide (Fig. 21A). In this experiment, cycloheximide pretreatment inhibited protein synthesis by the anterior pituitary by greater than 85% (Fig. 22A). The transcription of the Prl gene was also stimulated at 1 hour after injection of 16α-estradiol in animals pretreated with puromycin (Fig. 21B) at a dose which inhibited protein synthesis by greater than 90% (Fig. 22B). These data are consistent with those presented in previous sections of this review (Figs. 7–9, 13–16) and indicate that the induction of this initial phase of stimulated Prl gene transcription by estrogen does not require the synthesis of any intermediary protein or proteins by the anterior pituitary.

The induction of the second phase of stimulated Prl gene transcription was blocked by cycloheximide pretreatment (Fig. 23A). In this

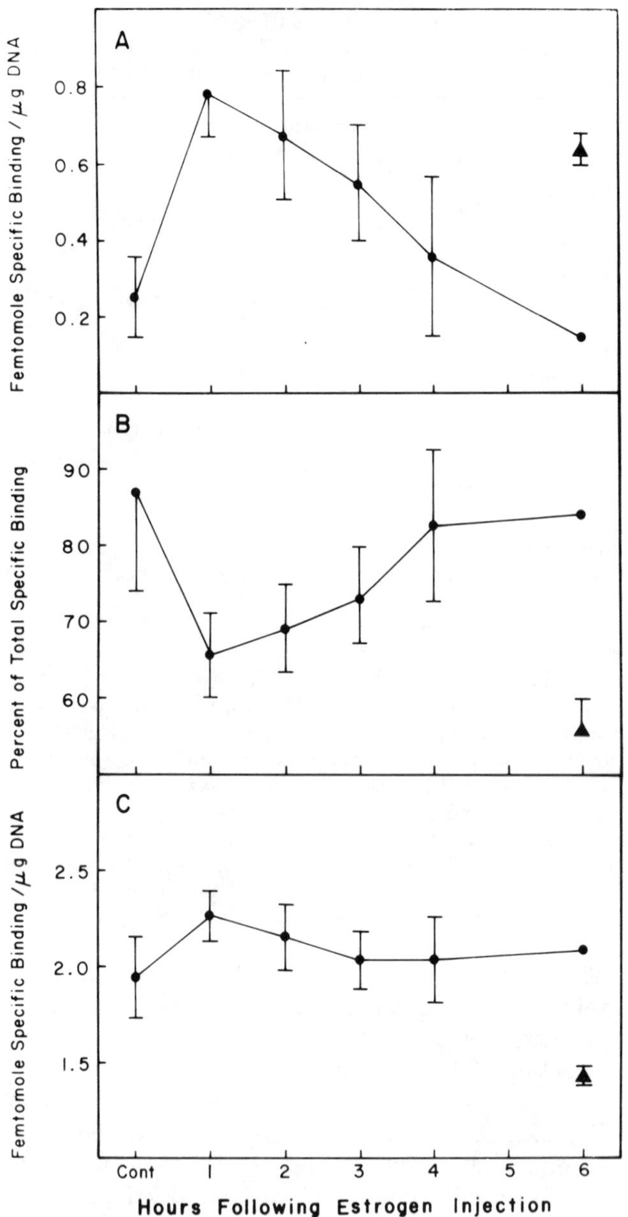

FIG. 20. Time course of transformation of the anterior pituitary estrogen receptor population following single injections of 16α-estradiol or 17β-estradiol. At the indicated times following a single injection of 16α-estradiol (●, 10 μg, ip) or 17β-estradiol (▲, 10 μg, ip) the animals (four per group) were sacrificed and the nuclear-form (A), cytosol-form (B), and total estrogen receptors (C) were assayed as described in Shull and Gorski (1985). The mean values and standard errors of the mean values are presented.

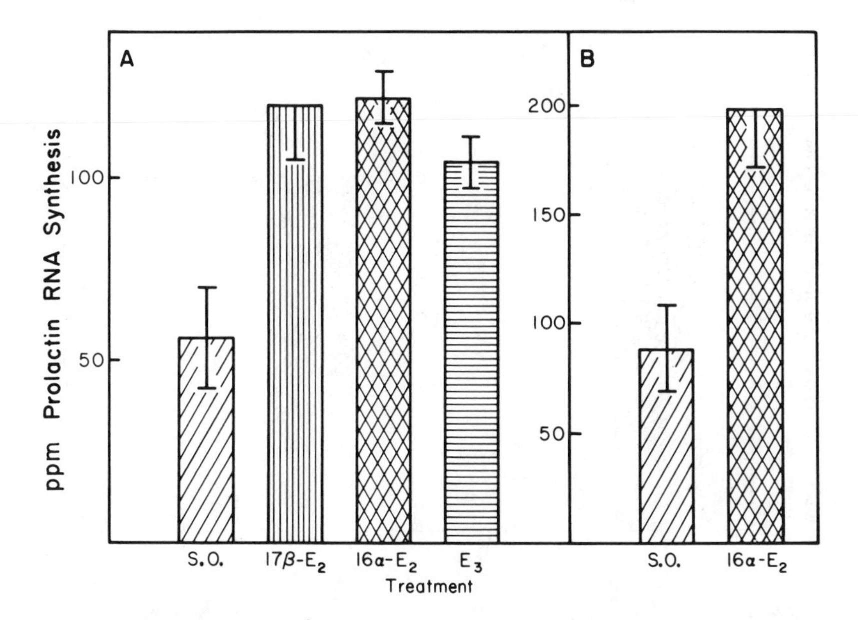

FIG. 21. The effect of inhibitors of pituitary protein synthesis on the induction of the first phase of stimulated prolactin gene transcription observed 1 hour following estrogen treatment. (A) Cycloheximide (3.33 mg/kg, ip) was injected 10 minutes prior to the indicated estrogen (10 μg, ip) or the sesame oil vehicle (S.O.). One hour following estrogen treatment, the animals were sacrificed, anterior pituitary nuclei were prepared, and prolactin gene transcription was assayed as described in Shull and Gorski (1985). (B) Puromycin (250 mg/kg, ip) was injected 10 minutes prior to 16α-estradiol (10 μg, ip) or the sesame oil vehicle. Procedures were as in (A).

experiment, cycloheximide was injected 10 minutes before and again 3 hours after 16α-estradiol. Pituitary protein synthesis was inhibited approximately 85% by cycloheximide in rats given either 16α-estradiol or its sesame oil vehicle (Fig. 24). Under these conditions the effect of 16α-estradiol on Prl gene transcription (1.17 $\pm$ 0.08-fold induction) was markedly reduced (Fig. 23A). The usual 1.5-fold induction of Prl gene transcription by 16α-estradiol was observed in control animals given saline (Fig. 23B). These data suggest that the synthesis of an intermediary protein by the anterior pituitary or another estrogen target tissue may be a prerequisite for the induction of this phase of stimulated Prl gene transcription by 16α-estradiol. However, we cannot exclude the possibility that cycloheximide interferes with other metabolic events potentially required for induction.

These data show that 16α-estradiol induces two temporally resolved phases of stimulated Prl gene transcription that differ in sensitivity to inhibitors of protein synthesis and strongly suggest that estrogen stim-

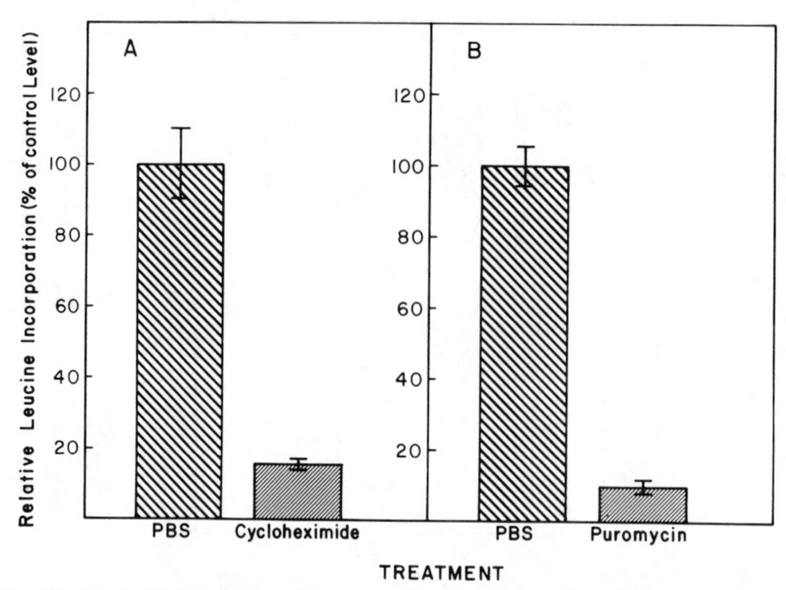

FIG. 22. The inhibitory effects of cycloheximide and puromycin on protein synthesis by the anterior pituitary, examined through a 1-hour time course. Male rats (three to five per group) were injected with (A) cycloheximide, 3.33 mg/kg, (B) puromycin, 250 mg/kg, or the PBS vehicle alone, and were injected ip 10 minutes later with [^{3}H]leucine (100 μCi per animal). The animals are sacrificed 1 hour later and the amount of leucine incorporated was assayed as described in Shull and Gorski (1985). Each data bar represents the level of [^{3}H]leucine incorporation, expressed as a percentage of the control level, and the standard error of this ratio.

ulates the transcription of the rat Prl gene *in vivo* through at least two independent mechanisms. Our observations that the initial phase of stimulated Prl gene transcription (Figs. 17 and 18) parallels the increase and subsequent decline in amount of nuclear-form pituitary estrogen receptor (Fig. 20) led us to propose that induction of the initial phase proceeds through a mechanism mediated by the nuclear-form receptor. Moreover, this mechanism is independent of protein synthesis (Figs. 21 and 22). It seems likely that this same mechanism must function in the induction of Prl gene transcription by 17β-estradiol. The difference between these two estrogens is that 16α-estradiol, with lower affinity for the estrogen receptor and reduced effectiveness in maintaining elevated levels of nuclear-form receptor (Fig. 20; Kassis and Gorski, 1981), induces an initial phase of stimulated Prl gene transcription of shorter duration than found with 17β-estradiol. Thus the two phases can be resolved in animals treated with 16α-estradiol, whereas they overlap in animals given 17β-estradiol (Fig. 25). The results of the cycloheximide experiment shown in Fig. 8 suggest that

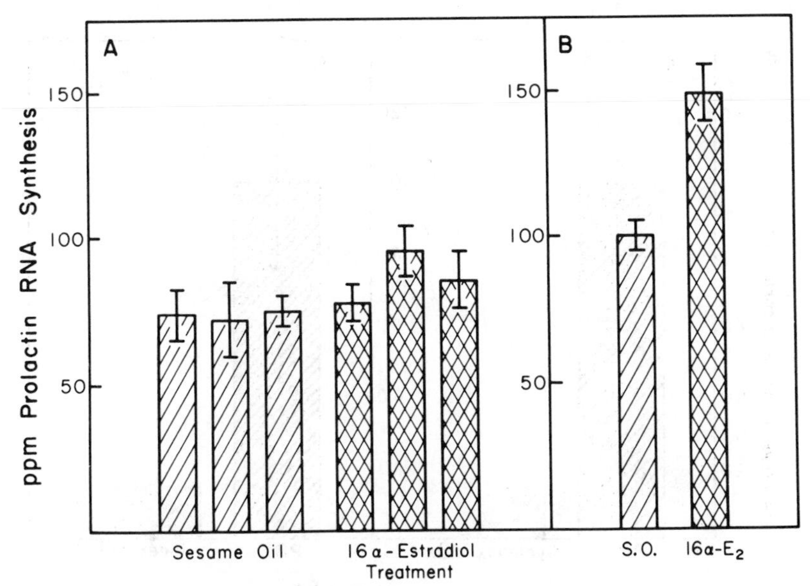

FIG. 23. The effect of cycloheximide on the induction of the second phase of stimulated prolactin gene transcription observed 6 hours following 16α-estradiol treatment. (A) Cycloheximide, 3.33 mg/kg, ip, or (B) its saline vehicle was injected 10 minutes prior to, and again 3 hours following, the injection of 16α-estradiol (10 μg, ip) or its sesame oil vehicle (S.O.). Six hours following hormone treatment, the animals were sacrificed, anterior pituitary nuclei were prepared, and prolactin gene transcription was assayed as described in Shull and Gorski (1985). Each bar represents the mean ($\pm$ standard error of the mean; $n = 3$) for the assay of RNA purified from a single *in vitro* transcription reaction which included nuclei isolated from 8–10 anterior pituitary glands.

the initial phase of stimulated transcription in 17β-estradiol-treated animals persists for at least 8 hours. Furthermore, increased amounts of nuclear-form receptor were detected for at least 6 hours after 17β-estradiol injection (Figs. 6 and 20) as opposed to 4 hours after 16α-estradiol (Fig. 20). Maurer recently showed that the rat estrogen receptor binds selectively to a region located 1.2–2.0 kb upstream from the transcription initiation site of the Prl gene. This region contains large tracts of alternating purine and pyrimidine residues that could possibly function in the formation of Z-DNA (Maurer, 1985). Further studies are required to evaluate the role of this potential regulatory domain in the regulation of transcription of the Prl gene by estrogen.

As we have discussed, it is possible that the second phase of stimulated Prl gene transcription in response to 16α-estradiol is the result of either an estrogen-induced alteration in the responsiveness of the cells of the anterior pituitary to another regulator of Prl gene transcription or an estrogen-induced alteration in the level of a second regulator

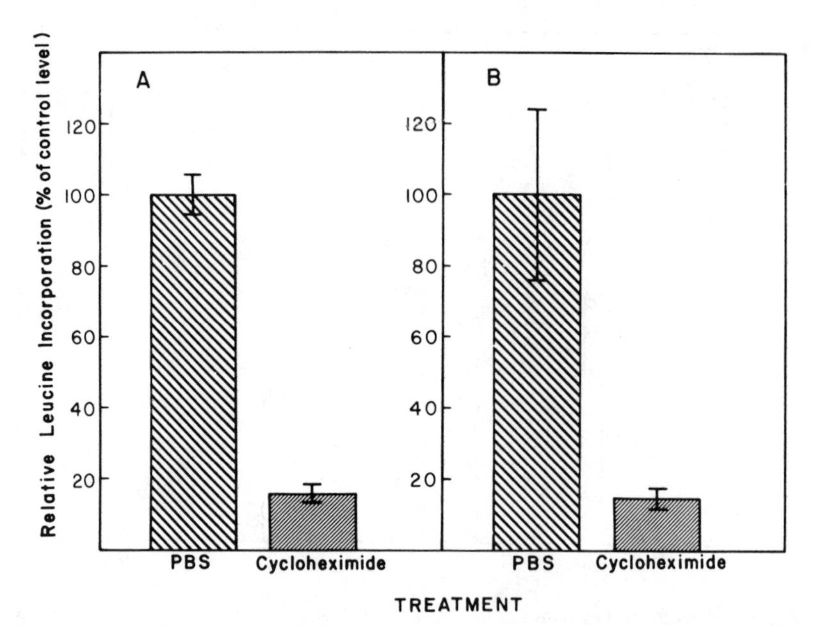

FIG. 24. The inhibitory effects of cycloheximide on protein synthesis by the anterior pituitary, examined through a 6-hour time course. Male rats (three to five per group) were injected with either cycloheximide (3.33 mg/kg) or the PBS vehicle 10 minutes prior to, and again 3 hours following, an injection of either sesame oil (A) or 16α-estradiol (B). [^{3}H]Leucine (100 μCi per injection) was injected 2 and 5 hours following treatment with the 16α-estradiol or its oil vehicle. At 6 hours relative to hormone treatment, the animals were sacrificed and the amount of leucine incorporated was assayed as described in Shull and Gorski (1985). Each data bar represents the level of [^{3}H]leucine incorporation, expressed as a percentage of the control level, and the standard error of this ratio.

reaching the cells of the anterior pituitary (Shull and Gorski, 1984, 1985). In the next section we discuss data favoring the second alternative.

3. *Pretreatment with α-Ergocryptine Blocks the Induction of the Second Phase of Stimulated Prolactin Gene Transcription by 16α-Estradiol*

Previous studies in our laboratory showed that pimozide, a dopamine antagonist, increases Prl synthesis (Maurer and Gorski, 1977) and Prl mRNA content (Stone *et al.*, 1977) *in vivo*. We found that pimozide stimulates the transcription of the Prl gene through a mechanism that is blocked by cycloheximide pretreatment (Shull *et al.*, 1984b). Furthermore, the effect on Prl gene transcription persists for

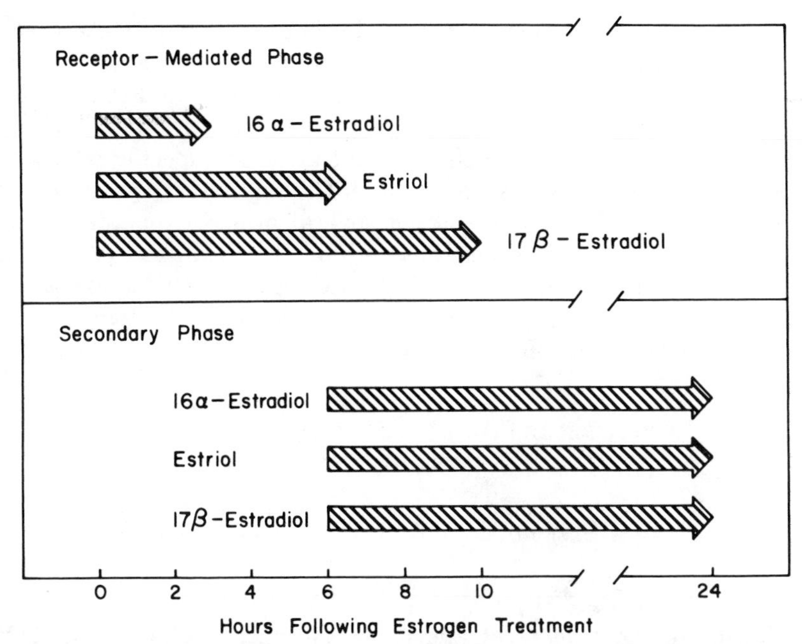

FIG. 25. A schematic representation of the two phases of stimulated prolactin gene transcription observed in response to various estrogens. The indicated duration of the receptor-mediated phase following 16α-estradiol was observed experimentally. We have approximated the duration of this phase in response to estriol and 17β-estradiol from data on the effects of these estrogens in maintaining elevated levels of nuclear-form estrogen receptors. We assume that estriol and 17β-estradiol also induce the secondary phase of stimulated Prl gene transcription within 6 hours of their injection as was observed experimentally in response to 16α-estradiol. This figure is included to illustrate our present concepts of how estrogen regulates Prl gene transcription *in vivo*.

24–48 hours after injection of pimozide. Since the effects of the dopamine antagonist pimozide resemble closely the effects of 16α-estradiol in the induction of the second phase of stimulated Prl gene transcription (Fig. 17), we hypothesized that estrogen may induce this second phase of stimulated transcription by reducing within 3–5 hours the amount of dopamine reaching the anterior pituitary gland.

α-Ergocryptine, a dopamine agonist, inhibited Prl gene transcription in cultured pituitary cells (Maurer, 1981) and *in vivo* (Shull *et al.*, 1984b). Pretreatment with α-ergocryptine blocked the induction of Prl gene transcription by pimozide. Pretreatment with α-ergocryptine also inhibited induction of the second phase of stimulated Prl gene transcription by 16α-estradiol without affecting induction of the initial phase of stimulated transcription by this estrogen (Shull *et al.*, 1984b).

The results of these experiments are admittedly difficult to interpret as little is known about the molecular mechanisms whereby dopamine agonists and antagonists affect the transcription of the Prl gene. It is possible that several regulators of Prl gene transcription may share a common mechanistic step such as modification of a specific regulatory protein. Therefore, the manipulation of the regulatory system by one factor may modulate the effects of several others. Nonetheless, the data discussed are fully consistent with our hypothesis. We recognize of course that the confirmation of this hypothesis will require the direct measure of dopamine in hypophysial portal blood during the initial hours after injection of estrogen.

IV. Regulation of Prolactin Synthesis by Other Factors: A Brief Discussion

A. Regulation by Steroid Hormones Other than Estrogen

1. *Androgen*

Pharmacological doses of androgens enhance Prl synthesis. Nine days after a 40-mg injection of testosterone enanthate, Prl synthesis was stimulated approximately six-fold in orchiectomized male rats (MacLeod *et al.*, 1969), while a 1-mg injection of testosterone propionate increased Prl synthesis 1.5-fold within 12 hours (Yamamoto *et al.*, 1975). The physiological significance of this is not clear, because orchiectomy did not significantly lower the level of Prl synthesis relative to that of intact males (Yamamoto *et al.*, 1975). In primary pituitary cell cultures, testosterone at 10^{-7} *M* stimulated Prl synthesis but 10^{-9} *M* did not (Lieberman *et al.*, 1978). The stimulatory effects of testosterone on Prl synthesis may be due to, among other possibilities, metabolic conversion of this androgen to estrogen (Baggett *et al.*, 1956) or the androgen binding to and functioning through the estrogen receptor (Ruh and Ruh, 1975).

2. *Progesterone*

The progestin 17α-hydroxyprogesterone did not affect Prl synthesis in intact male rats (MacLeod *et al.*, 1969), and progesterone was without effect in primary cultures of rat (Lieberman *et al.*, 1978) or ovine (Vician *et al.*, 1979) pituitary cells. Chen and Meites (1970) reported that progesterone inhibited the estrogen-induced increase in pituitary Prl. In cultured ovine pituitary cells, progesterone inhibited the estrogen induction of Prl mRNA and Prl synthesis (Vician *et al.*, 1979).

These reports suggested that progestins regulate Prl synthesis indirectly by altering the ability of estrogens to stimulate Prl synthesis. Progesterone inhibited estrogen receptor recycling in the rat uterus (Hsueh *et al.*, 1976). It is possible that a similar mechanism in the pituitary might lower the responsiveness of this tissue to estrogen.

3. *Glucocorticoids*

Hydrocortisone (5 μM) reduced Prl synthesis 50–80 % in GH_3 cells cultured for 7 days (Dannies and Tashjian, 1973). Similar results have been reported by Perrone *et al.* (1980). In cultured GH_4 cells, 0.3 μM dexamethasone reduced the levels of Prl mRNA and a 1.8-kb Prl RNA precursor (examined by RNA blotting procedures) within 48 hours (Potter *et al.*, 1981). Dexamethasone (1 μM) inhibited transcription of the Prl gene in cultured G/C cells by approximately 50% within 1 hour (Evans *et al.*, 1982). However, in primary cultures of rat pituitary cells, corticosterone at 10^{-9} to 10^{-7} M did not affect Prl synthesis (Lieberman *et al.*, 1978). Furthermore, at 10^{-7} M the glucocorticoid was without effect in cultures of ovine pituitary cells (Vician *et al.*, 1979). These reports clearly show that glucocorticoids inhibit Prl synthesis in cultured pituitary tumor cells and that this inhibition is most likely mediated through a reduction in Prl gene transcription. It appears that this glucocorticoid effect may be unique to these pituitary tumor cell lines, since inhibition of Prl synthesis has not been found in primary pituitary cell cultures.

4. *Vitamin D_3*

The active metabolite of vitamin D, 1α,25-dihydroxyvitamin D_3 [1,25-$(OH)_2D_3$], inhibited the basal level of Prl synthesis in cultured GH_4 cells but potentiated the stimulation of Prl synthesis by thyrotropin-releasing hormone (Murdoch and Rosenfeld, 1981). In these experiments, the ED_{50} for each response was 6×10^{-9} M. In primary cultures of rat anterior pituitary cells, 1,25-$(OH)_2D_3$ at a concentration of 5×10^{-8} M stimulated Prl synthesis by approximately 60% (Vician and Mellon, 1982). The stimulatory effect of 1,25-$(OH)_2D_3$ was additive, with an approximate 3.5-fold increase in Prl synthesis in response to 17β-estradiol at 10^{-8} M. Wark and Tashjian (1982) reported that 1,25-$(OH)_2D_3$ stimulated the synthesis of Prl (assayed by quantitating the levels of Prl accumulation in the media) by GH_4C_1 cells cultured under serum-free conditions. A small but significant 1.8-fold stimulation was observed in the initial 48 hours of treatment, while a larger 3.7-fold stimulation was observed in response to 1,25-$(OH)_2D_3$ treatment during the second 48 hours (Wark and Tashjian, 1982). Thus, both inhibitory and stimulatory effects of 1,25-$(OH)_2D_3$ on Prl synthesis have been reported.

B. Regulation by Dopamine

Dopamine is synthesized in the tuberoinfundibular neurons of the hypothalamus, released into the hypophysial portal blood system, and transported to the anterior pituitary in quantities sufficient to inhibit Prl secretion (Gibbs and Neill, 1978). This inhibitory action has been reviewed recently (Leong *et al.,* 1983; Gunnet and Freeman, 1983).

Dopamine and the dopamine agonist α-ergocryptine reduced the level of Prl mRNA in cultured pituitary cells and consequently inhibited Prl synthesis (Maurer, 1980b). Maximally inhibited levels of Prl synthesis were observed with 3–4 days of ergocryptine treatment (Maurer, 1980b). Similar results were observed *in vivo* in response to twice daily injections of the dopamine agonist 2-bromo-α-ergocryptine (Brocas *et al.,* 1981). Maurer (1981) showed that ergocryptine inhibits transcription of the Prl gene by 70–80% within 45 minutes of addition to cultured cells. Ergocryptine inhibited Prl gene transcription *in vivo* by 50–80% within 1 hour of injection (Shull *et al.,* 1984b). In contrast, pimozide, a dopamine antagonist, rapidly stimulated Prl gene transcription *in vivo* (Shull *et al.,* 1984b), resulting in increased Prl mRNA (Stone *et al.,* 1977) and Prl synthesis (Maurer and Gorski, 1977). These rapid effects of dopamine agonists and antagonists on Prl gene transcription and delayed effects on Prl mRNA and Prl synthesis suggest that Prl mRNA is quite stable, with a half-life of approximately 48 hours.

C. Regulation by Thyrotropin-Releasing Hormone

Thyrotropin-releasing hormone (THR) is a tripeptide hormone (pyroglutamyl-histidyl-proline-NH_2) synthesized in the hypothalamus (Schally *et al.,* 1978). High-affinity receptors for TRH exist in the anterior pituitary and appear to reside on the cytoplasmic membrane (Hinkle and Tashjian, 1973; Halpern and Hinkle, 1981). TRH at a concentration of 28 n*M* stimulated Prl synthesis approximately 2.5-fold in cultured GH_3 cells (Dannies and Tashjian, 1973). This increased rate of Prl synthesis is caused by an increase in Prl mRNA, as assayed by cell-free translation (Dannies and Tashjian, 1976; Evans *et al.,* 1978) and hybridization to a Prl cDNA probe (Evans *et al.,* 1978; Evans and Rosenfeld, 1979; Potter *et al.,* 1981; Biswas *et al.,* 1982; White and Bancroft, 1983). Using techniques similar to those described in this

review (Fig. 3), Murdoch *et al.* (1983) found that TRH (3×10^{-7} *M*) stimulated the transcription of the Prl gene 7- to 10-fold within minutes of addition to cultured GH_4 cells. After 1 hour the stimulation of Prl gene transcription began to decline; Prl gene transcription remained stimulated approximately twofold at 36 hours (Murdoch *et al.*, 1983).

An intensive effort is being directed toward understanding the mechanisms through which TRH regulates Prl gene expression. TRH induces the phosphorylation of a number of cytoplasmic proteins in cultured GH_3 and GH_4C_1 cells (Drust *et al.*, 1982; Drust and Martin, 1982; Sobel and Tashjian, 1983; Drust and Martin, 1984). Furthermore, the phosphorylation of certain cytoplasmic proteins appears linked to Prl release from the cells while phosphorylation of others appears linked to Prl synthesis (Sobel and Tashjian, 1983). Phosphorylation of a nuclear protein correlated with the stimulation of Prl gene transcription by TRH in cultured GH_4 cells (Murdoch *et al.*, 1983). White and Bancroft (1983) found that EGTA blocks the TRH induction of Prl mRNA in GH_3 cells, suggesting that calcium may be a second messenger for TRH regulation of Prl synthesis. Further experiments are required to identify the mechanisms involved and to determine whether phosphorylation of specific cytoplasmic and nuclear proteins is obligatory in TRH action.

D. Regulation by Epidermal Growth Factor

Epidermal growth factor (EGF) interacts specifically with a receptor on the surface of GH_3D6 cells (Johnson *et al.*, 1980). In this strain of pituitary tumor cells, EGF (25 ng/ml) induced Prl synthesis by 5.7-fold (Johnson *et al.*, 1980). In GH_4C_1 cells, treatment for 2–6 days with EGF (10^{-8} *M*) caused 5- to 9-fold stimulation of Prl synthesis (Schonbrunn *et al.*, 1980). Furthermore, these authors showed that the effects of EGF on stimulation of Prl synthesis were quantitatively different (although qualitatively similar) from effects of TRH (Schonbrunn *et al.*, 1980). EGF (5×10^{-8} *M*) rapidly stimulated transcription of the Prl gene in cultured GH_4 cells, yielding increased amounts of Prl precursor RNA and mature Prl mRNA (Murdoch *et al.*, 1982b). The fusion of 5′ flanking sequences from the rat Prl gene to structural and intervening sequences from the rat GH gene produced a chimeric gene whose transcription was enhanced by EGF upon introduction into human A431 cells possessing EGF receptors. Thus the 5′ flanking region of the Prl gene contains the sequences required for transcriptional regulation by EGF (Supowit *et al.*, 1984). In GH_3 cells cultured with EGTA to chelate calcium ions, EGF (10 n*M*) induced a fourfold increase in Prl mRNA; in cultures containing calcium (0.4 m*M*) EGF increased Prl mRNA content 66-fold (White and Bancroft, 1983). These data suggest that EGF stimulates Prl gene transcription through a mechanism requiring calcium, and thereby increases Prl mRNA content and Prl synthesis. The physiological importance of this regulation by EGF remains to be determined.

E. Regulation by Thyroid Hormones

L-Triiodothyronine (T_3) inhibits Prl synthesis in primary cultures of rat anterior pituitary cells; Prl synthesis was reduced by approximately 75% with 6 days of treatment with T_3 (10 n*M*) (Maurer, 1982d). L-Thyroxine (T_4) inhibited Prl synthesis as well, but with a potency one-tenth that of T_3 (Maurer, 1982d). It was also shown that the T_3-mediated decrease in Prl synthesis paralleled a decrease in Prl mRNA content (Maurer, 1982d). It is of interest to note that 17β-estradiol (10^{-9} *M*) did not block T_3 inhibition of Prl synthesis as it did the effect of ergocryptine (Maurer, 1982b). Contrasting effects of T_3 on Prl synthesis were observed in GH_3 cells; Prl synthesis was increased approximately twofold following 6 days of T_3 treatment at 50 n*M* (Perrone *et al.*, 1980). Prl synthesis in GH_1 cells was reduced by approximately 50% by 48-hour treatment with 0.5 n*M* T_3 (Stanley and Samuels, 1984). In cells pretreated with *n*-butyrate, however, T_3 increased Prl synthesis and Prl mRNA (Stanley and Samuels, 1984). The authors suggested that the reversal in T_3 action on Prl synthesis may be due to *n*-butyrate-induced alterations in the acetylation of chromatin proteins. These studies suggest thyroid hormones are physiological regulators of Prl gene expression.

F. Regulation by Platelet-Derived Growth Factor

Platelet-derived growth factor (PDGF) inhibited the production (release of Prl into the culture medium) of Prl by cultured GH_3 and GH_4C_1 cells (Sullivan and Tashjian, 1983). This inhibition was likely due to a reduction in Prl synthesis. In this study, PDGF at a concentration of 50 ng/ml maximally inhibited Prl production by approximately 50% with 4–7 days of treatment. The physiological importance of PDGF in regulating Prl gene expression is not known at this time (Sullivan and Tashjian, 1983).

G. Regulation by Vasoactive Intestinal Peptide

Vasoactive intestinal peptide (VIP) effected an increase in Prl mRNA and putative precursors of Prl mRNA in GH_3 cells (Carillo *et al.*, 1985). The increase in Prl mRNA observed at 25 hours with VIP at 2×10^{-7} to 2×10^{-8} M paralleled increased Prl release into the culture medium (Carillo *et al.*, 1985). VIP regulates Prl gene expression at a pretranslational level, likely through stimulation of Prl gene transcription. VIP is released by the hypothalamus into hypophysial portal blood (Said and Porter, 1979; Shimatsu *et al.*, 1981). Therefore, it is possible that VIP is a physiological regulator of Prl gene expression.

H. Regulation by Prolactin

Prolactin regulates its own expression. This action is mediated, at least in part, at the level of the hypothalamus through induction of dopamine release into the hypophysial portal blood (Gudelsky and Porter, 1980). At the pituitary level Prl does not appear to regulate its expression; ovine Prl did not alter the rate of either Prl synthesis or Prl secretion by rat anterior pituitary cells in primary culture (Vician *et al.*, 1982).

I. Regulation by Adenosine 3′, 5′-Monophosphate

Adenosine 3′,5′-monophosphate (cAMP) is often considered an intracellular mediator of hormone action. Dopamine inhibited adenylate cyclase activity in the rat anterior pituitary (Giannattasio *et al.*, 1981) and depressed cAMP levels in cultured pituitary cells (Swennen and Denef, 1982). In contrast, TRH increased cAMP levels in cultured GH_4C_1 cells (Dannies *et al.*, 1976).

Ergocryptine, a dopamine agonist, inhibited in parallel cAMP production and Prl synthesis by cultured pituitary cells (Maurer, 1982c). An analog of cAMP, monobutyryl cAMP, antagonized in a dose-dependent manner this inhibitory effect of ergocryptine; Prl synthesis and mRNA content were restored to basal levels in cultures treated with both ergocryptine and the cAMP analog (Maurer, 1982c). The antagonistic effects of monobutyryl cAMP with respect to ergocryptine inhibition of Prl synthesis appeared to be mediated at the level of Prl gene transcription (Maurer, 1981).

In cultured GH_4 cells, cAMP analogs stimulated Prl gene transcription within 20 minutes (Murdoch *et al.*, 1982a). The transcription of the Prl gene was also stimulated within minutes by forskolin, a compound which activates adenylate cyclase, and this caused an increase in Prl mRNA content (Murdoch *et al.*, 1982a). Forskolin treatment also increased phosphorylation of a basic chromatin-associated protein (Murdoch *et al.*, 1982a). Increased phosphorylation of this protein has been observed in GH_4 cells in response to TRH (Murdoch *et al.*, 1983), EGF, and phorbol esters (Murdoch *et al.*, 1985). It has been suggested that the increased phosphorylation of this protein may be a necessary step in the stimulation of Prl gene transcription by these compounds (Murdoch *et al.*, 1982a).

In other studies cAMP has not affected Prl synthesis. In cultured GH_1 cells, forskolin increased cAMP levels 400-fold without effect on Prl synthesis (Stanley and Samuels, 1984). Monobutyryl cAMP alone did not stimulate Prl synthesis in primary cultures of anterior pituitary cells although this analog did antagonize the inhibition of Prl synthesis by ergocryptine (Maurer, 1982c).

The data discussed in this section suggest that cAMP may be involved in the regulation of Prl gene expression by certain hormones, but its precise function is unknown. One question to be answered is whether the phosphorylation of the basic chromatin-associated protein observed by Murdoch *et al.* (1982a) is a requisite step in activating Prl gene transcription.

V. Possible Estrogenic Modulation of Regulation of Prolactin Synthesis by Other Factors

A. Effects of Estrogen on Regulation by Dopamine

The mechanisms controlling dopamine release into the hypophysial portal blood are not entirely understood. (For a recent review of the regulation of catecholamine metabolism in the hypothalamus see Barraclough and Wise, 1982.) Estrogen receptors have been localized in dopaminergic neurons of the tuberoinfundibular system (Sar, 1984), but the effect of estrogen on dopamine release from these neurons is not clear.

17β-Estradiol (50 μg) blocked the usual increase in dopamine concentration in the hypophysial portal plasma of cycling female rats between proestrus and estrus (Cramer *et al.*, 1979). In this study, the authors concluded that 17β-estradiol acutely suppresses release of dopamine into hypophysial portal blood from the hypothalamus. In contrast, 5 daily injections of estradiol benzoate (25 μg/kg) caused a 2.5-fold increase in dopamine concentration in hypophysial portal plasma (Gudelsky *et al.*, 1981). However, this treatment also significantly increased Prl in the circulation (Gudelsky *et al.*, 1981). The same group showed that Prl, injected intracerebroventricularly, increases dopamine concentration in hypophysial portal plasma (Gudelsky and Porter, 1980). Therefore, it is possible that the effect of chronic estrogen treatment on dopamine release from the hypothalamus is mediated by Prl (Gudelsky *et al.*, 1981).

A specific interaction between dopamine and a receptor in the membrane fraction of anterior pituitary cells has been described (Caron *et al.*, 1978; Cronin *et al.*, 1978; De Lean *et al.*, 1982; Sibley *et al.*, 1982). The affinity of a number of dopamine agonists for this receptor correlated highly with potency of these agonists in inhibiting Prl secretion, and the affinity of antagonists correlated with potency in blocking the inhibitory effect of dopamine (Caron *et al.*, 1978). These reports strongly suggest that dopamine functions through this receptor in regulating Prl gene expression.

Recent studies have suggested that the number of anterior pituitary dopamine receptors is regulated. In cycling female rats dopamine binding capacity was greatest on the afternoon of proestrus, decreased through estrus and diestrus I, and was lowest on diestrus II through the morning of proestrus (Heiman and Ben-Jonathan, 1982a). The effect of estrogen on the dopamine receptor is not clear. In ovariectomized female rats, 5 daily injections of estradiol benzoate (5 or 25 μg/kg) reduced the number of anterior pituitary dopamine receptors by 30 or 50%, respectively, without altering their affinity for ligand (Heiman and Ben-Jonathan, 1982b). In contrast, twice daily injections of 17β-estradiol (10 μg) for 7 days did not affect dopamine receptor level in the anterior pituitary of ovariectomized female rats (Di Paolo *et al.*, 1979). In ovariectomized rats implanted for 48–54 hours or 72–78 hours with silastic capsules containing 17β-estradiol, the dopamine receptor number was similar to that observed in control animals (Pilotte *et al.*, 1984). It is possible that varying results from study to study may reflect the dose of estrogen administered.

The reports discussed in this section indicate that dopamine is a physiological regulator of Prl gene expression. Points at which the inhibitory effects of dopamine might be modulated by estrogen have been discussed. Interestingly, estrogen partially antagonizes dopamine inhibition of Prl secretion (Raymond *et al.*, 1978) and Prl synthesis (Maurer, 1982b) by cultured pituitary cells. At present, the mechanism of this antagonism remains unknown.

B. Effects of Estrogen on Regulation by Thyrotropin-Releasing Hormone

The interaction of TRH with a specific receptor on the cytoplasmic membrane enhances Prl gene transcription, accumulation of Prl mRNA, and the rate of Prl synthesis (Section IV,C). The number of TRH receptors in the anterior pituitary varies during the estrous cycle of the female rat; minimal TRH binding capacity is observed on the morning of diestrus II while maximal binding capacity develops on the evening of proestrus (De Lean *et al.,* 1977a). Daily injections of estradiol benzoate (25 μg) to male rats significantly increased TRH binding capacity after 4 injections, while 7–10 injections produced maximal increases of 2.5- to 3-fold (De Lean *et al.,* 1977b). Estradiol benzoate also increased TRH binding capacity in the anterior pituitary of the female rat without affecting affinity of the binding sites for TRH (De Lean *et al.,* 1977b). 17β-Estradiol induced the release of TRH from the hypothalamus; hypothalamic tissue removed from ovariectomized female rats implanted with silastic capsules containing 17β-estradiol released threefold more TRH into the incubation medium than tissue from control animals (Franks *et al.,* 1984). Thus, estrogen may indirectly affect Prl gene expression *in vivo* by increasing TRH release from the hypothalamus and by increasing the responsiveness of the anterior pituitary to TRH by increasing the number of TRH receptors.

VI. Summary

We have reviewed the evidence that estrogen stimulates the transcription of the rat Prl gene *in vivo* through at least two independent mechanisms. One mechanism does not require synthesis of any intermediary protein by the anterior pituitary and appears to be mediated directly by the estrogen receptor. The second mechanism is as yet undefined but may be mediated through a reduction in amount of dopamine (an inhibitor of Prl gene transcription) reaching the cells of the anterior pituitary. These mechanisms, as well as other points at which estrogen might modulate Prl gene transcription *in vivo,* are represented in Fig. 26.

An initial goal of our study was to determine the effects of a single pulse of estrogen on the transcription of the Prl and GH genes. Our observations that estrogen stimulates Prl gene transcription through two mechanisms, which can be temporally resolved, illustrate the importance of time in determining hormone effect. Further studies indicated the dose of administered estrogen was also important; doses yielding near-physiological levels of circulating estrogen gave maxi-

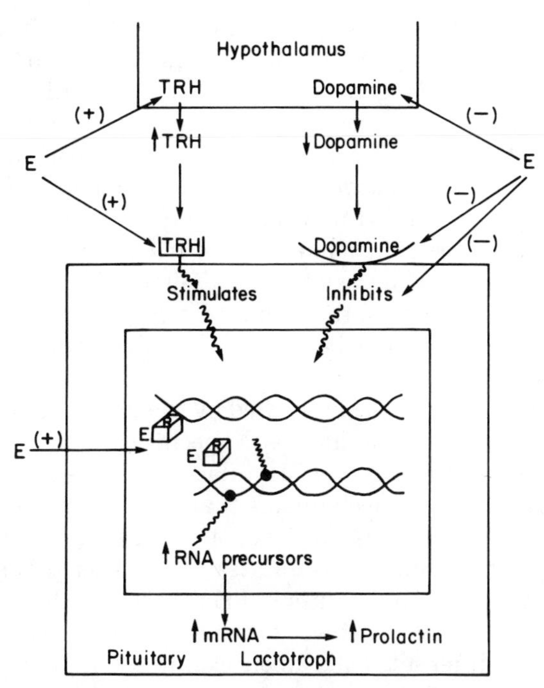

FIG. 26. An illustration of the pathways through which estrogen might regulate prolactin gene transcription *in vivo*. Estrogen acts directly on the cells of the anterior pituitary and stimulates Prl gene transcription through a mechanism which is independent of pituitary protein synthesis and which appears to be mediated by the nuclear form of the estrogen receptor. Our data also suggest the possibility that estrogen may exert a stimulatory effect by reducing the level of dopamine reaching the cells of the anterior pituitary. At the present time this hypothesis is unconfirmed. Other possible mechanisms through which estrogen might modulate the regulation of Prl gene transcription by other factors include (1) increasing TRH release from the hypothalamus, (2) increasing pituitary TRH receptors, (3) decreasing pituitary dopamine receptors, and (4) decreasing the responsiveness of the pituitary to dopamine. See text for further discussion.

mal stimulation of the initial phase of the biphasic response while hyperphysiological doses failed to stimulate this initial phase of Prl gene transcription (J. D. Shull and J. Gorski, unpublished observations). Therefore, in our review, we have indicated doses of estrogen administered and times at which levels of Prl synthesis, mRNA, or gene transcription were measured.

As a model system for our studies, we have chosen the intact male rat. Similar effects of estrogen on Prl gene transcription have been observed in ovariectomized female rats (Maurer, 1982a). In addition, our studies have shown that cultured anterior pituitary cells derived from intact male or female rats respond to estrogen in a similar manner. The synthesis (Ieiri *et al.*, 1971) and secretion (Butcher *et al.*, 1974) of Prl appear to vary during the estrous cycle. A single injection of estrogen stimulates Prl gene transcription for 48–72 hours and the mRNA for Prl appears to be very stable. In combination these observations suggest either that Prl synthesis is regulated throughout the estrous cycle at a point subsequent to transcription or that a factor or factors exist in intact female rats which would serve in the attenuation of the transcriptional response to estrogen. In cultured pituitary cells, the level of Prl synthesis invariably parallels the level of Prl mRNA, implying that regulation of this gene is solely transcriptional. Although the same may prove to be true *in vivo,* we should not make this assumption hastily.

In vivo studies are clearly complicated by the multitude of pathways through which a hormone might alter a specific cellular response (Fig. 26). A transitory pulse of estrogen stimulates Prl gene transcription *in vivo* through at least two mechanisms that increase Prl synthesis. In cultured pituitary cells a constant level of estrogen, likely functioning through a single mechanism, stimulates the transcription of the Prl gene and also results in an increase in Prl synthesis. Although the end results may be similar, the pathways through which these results were elicited are quite different. Only upon examination at the transcriptional level do these differences become apparent. In most cell culture systems we generally examine the effects of constant levels of regulatory factors over relatively long periods of time. However, in the intact organism, hormone concentrations are dynamic and seldom, if ever, constant. We can now examine within minutes of treatment the effects of hormones on the transcription of specific genes. These capabilities should aid greatly in our attempts to identify the biochemical events required for the regulation of gene expression by hormones.

ACKNOWLEDGMENT

This work was supported by the College of Agricultural and Life Sciences, University of Wisconsin–Madison: NIH Grants HD-08192 and CA-18110 to J. Gorski; NIH Training Grant 5-T32-HD-07007-05; and a Steenbock Predoctoral Fellowship to J. D. Shull. We extend our thanks to Julie Busby for her aid in preparing the manuscript.

REFERENCES

Amara, J. F., and Dannies, P. S. (1983). 17β-Estradiol has a biphasic effect on GH cell growth. *Endocrinology* **112,** 1141–1143.

Baggett, B., Engel, L. L., Savard, K., and Dorfman, R. L. (1956). The conversion of testosterone-3-C^{14} to C^{14}-estradiol-17β by human ovarian tissue. *J. Biol. Chem.* **221,** 931–941.

Baker, B. L., Clark, R. H., and Hunter, R. L. (1963). Starch gel electrophoresis of rat hypophysis in relation to prolactin activity. *Proc. Soc. Exp. Biol. Med.* **114,** 251–255.

Barraclough, C. A., and Wise, P. M. (1982). The role of catecholamines in the regulation of pituitary luteinizing hormone and follicle-stimulating hormone secretion. *Endocr. Rev.* **3,** 91–119.

Bartke, A. (1980). Role of prolactin in reproduction in male mammals. *Fed. Proc., Fed. Am. Soc. Exp. Biol.* **39,** 2577–2581.

Biswas, D. K., Hanes, S. D., and Brennessel, B. A. (1982). Mechanism of induction of prolactin synthesis in GH cells. *Proc. Natl. Acad. Sci. U.S.A.* **79,** 66–70.

Brocas, H., Coevorden, A. V., Seo, H., Refetoff, S., and Vassart, G. (1981). Dopaminergic control of prolactin mRNA accumulation in the pituitary of the male rate. *Mol. Cell Endocrinol.* **22,** 25–30.

Butcher, R. L., Collins, W. E., and Fugo, N. W. (1974). Plasma concentrations of LH, FSH, prolactin, progesterone and estradiol-17β throughout the 4-day estrous cycle of the rat. *Endocrinology* **94,** 1704–1708.

Caron, M. G., Beaulieu, M., Raymond, V., Gagne, B., Drouin, J., Lefkowitz, R. J., and Labrie, F. (1978). Dopaminergic receptors in the anterior pituitary gland. *J. Biol. Chem.* **253,** 2244–2253.

Carrillo, A. J., Pool, T. B., and Sharp, Z. D. (1985). Vasoactive intestinal peptide increases prolactin messenger ribonucleic acid content in GH_3 cells. *Endocrinology* **116,** 202–206.

Chen, C. L., and Meites, J. (1970). Effects of estrogen and progesterone on serum and pituitary prolactin levels in ovariectomized rats. *Endocrinology* **86,** 503–508.

Chien, Y.-H, and Thompson, E. B. (1980). Genomic organization of rat prolactin and growth hormone genes. *Proc. Natl. Acad. Sci. U.S.A.* **77,** 4583–4587.

Clemens, J. A., and Shaar, C. J. (1980). Control of prolactin secretion in mammals. *Fed. Proc., Fed. Am. Soc. Exp. Biol.* **39,** 2588–2592.

Cooke, N. E., and Baxter, J. D. (1982). Structural analysis of the prolactin gene suggests a separate origin for its 5′ end. *Nature (London)* **297,** 603–606.

Cramer, O. M., Parker, C. R., and Porter, J. C. (1979). Estrogen inhibition of dopamine release into hypophysial portal blood. *Endocrinology* **104,** 419–422.

Cronin, M. J., Roberts, J. M., and Weiner, R. I. (1978). Dopamine and dihydroergocryptine binding to the anterior pituitary and other brain areas of the rat and sheep. *Endocrinology* **103,** 302–309.

Dannies, P. S., and Tashjian, A. H., Jr. (1973). Effects of thyrotropin-releasing hormone and hydrocortisone on synthesis and degradation of prolactin in a rat pituitary cell strain. *J. Biol. Chem.* **248,** 6174–6179.

Dannies, P. S., and Tashjian, A. H., Jr. (1976). Thyrotropin-releasing hormone increases prolactin mRNA activity in the cytoplasm of GH cells as measured by translation in a wheat germ cell-free system. *Biochem. Biophys. Res. Comm.* **70,** 1180–1189.

Dannies, P. S., Gautvik, K. M., and Tashjian, A. H., Jr. (1976). A possible role of cyclic AMP in mediating the effects of thyrotropin-releasing hormone on prolactin release and on prolactin and growth hormone synthesis in pituitary cells in culture. *Endocrinology* **98,** 1147–1159.

De Lean, A., Ferland, L., Drouin, J., Kelly, P. A., and Labrie, F. (1977a). Modulation of pituitary thyrotropin releasing hormone receptor levels by estrogens and thyroid hormones. *Endocrinology* **100,** 1496–1504.

De Lean, A., Garon, M., Kelly, P. A., and Labrie, F. (1977b). Changes of pituitary thyrotropin releasing hormone (TRH) receptor level and prolactin response to TRH during the rat estrous cycle. *Endocrinology* **100,** 1505–1510.

De Lean, A., Kilpatrick, B. F., and Caron, M. G. (1982). Guanine nucleotides regulate both dopaminergic agonist and antagonist binding in porcine anterior pituitary. *Endocrinology* **110,** 1064–1066.

DiPaolo, T., Carmichael, R., Labrie, F., and Raynaud, J. P. (1979). Effects of estrogens on the characteristics of [^{3}H]spiroperidol and [^{3}H]RU24213 binding in rat anterior pituitary gland and brain. *Mol. Cell. Endocrinol.* **16,** 99–112.

Drust, D. S., and Martin, T. F. J. (1982). Thyrotropin-releasing hormone rapidly and transiently stimulates cytosolic calcium-dependent protein phosphorylation in GH_3 pituitary cells. *J. Biol. Chem.* **257,** 7566–7573.

Drust, D. S., and Martin, T. F. J. (1984). Thyrotropin-releasing hormone rapidly activates protein phosphorylation in GH_3 pituitary cells by a lipid-linked, protein kinase C-mediated pathway. *J. Biol. Chem.* **259,** 14520–14530.

Drust, D. S., Sutton, C. A., and Martin, T. F. J. (1982). Thyrotropin releasing hormone and cyclic AMP activate distinctive pathways of protein phosphorylation in GH pituitary cells. *J. Biol. Chem.* **257,** 3306–3312.

Durrin, L. K., Weber, J. L., and Gorski, J. (1984). Chromatin structure, transcription and methylation of the prolactin gene domain in pituitary tumors of Fischer 344 rats. *J. Biol. Chem.* **259,** 7086–7093.

Emerson, B. M., Lewis, C. D., and Felsenfeld, G. (1985). Interaction of specific nuclear factors with the nuclease-hypersensitive region of the chicken adult β-globin gene: Nature of the binding domain. *Cell* **41,** 21–30.

Evans, G. A., and Rosenfeld, M. G. (1976). Cell-free synthesis of a prolactin precursor directed by mRNA from cultured rat pituitary cells. *J. Biol. Chem.* **251,** 2842–2847.

Evans, G. A., and Rosenfeld, M. G. (1979). Regulation of prolactin mRNA analyzed using a specific cDNA probe. *J. Biol. Chem.* **254,** 8023–8030.

Evans, G. A., David, D. N., and Rosenfeld, M. G. (1978). Regulation of prolactin and somatotropin mRNAs by thyroliberin. *Proc. Natl. Acad. Sci. U.S.A.* **75,** 1294–1298.

Evans, R. M., Birnberg, N. C., and Rosenfeld, M. G. (1982). Glucocorticoid and thyroid hormones transcriptionally regulate growth hormone gene expression. *Proc. Natl. Acad. Sci. U.S.A.* **79,** 7659–7663.

Franks, S., Mason, H. D., Shennan, K. I. J., and Sheppard, M. C. (1984). Stimulation of prolactin secretion by oestradiol in the rat is associated with increased hypothalamic release of thyrotropin-releasing hormone. *J. Endocrinol.* **103,** 257–261.

Giannattasio, G., DeFerrari, M. E., and Spada, A. (1981). Dopamine-inhibited adenylate cyclase in female rat adenohypophysis. *Life Sci.* **28,** 1605–1612.

Gibbs, D. M., and Neill, J. D. (1978). Dopamine levels in hypophysial stalk blood in the rat are sufficient to inhibit prolactin secretion *in vivo*. *Endocrinology* **102,** 1895–1900.

Gorski, J., and Gannon, F. (1976). Current models of steroid hormone action: A critique. *Annu. Rev. Physiol.* **38,** 425–450.

Gorski, J., Welshons, W., and Sakai, D. (1984). Remodeling the estrogen receptor model. *Mol. Cell. Endocrinol.* **36,** 11–15.

Gubbins, E. J., Maurer, R. A., Lagrimini, M., Erwin, C. R., and Donelson, J. E. (1980). Structure of the rat prolactin gene. *J. Biol. Chem.* **255,** 8655–8662.

Gudelsky, G. A., and Porter, J. C. (1980). Release of dopamine from tuberoinfundibular neurons into pituitary stalk blood after prolactin or haloperidol administration. *Endocrinology* **106,** 526–529.

Gudelsky, G., Nansel, D. D., and Porter, J. C. (1981). Role of estrogen in the dopaminergic control of prolactin secretion. *Endocrinology* **108,** 440–444.

Gunnet, J. W., and Freeman, M. E. (1983). The mating-induced release of prolactin: A unique neuroendocrine response. *Endocr. Rev.* **4,** 44–61.

Halpern, J., and Hinkle, P. M. (1981). Direct visualization of receptors for thyrotropin-releasing hormone with a fluorescein-labeled analog. *Proc. Natl. Acad. Sci. U.S.A.* **78,** 587–591.

Heiman, M. L., and Ben-Jonathan, N. (1982a). Dopaminergic receptors in the rat anterior pituitary change during the estrous cycle. *Endocrinology* **111,** 37–41.

Heiman, M. L., and Ben-Jonathan, N. (1982b). Rat anterior pituitary dopaminergic receptors are regulated by estradiol and during lactation. *Endocrinology* **111,** 1057–1060.

Hinkle, P. M., and Tashjian, A. H., Jr. (1973). Receptors for thyrotropin-releasing hormone in prolactin producing rat pituitary cells in culture. *J. Biol. Chem.* **248,** 6180–6186.

Hoffman, L. M., Fritsch, M. K., and Gorski, J. (1981). Probable nuclear precursors of preprolactin mRNA in rat pituitary cells. *J. Biol. Chem.* **256,** 2597–2600.

Horrobin, D. F. (1980). Prolactin as a regulator of fluid and electrolyte metabolism in mammals. *Fed. Proc., Fed. Am. Soc. Exp. Biol.* **39,** 2567–2570.

Hsueh, A. J. W., Peck, E. J., Jr., and Clark, J. H. (1976). Control of uterine estrogen receptor level by progesterone. *Endocrinology* **98,** 438–444.

Hymer, W. C., Snyder, J., Wilfinger, W., Swanson, N., and Davis, J. A. (1974). Separation of pituitary mammotrophs from the female rat by velocity sedimentation at unit gravity. *Endocrinology* **95,** 107–122.

Ieiri, T., Akikusa, Y., and Yamamoto, K. (1971). Synthesis and release of prolactin and growth hormone *in vitro* during the estrous cycle of the rat. *Endocrinology* **89,** 1533–1537.

Johnson, L. K., Baxter, J. D., Vlodavsky, I., and Gospodarowicz, D. (1980). Epidermal growth factor and expression of specific genes: Effects on cultured rat pituitary cells are dissociable from the mitogenic response. *Proc. Natl. Acad. Sci. U.S.A.* **77,** 394–398.

Kassis, J. A., and Gorski, J. (1981). Estrogen receptor replenishment. *J. Biol. Chem.* **256,** 7378–7382.

Kassis, J. A., and Gorski, J. (1983). On the mechanism of estrogen receptor replenishment: Recycling, resynthesis and/or processing. *Mol. Cell. Biochem.* **52,** 27–36.

Kelly, P. A., Djian, J., Katoh, M., Ferland, L. H., Houdebine, L. M., Teyssot, B., and Dusanter-Fourt, I. (1984). The interaction of prolactin with its receptors in target tissues and its mechanism of action. *Recent Prog. Horm. Res.* **40,** 379–439.

King, W. J., and Greene, G. L. (1984). Monoclonal antibodies to estrogen receptor localize receptor in the nucleus of target cells. *Nature (London)* **307,** 745–747.

Leong, D. A., Frawley, L. S., and Neill, J. D. (1983). Neuroendocrine control of prolactin secretion. *Annu. Rev. Physiol.* **45,** 109–127.

Levy-Wilson, B. (1983). Modulations of prolactin and growth hormone gene expression and chromatin structure in cultured rat pituitary cells. *Nucleic Acids Res.* **11,** 823–835.

Lieberman, M. E., Maurer, R. A., and Gorski, J. (1978). Estrogen control of prolactin synthesis *in vitro*. *Proc. Natl. Acad. Sci. U.S.A.* **75,** 5946–5949.

Lieberman, M. E., Maurer, R. A., Claude, P., and Gorski, J. (1982). Prolactin synthesis in primary cultures of pituitary cells: Regulation by estradiol. *Mol. Cell. Endocrinol.* **25,** 277–294.

Lin, S.-Y., and Riggs, A. D. (1972). Lac repressor binding to nonoperator DNA: Detailed studies and a comparison of equilibrium and rate competition methods. *J. Mol. Biol.* **72,** 671–690.

MacLeod, R. M., Abad, A., and Eidson, L. L. (1969). *In vivo* effect of sex hormones on the *in vitro* synthesis of prolactin and growth hormone in normal and pituitary tumor-bearing rats. *Endocrinology* **84,** 1475–1483.

Maurer, R. A. (1980a). Immunochemical isolation of prolactin messenger RNA. *J. Biol. Chem.* **255,** 854–859.

Maurer, R. A. (1980b). Dopaminergic inhibition of prolactin synthesis and prolactin messenger RNA accumulation in cultured pituitary cells. *J. Biol. Chem.* **255,** 8092–8097.

Maurer, R. A. (1981). Transcriptional regulation of the prolactin gene by ergocryptine and cyclic AMP. *Nature (London)* **294,** 94–97.

Maurer, R. A. (1982a). Estradiol regulates the transcription of the prolactin gene. *J. Biol. Chem.* **257,** 2133–2136.

Maurer, R. A. (1982b). Relationship between estradiol, ergocryptine, and thyroid hormone: Effects on prolactin synthesis and prolactin messenger ribonucleic acid levels. *Endocrinology* **110,** 1515–1520.

Maurer, R. A. (1982c). Adenosine 3′,5′-monophosphate derivatives increase prolactin synthesis and prolactin messenger ribonucleic acid levels in ergocryptine-treated pituitary cells. *Endocrinology* **110,** 1957–1963.

Maurer, R. A. (1982d). Thyroid hormone specifically inhibits prolactin synthesis and decreases prolactin messenger ribonucleic acid levels in cultured pituitary cells. *Endocrinology* **110,** 1507–1514.

Maurer, R. A. (1985). Selective binding of the estradiol receptor to a region at least one kilobase upstream from the rat prolactin gene. *DNA* **4,** 1–9.

Maurer, R. A., and Gorski, J. (1977). Effect of estradiol-17β and pimozide on prolactin synthesis in male and female rats. *Endocrinology* **101,** 76–84.

Maurer, R. A., Stone, R., and Gorski, J. (1976). Cell-free synthesis of a large translation product of prolactin messenger RNA. *J. Biol. Chem.* **25,** 2801–2807.

Maurer, R. A., Gorski, J., and McKean, D. J. (1977). Partial amino acid sequence of rat pre-prolactin. *Biochem. J.* **161,** 189–192.

Maurer, R. A., Gubbins, E. J., Erwin, C. R., and Donelson, J. E. (1980). Comparison of potential nuclear precursors for prolactin and growth hormone messenger RNA. *J. Biol. Chem.* **255,** 2243–2246.

Maurer, R. A., Erwin, C. R., and Donelson, J. E. (1981). Analysis of 5′ flanking sequences and intron–exon boundaries of the rat prolactin gene. *J. Biol. Chem.* **256,** 10524–10528.

Miller, W. L., and Eberhardt, N. L. (1983). Structure and evolution of the growth hormone gene family. *Endocr. Rev.* **4,** 97–130.

Murdoch, G. H., and Rosenfeld, M. G. (1981). Regulation of pituitary function and prolactin production in the GH_4 cell line by vitamin D. *J. Biol. Chem.* **256,** 4050–4055.

Murdoch, G. H., Rosenfeld, M. G., and Evans, R. M. (1982a). Eukaryotic transcriptional regulation and chromatin-associated protein phosphorylation by cyclic AMP. *Science* **218,** 1315–1317.

Murdoch, G. H., Potter, E., Nicolaisen, A. K., Evans, R. M., and Rosenfeld, M. G. (1982b). Epidermal growth factor rapidly stimulates prolactin gene transcription. *Nature (London)* **300,** 192–195.

Murdoch, G. H., Franco, R., Evans, R. M., and Rosenfeld, M. G. (1983). Polypeptide hormone regulation of gene expression. *J. Biol. Chem.* **258,** 15329–15335.

Murdoch, G. H., Evans, R. M., and Rosenfeld, M. G. (1985). Polypeptide hormone regulation of prolactin gene transcription. *Biochem. Act. Horm.* **12,** 37–68.

Neill, J. D., and Frawley, L. S. (1983). Detection of hormone release from individual cells in mixed populations using a reverse hemolytic plaque assay. *Endocrinology* **112,** 1135–1137.

Neill, J. D., Freeman, M. E., and Tillson, S. A. (1971). Control of the proestrus surge of prolactin and luteinizing hormone secretion by estrogens in the rat. *Endocrinology* **89,** 1448–1453.

Nicoll, C. S. (1980). Ontogeny and evolution of prolactin's functions. *Fed. Proc., Fed. Am. Soc. Exp. Biol.* **39,** 2563–2566.

Payvar, F., DeFranco, D., Firestone, G. L., Edgar, B., Wrange, O., Okret, S., Gustafsson, J.-A., and Yamamoto, K. (1983). Sequence-specific binding of glucocorticoid receptor to MTV DNA at sites within and upstream of the transcribed region. *Cell* **35,** 381–392.

Perrone, M. H., Greer, T. L., and Hinkle, P. M. (1980). Relationship between thyroid hormone and glucocorticoid effects in GH3 pituitary cells. *Endocrinology* **106,** 600–605.

Phelps, C., and Hymer, W. C. (1983). Characterization of estrogen-induced adenohypophysial tumors in the Fischer 344 rat. *Neuroendocrinology* **37,** 23–31.

Pilotte, N. S., Burt, D. R., and Barraclough, C. A. (1984). Ovarian steroids modulate the release of dopamine into hypophysial portal blood and the density of anterior pituitary [^{3}H]spiperone-binding sites in ovariectomized rats. *Endocrinology* **114,** 2306–2311.

Potter, E., Nicolaisen, A. K., Ong, E. S., Evans, R. M., and Rosenfeld, M. G. (1981). Thyrotropin-releasing hormone exerts rapid nuclear effects to increase production of the primary prolactin mRNA transcript. *Proc. Natl. Acad. Sci. U.S.A.* **78,** 6662–6666.

Raymond, V., Beaulieu, M., Labrie, F., and Boissier, J. (1978). Potent antidopaminergic activity of estradiol at the pituitary level on prolactin release. *Science* **200,** 1173–1175.

Rillema, J. A. (1980). Mechanism of prolactin action. *Fed. Proc., Fed. Am. Soc. Exp. Biol.* **39,** 2593–2598.

Ringold, G. M., Yamamoto, K. R., Bishop, J. M., and Varmus, H. E. (1977). Glucocorticoid-stimulated accumulation of mouse mammary tumor virus RNA: Increased rate of synthesis of viral RNA. *Proc. Natl. Acad. Sci. U.S.A.* **74,** 2879–2883.

Ruh, T. S., and Ruh, M. F. (1975). Androgen induction of a specific uterine protein. *Endocrinology* **97,** 1144–1150.

Ryan, R., Shupnik, M. A., and Gorski, J. (1979). Effect of estrogen on preprolactin messenger ribonucleic acid sequences. *Biochemistry* **18,** 2044–2048.

Said, S. I., and Porter, J. C. (1979). Vasoactive intestinal polypeptide: Release into hypophysial portal blood. *Life Sci.* **24,** 227–230.

Sar, M. (1984). Estradiol is concentrated in tyrosine hydroxylase-containing neurons in the hypothalamus. *Science* **223,** 938–940.

Schally, A. O., Coy, D. H., and Meyers, C. A. (1978). Hypothalamic regulatory hormones. *Annu. Rev. Biochem.* **47,** 89–128.

Schonbrunn, A., Krasnoff, M., Westendorf, J. M., and Tashjian, A. H., Jr. (1980). Epidermal growth factor and thyrotropin-releasing hormone act similarly on a clonal pituitary cell strain. *J. Cell Biol.* **85,** 786–797.

Schuler, L. A., Weber, J. L., and Gorski, J. (1983). Polymorphism near the rat prolactin gene caused by insertion of an Alu-like element. *Nature (London)* **305,** 159–160.

Seo, H., Refetoff, S., Vassart, G., and Brocas, H. (1979a). Comparison of primary and secondary stimulation of male rats by estradiol in terms of prolactin synthesis and mRNA accumulation in the pituitary. *Proc. Natl. Acad. Sci. U.S.A.* **76,** 824–828.

Seo, H., Refetoff, S., Martino, E., Vassart, G., and Brocas, H. (1979b). The differential stimulatory effect of thyroid hormone on growth hormone synthesis and estrogen on prolactin synthesis due to accumulation of specific messenger ribonucleic acids. *Endocrinology* **104,** 1083–1090.

Shimatsu, A., Kato, Y., Matsushita, N., Katakami, H., Yanaihara, N., and Imura, H. (1981). Immunoreactive vasoactive intestinal polypeptide in rat hypophysial portal blood. *Endocrinology* **108,** 395–398.

Shull, J. D., and Gorski, J. (1982). The effect of estradiol on the synthesis of prolactin RNA in isolated rat pituitary nuclei. *Endocrinology* **110** (Suppl.), 292.

Shull, J. D., and Gorski, J. (1983). Prolactin gene transcription: Two stages of regulation by estrogen. *Fed. Proc., Fed. Am. Soc. Exp. Biol.* **42,** 206.

Shull, J. D., and Gorski, J. (1984). Estrogen stimulates prolactin gene transcription by a mechanism independent of pituitary protein synthesis. *Endocrinology* **114,** 1550–1557.

Shull, J. D., and Gorski, J. (1985). Estrogen regulates the transcription of the rat prolactin gene *in vivo* through at least two independent mechanisms. *Endocrinology* **116,** 2456–2462.

Shull, J. D., Walent, J. H., Lieberman, M. E., and Gorski, J. (1984a). Estrogen stimulates prolactin gene transcription in primary pituitary cell cultures. *Abstr. 7th, Int. Congr. Endocrinol., Quebec,* p. 2139.

Shull, J. D., Mellon, S. R., and Gorski, J. (1984b). Regulation of prolactin gene transcription *in vivo:* Roles of estrogen and dopamine. *Abstr. 7th, Int. Congr. Endocrinol., Quebec,* p. 2140.

Sibley, D. R., De Lean, A., and Creese, I. (1982). Anterior pituitary dopamine receptors. Demonstration of interconvertible high and low affinity states of the D-2 dopamine receptor. *J. Biol. Chem.* **257,** 6351–6361.

Smith, M. S. (1980). Role of prolactin in regulating gonadotropin secretion and gonad function in female rats. *Fed. Proc., Fed. Am. Soc. Exp. Biol.* **39,** 2571–2576.

Sobel, A., and Tashjian, A. H., Jr. (1983). Distinct patterns of cytoplasmic protein phosphorylation related to regulation of synthesis and release of prolactin by GH cells. *J. Biol. Chem.* **258,** 10312–10324.

Stack, G. E. (1983). Estrogen stimulation of DNA synthesis in the prepuberal rat uterus. Ph.D. thesis, University of Wisconsin, Madison.

Stanley, F., and Samuels, H. H. (1984). *n*-Butyrate effects thyroid hormone stimulation of prolactin production and mRNA levels in GH_1 cells. *J. Biol. Chem.* **259,** 9768–9775.

Stone, R. T., Maurer, R. A., and Gorski, J. (1977). Effect of estradiol-17β on preprolactin messenger ribonucleic acid activity in the rat pituitary gland. *Biochemistry* **16,** 4915–4921.

Sullivan, N. J., and Tashjian, A. H., Jr. (1983). Platelet-derived growth factor selectively decreases prolactin production in pituitary cells in culture. *Endocrinology* **113,** 639–645.

Supowit, S. C., Potter, E., Evans, R. M., and Rosenfeld, M. G. (1984). Polypeptide hormone regulation of gene transcription: Specific 5′ genomic sequences are required for epidermal growth factor and phorbol ester regulation of prolactin gene expression. *Proc. Natl. Acad. Sci. U.S.A.* **81,** 2975–2979.

Swennen, L., and Denef, C. (1982). Physiological concentrations of dopamine decrease adenosine 3′,5′-monophosphate levels in cultured rat anterior pituitary cells and enriched populations of lactotrophs: Evidence for a causal relationship to inhibition of prolactin release. *Endocrinology* **111,** 398–405.

Truong, A. T., Duez, C., Belayew, A., Renard, A., Pictet, R., Bell, G. I., and Martial, J. A. (1984). Isolation and characterization of the human prolactin gene. *EMBO J.* **3,** 429–437.

Vale, W., Grant, G., Amoss, M., Blackwell, R., and Guillemin, R. (1972). Culture of enzymatically dispersed pituitary cells: Functional validation of a method. *Endocrinology* **91,** 562–571.

Vician, L., and Mellon, W. S. (1982). Stimulatory effects of 1,25-dihydroxy-vitamin D_3 on prolactin synthesis in primary cultures of rat pituitary cells. *Endocrinology* **110** (Suppl.), 304.

Vician, L., Shupnik, M. A., and Gorski, J. (1979). Effect of estrogen on primary ovine pituitary cell cultures. Stimulation of prolactin secretion, synthesis and preprolactin messenger ribonucleic acid activity. *Endocrinology* **104,** 736–743.

Vician, L., Lieberman, M. E., and Gorski, J. (1982). Evidence that autoregulation of prolactin production does not occur at the pituitary level. *Endocrinology* **110,** 722–726.

Wark, J. D., and Tashjian, A. H., Jr. (1982). Vitamin D stimulates prolactin synthesis by GH_4C_1 cells incubated in chemically defined medium. *Endocrinology* **111,** 1755–1757.

Wark, J. D., and Tashjian, A. H., Jr. (1983). Regulation of prolactin mRNA by 1,25-dihydroxyvitamin D_3 in GH_4C_1 cells. *J. Biol. Chem.* **258,** 12118–12121.

Weber, J. L., Durrin, L. K., and Gorski, J. (1985). Repetitive DNA sequences within and around the rat prolactin gene. *Mol. Cell. Biochem.* **65,** 171–179.

Weintraub, H., and Groudine, M. (1976). Chromosomal subunits in active genes have an altered conformation. *Science* **193,** 848–856.

Welshons, W. V., Lieberman, M. E., and Gorski, J. (1984). Nuclear localization of unoccupied estrogen receptors: Cytochalasin enucleation of GH_3 cells. *Nature (London)* **370,** 747–749.

White, B. A., and Bancroft, F. C. (1983). Epidermal growth factor and thyrotropin-releasing hormone interact synergistically with calcium to regulate prolactin mRNA levels. *J. Biol. Chem.* **258,** 4618–4622.

Wiklund, J., Wertz, N., and Gorski, J. (1981). A comparison of estrogen effects on uterine and pituitary growth and prolactin synthesis in F344 and Holtzman rats. *Endocrinology* **109,** 1700–1707.

Yamamoto, K., Kasai, K., and Ieiri, T. (1975). Control of pituitary functions of synthesis and release of prolactin and growth hormone by gonadal steroids in male and female rats. *Jpn. J. Physiol.* **25,** 645–658.

Hormonal Regulation in *in Vitro* Fertilization

GARY D. HODGEN

The Howard and Georgeanna Jones Institute for Reproductive Medicine,
Department of Obstetrics and Gynecology,
Eastern Virginia Medical School,
Norfolk, Virginia 23507

I. Introduction

In order to gain appropriate perspective on the current status of human *in vitro* fertilization and embryo transfer (Fig. 1), its caveat procedures, and research directions, we must see this novel medical therapy in the context of the larger ongoing reproductive revolution. We are living in the midst of a most dynamic shift in the modes and means for manipulating (suppression or enhancement) the reproductive potential of men and women. Indeed, the ramifications of the new reproductive technology are indelibly affecting the social, economic, political and ecologic status of mankind across the planet. The drive for quality of human life, threatened for the masses by overpopulation or for individuals through disadvantages of infertility or heritable defects, is challenging the ancient inexorable drive to reproduce as the race competes for living space, finite resources, and choice of life-styles. Effective family planning may be the ultimate solution for starving nations, and among "developed" countries, it has enhanced educational and career opportunities for millions of young women. Reproductive technology is the new hope for progress in antenatal diagnostics and *in utero* treatment for the unborn; now, the fetus, too, is a patient even before achieving legal status as a person. These examples are among the many social and health issues that depend on the new technology. *In vitro* fertilization and embryo transfer represents only one of the rapidly emerging applied advances in reproductive medicine beginning in the late 1950s; these include "the pill" and the IUD for contraception, and hormones for the infertile requiring gonadal stimulation by gonadotropins, clomiphene citrate, or bromocryptine, to mention only a few.

But from where and when did the biological basis for these sweeping changes derive? Virtually all of the recent applications grew out of imaginative basic research spawned in the 1920s and 1930s with the identification and characterization of vitamins and hormones. Indeed,

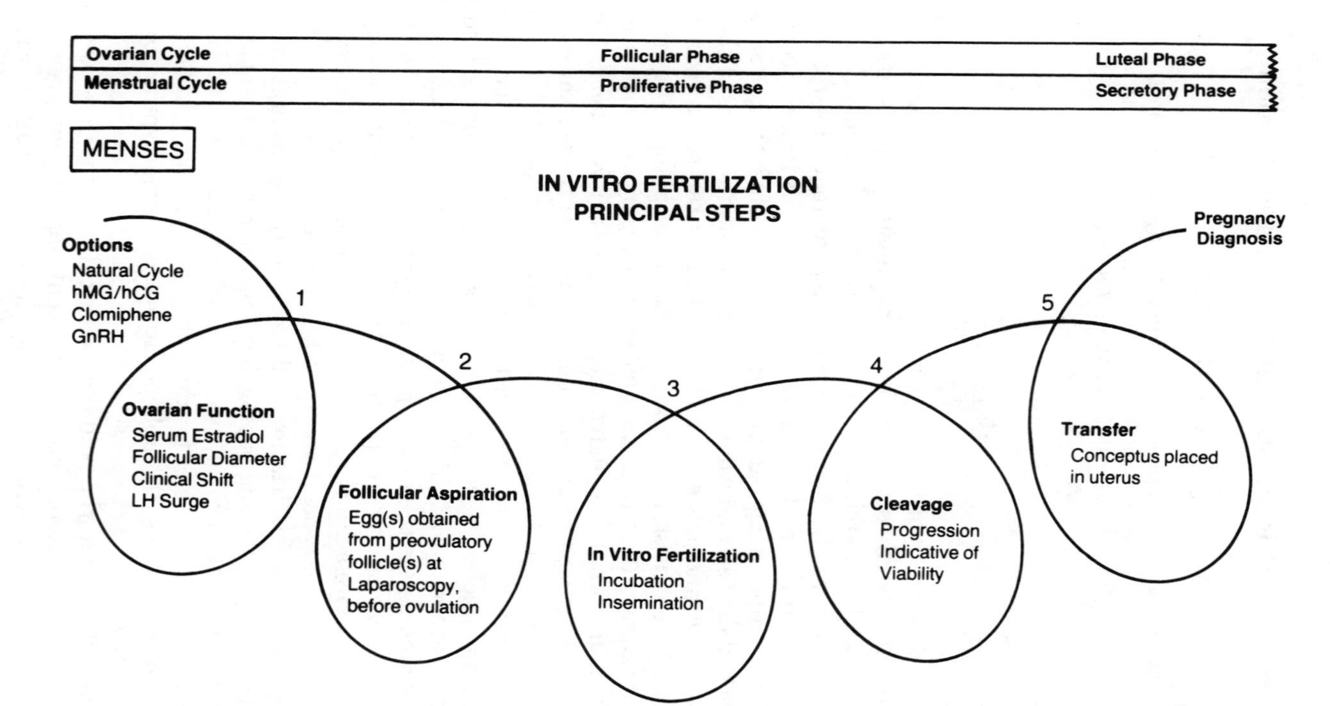

FIG. 1. The five principal steps of *in vitro* fertilization and embryo transfer procedures.

the history of early endocrinology is tightly wrapped in nutrition and growth studies. It is fitting that this volume cite and acknowledge the essential nature of these early findings as a foundation for the success of *in vitro* fertilization and embryo transfer today. And, too, the fundamental animal studies which taught us nature's axioms for gametogenesis, fertilization, development, and differentiation (Chang, 1971).

Millions are now seeking voluntary manipulation of their intrinsic reproductive capabilities to gain quality of life benefits for themselves and their children. Although not universal, the popularity of such options sparked industrial investment, governmental policies, and international agencies to promote development of safer, more effective drugs and devices. Increased advocacy toward aggressive treatment for infertile couples was a spontaneous outgrowth of this movement. Thus the right of individuals to procreate, even to pursue the extraordinary means required, arose from the diverse events of the nascent reproductive revolution.

II. Impetus from the First Success

During the late 1960s Bob Edwards and colleagues developed the thesis that *in vitro* fertilization and embryo transfer in humans would provide enormous therapeutic and scientific opportunities. Although not espousing a radical new idea, he, along with the clinician Patrick Steptoe, was the first to persevere in the face of both peer and public ridicule, as well as seemingly insurmountable technical problems. We should recall that initially public tolerance for such endeavors was slight indeed. The situation changed dramatically in the summer of 1978 with the birth of Louise Brown in Oldham, England. At last, Edwards and Steptoe had succeeded in one case with *in vitro* fertilization and embryo transfer. While we were all amazed (some were skeptical; others were dubious) at this great achievement, it had arrived, not unlike most medical advances, through years of preliminary animal and human studies, ultimately brought to clinical application through heroic effort and rigorous scientific study. But these events are best recorded by Edwards himself (Edwards and Purdy, 1982). Even so, it must be noted that practical utility of *in vitro* fertilization and embryo transfer on a broad scale required radical revisions of the initial procedures in order to achieve anything approaching a reliable treatment (see below).

In less than 7 years, more than 1000 children worldwide were born to couples treated by *in vitro* fertilization and embryo transfer. Although exact statistics are difficult to compile, surely several hundred more pregnancies have derived from extracorporeal fertilization. The utility of this procedure and its problems are increasing. *In vitro* fertilization and embryo transfer is no longer an experimental technique; rather, it is a recognized medical procedure. Indeed, some states require health insurance carriers to offer coverage specifically designed for *in vitro* fertilization and embryo transfer treatment. Although federal guidelines for this treatment have lagged since the HEW Ethics Advisory Board Report (1979), many states and local institutional review boards have adopted regulatory standards and oversight committees for both clinical service and research involving *in vitro* fertilization and embryo transfer. Moreover, professional societies and organizations concerned with reproductive health have made specific recommendations on ethical and legal issues surrounding *in vitro* fertilization and embryo transfer and some of its caveat procedures. The moral debate continues, gathering balance and perspective by the collective input of widely divergent opinions (Hodgen, 1984). At the epicenter of this controversy are research objectives that require access to human embryonic tissue in order to find new discoveries for treatment or prevention of disease versus primordial feelings of intrusion upon the very essence of being human. The choices are difficult at best.

III. Indications for *in Vitro* Fertilization

In vitro fertilization was first applied to patients with uncorrectable tubal disease; now the indications extend to a variety of disorders (Table I). Much of this presentation is taken from the work of Howard Jones, Jr. (H. W. Jones, 1985) and his colleagues, who pioneered this work in the United States.

A. Tubal Disease

Some 615 of the first 825 treatment cycles (75%) at the Eastern Virginia Medical School (EVMS), Norfolk, Virginia were for tubal disease. Essentially all patients had failed conventional therapy and many had had multiple laparotomies. All eggs were harvested by laparoscopy. It is of significance that the pregnancy rate by cycle (18.4%) (excluding the male factor) and by transfer (22.3%) was the lowest for the tubal disease group among the five major indications for therapy in the EVMS series. Furthermore, the transfer rate (82%), excluding the

TABLE I
INDICATIONS FOR PATIENT SELECTION AT NORFOLK[a]

Generally healthy husband and wife
Accessible ovaries
A normally functioning uterus
Normal or correctable menstrual function
Under age 40
An uncorrected problem
- Tubal
- Inadequate sperm for normal reproduction but not azospermia
- Endometriosis
- Undiagnosed by available methods
- Diethylstilbestrol exposure
- Cervical hostility
- Immunological
- Anovulation
- Other

[a] From H. W. Jones (1985).

male fertility problem, was the lowest of the major diagnostic categories (Table II).

This low rate probably reflects the extent of pelvic disease. Some 122 cycles (20%) represented patients who had only one remaining ovary or had undergone partial ovariectomy. Seventy-two cycles represented patients with a secondary diagnosis that of itself could have caused infertility. However, neither a single remaining ovary nor a secondary diagnosis, nor a combination of the two, seemed to influence the pregnancy rate.

TABLE II
FIRST TREATMENT GROUP AT NORFOLK, JANUARY 1981 TO SEPTEMBER 1984 (SERIES 1–16)[a]

Category of infertility	Number of cycles	Number of transfers	Transfers per cycle (%)	Number of pregnancies	Pregnancy rate by cycle (%)	Pregnancy rate by transfer (%)
Tubal	615	504	82	113	18.4	22.3
Male	65	32	49	11	16.9	34.3
Endometriosis	55	48	87	14	25.5	29.2
Undiagnosed	37	32	86	11	29.7	34.3
DES	33	30	91	8	24.2	26.6
Cervical	9	8	89	1	11.1	12.5
Immunological	7	6	86	2	28.6	33.3
Anovulation	4	4	100	1	25.0	25.0

[a] From H. W. Jones (1985).

B. Male Infertility

There are still no absolute criteria for semen characteristics that define infertility. Nevertheless, most patients in this category show repeatedly sperm counts of less than 20 million. However, good motility seems to be an essential requirement as penetration of the zona seems impossible without it.

Screening of two to three samples prior to admission into the program is helpful. Continuing pregnancies have developed from specimens yielding 1.5 million actively motile sperm after swim-up. There has also been a good correlation with pregnancy with a positive hamster penetration test (Van Uem *et al.*, 1985). Although we have found that fertilization can occur with as few as 12,500 sperm from a euspermic man, present evidence suggests that this number may be far too few for an oligospermic specimen.

Presently, there are no completely reliable criteria to discriminate effective from ineffective oligoasthenospermic specimens. Nevertheless, *in vitro* fertilization offers the only opportunity for fatherhood for some oligoasthenospermic men. Among the first 65 couples treated at EVMS whose primary problem seemed to rest with the male, in 41 (63%) there was a contributing problem in the female as well. As with tubal ligation, the secondary factor did not seem to influence the end result.

Couples with a male factor experienced a very low rate of transfer (49%) compared to other diagnostic categories (Table III). However, if the procedure reached the transfer stage the pregnancy rate was quite comparable to that in other groups. Among the male group, the total number of eggs harvested was quite comparable to other groups. However, the number of eggs transferred in the group was the lowest of any category, suggesting that even when fertilization occurred it did so with a lesser efficiency than in other groups (Tables II and III).

TABLE III
Male Factor Treatment Group at Norfolk, January 1981 to September 1984[a]

Category	Number of cycles	Number of transfers	Number of pregnancies	Pregnancy rate by cycle (%)	Pregnancy rate by transfer (%)
All	65	32	11	16.9	34.3
Single diagnosis	24	10	3	12.5	30.0
With secondary diagnosis	41	22	8	19.5	36.4

[a] From H. W. Jones (1985).

C. Endometriosis

All patients in this category have undergone prior endocrinological and/or surgical therapy without achieving pregnancy. At EVMS, among 55 aspirates from patients with a diagnosis of primary endometriosis, 38 were from cases with the sole diagnosis of endometriosis while 17 cases showed additional secondary problems. However, the transfer and pregnancy rates by cycle or by transfer were not influenced by the secondary factor (Table IV). There were only minor differences in the number of eggs collected and transferred between the two categories or between endometriosis patients and patients in other categories.

Evaluation of the utility of *in vitro* fertilization for patients with endometriosis is plagued by a problem of classification. A review of the problem based upon EVMS material through June 1984, reported by Chillik *et al.* (1985), yielded two groups. One comprised patients previously treated for endometriosis, but at harvest laparoscopy showed no active disease. None had become pregnant after the original treatment for endometriosis. There were 15 such cycles with 12 transfers and five pregnancies (33% by cycle, 42% by transfer). The second group, 14 patients previously treated for endometriosis, showed at the time of laparoscopy considerable residual active disease. There was but one pregnancy, ending in a first trimester abortion, among 14 cycles with 11 transfers (7% by cycle, 9% by transfer). Chillik and associates (1985) found 10 additional cycles among patients originally classified as undiagnosed infertility on the basis of a previous work-up who had minimal endometriosis at the time of harvest laparoscopy. All 10 underwent transfer and there were six pregnancies (60% by cycle, 60% by transfer). Thus, a detailed categorization of patients is essential to understand the indication for *in vitro* fertilization among patients with endometriosis.

TABLE IV
Endometriosis Treatment Group at Norfolk, January 1981 to September 1984[a]

Category	Number of cycles	Number of transfers	Number of pregnancies	Pregnancy rate by cycle (%)	Pregnancy rate by transfer (%)
All	55	48	14	25.5	29.2
Single diagnosis	38	34	10	26.3	29.4
With secondary diagnosis	17	14	4	23.5	28.6

[a] From H. W. Jones (1985).

In view of the success with *in vitro* fertilization among patients with minimal endometriosis and the success of *in vitro* fertilization in patients above the age of 35 (see below) it is possible that *in vitro* fertilization should be considered primary therapy for patients above the age of 35 with minimal endometriosis. The situation with active disease among patients above the age of 35 is less clear.

D. Undiagnosed

By definition, these patients have undergone testing by contemporary techniques without discovery of a cause for infertility. All patients must have had examinations of the semen, postcoital tests, hysterosalpingograms, timed endometrial biopsies with basal temperature charts, and laparoscopic examinations showing no abnormality. All patients (husband and wife) must have had a negative examination for antisperm antibodies.

While the number of patients is small, the results in the undiagnosed group at EVMS were higher than for any other diagnostic category (29.7% by cycle, 34.3% by transfer cycle). This success probably reflects the fact that this group showed a larger number of eggs transferred per cycle than any other diagnostic category (Table II).

E. Diethylstilbestrol

Exposure to diethylstilbestrol (DES), almost exclusively a problem confined to the United States, causes development of anomalies at various points along the mullerian ducts. Many of these patients have had ectopic pregnancies and salpingectomies, some bilateral, due to deformities of the fallopian tubes. Many have some degree of deformity in the endometrial cavity. Some have deformities of the cervix.

Overall, the results at EVMS (24.2% by cycle, 26.6% by transfer) were comparable to the other groups. Because of the deformity of the uterine cavity, a high miscarriage rate was anticipated. However, of eight pregnancies, only one terminated prior to viability.

The number of eggs transferred in this group was comparable to that of other groups. Mausher *et al.* (1984) have reported these cases in detail.

F. Cervical Factors

In some patients the sperm of the husband or donor is immobilized and there is no satisfactory explanation for this; no antisperm antibodies have been found in the serum of these women or their husbands. Insemination with washed sperm does not often achieve a pregnancy. Nevertheless, by *in vitro* fertilization one such patient at EVMS became pregnant.

G. Immunological

As used herein, the term *immunological infertility* is meant to imply that the female partner has antisperm antibodies in the serum. In one patient at EVMS, the follicular fluid was tested and found to contain antisperm antibodies in a concentration comparable to the peripheral serum. This patient nevertheless became pregnant and has delivered. One other patient became pregnant, but aborted.

H. Anovulation

Anovulatory patients refractory to standard methods of ovulation induction can be treated successfully by *in vitro* fertilization.

IV. Indications for Variations in the Basic Procedure

A. The Use of Donor Sperm

Insemination of normal females with donor sperm is a procedure used for many years to treat infertility due to inadequate sperm. The same can be done in a program of *in vitro* fertilization. However, the indications for this require some abnormality in the female which can be overcome only by *in vitro* fertilization.

Several programs have used this technique but the strict indications noted will limit its applicability in this instance.

B. The Use of Donor Eggs

Several abnormalities obviate harvesting of eggs from the female partner. These include congenital absence of the ovaries (streak gonads), premature menopause (perhaps even a normal menopause), or bilateral oophorectomy for whatever reason. Patients with blocked pelves obstructing laparoscopic harvest not amenable to surgical correction may be candidates for ultrasonic guided egg harvest, but even some of these may need and benefit from a donor egg.

Patients lacking oocytes require suitable treatment with estrogen and progesterone to mimic normal ovarian function. This has been achieved in both monkeys and women.

If the recipient has normal ovarian function, synchronization of donor and recipient is required. This has been done in monkeys (Hodgen, 1983) and women (Van Uem *et al.,* 1985) in the program at EVMS.

V. The Problem of Ovarian Inaccessibility

Some patients have pelvic disease so extensive that the ovaries are either partially or totally inaccessible to laparoscopic egg harvest. Minor avascular adhesions can be released by laparoscopic techniques either at the time of a preliminary screen or at the time of egg harvest. Other patients may be suitable candidates for ultrasonic guided transvesical or transvaginal egg harvest. However, until these techniques yield pregnancy rates equal to those available with laparoscopic harvest, preliminary laparotomy is useful to make available ovaries for laparoscopic harvest.

In properly selected patients, the results of such a procedure are acceptable. Such a procedure involves ovarian liberation, the removal of the tubes, if any, and suspension of the ovaries by severing the uteroovarian ligaments and suturing them to the round ligaments so that the ovary rests on the uterus more or less at the site of the excised tube. Finally, it is usually necessary to suspend the uterus. In the event adhesions reform to obstruct a subsequent laparoscopic approach, the ovaries should be ideally situated for a transvesical ultrasound guided approach.

By September 1984 in the program at EVMS, 54 patients had undergone such a preliminary laparotomy. At the time of writing, 37 of these had come to subsequent laparotomy (Garcia *et al.,* 1985). Fourteen of these patients became pregnant (38.8%). However, a total of 55 laparoscopies were required among these 37 patients. As one patient became pregnant twice, the pregnancy rate per laparoscopy was 15/55 (27%).

VI. Effect of Age

It has been recognized for years that natural fertility decreases with age and substantially so beginning at about age of 35 (Guttmacher, 1952). Therefore, it has been customary practice to withold surgery in patients beyond age 35. Many programs of *in vitro* fertilization, includ-

TABLE V
AGE GROUPS OF FIRST TREATMENT GROUP AT NORFOLK, JANUARY 1981 TO SEPTEMBER 1984[a]

Age	Pregnancies per transfer cycle (%)	Abortions per pregnancy (%)
<26	0/3 (0)	—
26–30	35/153 (23)	8/35 (23)
31–35	80/352 (23)	26/80 (32)
36–39	40/132 (30)	12/40 (30)
>40	6/27 (22)	2/6 (33)
Total	161/667 (24)	50/161 (31)

[a] From H. W. Jones (1985).

ing the ones at EVMS, began under the same restraints. This restriction is gradually eroding and at EVMS analysis showed that the pregnancy rate for patients aged 36–39 was better than that for other ages. Indeed, pregnancies have developed beyond age 40 and our oldest mother was 42 at delivery. Of significance is the finding that in the small series of patients age 40 and above the abortion rate was no greater than for the younger age group (Table V). Edwards and Steptoe (1983), however, have found that among patients beyond 40 the expectancy of pregnancy is diminished and associated with a high abortion rate. Thus, it seems that there is uncertainty about the application of *in vitro* fertilization to patients at or about the age of 40 years. With this caveat in regard to age, some self-evident criteria and indications based on the EVMS experience are stated in Table V.

VII. PROCEDURES OF *in Vitro* FERTILIZATION

The initial success with *in vitro* fertilization began with collection of one egg from the single dominant follicle of the natural ovarian/menstrual cycle (Fig. 1). It soon became evident that increasing pregnancy rates to practically useful levels would require aspiration of several preovulatory eggs from each patient (Garcia *et al.*, 1983; Leung *et al.*, 1983; Laufer *et al.*, 1983). This change has had more to do with improving *in vitro* results than any other primary revision in procedures. This change led to transfer of multiple embryos, which in turn, enhanced chances for achieving viable pregnancies (Fig. 2).

No. of Embryos Transferred	Pregnancy Rate/ Transfer Cycle	Multiple Pregnancy Rate
1	14%	1%
2	22%	4%
3	29%	9%
4	31%	15%
5	33%	21%
6	35%	28%

FIG. 2. With *in vitro* fertilization, multiple pregnancy rates rise along with the pregnancy rate as the number of embryos transferred increases.

A. METHODS OF OVARIAN STIMULATION

The number of stimulation protocols tested for *in vitro* fertilization patients is too great to permit description of each. Accordingly, I have drawn heavily from a recent summary by Georgeanna Seegar Jones in grouping comparisons of various procedures (G. S. Jones, 1984), several of which have been used successfully worldwide by *in vitro* fertilization and embryo transfer teams.

Three basic methods have been used for stimulation of multiple oocyte retrieval: (1) clomiphene citrate with or without human chorionic gonadotropin (hCG), (2) clomiphene citrate plus human menopausal gonadotropin (hMG) plus hCG, and (3) hMG plus hCG. At the present time, most *in vitro* fertilization programs have abandoned the use of clomiphene citrate alone because the number of oocytes obtained and the pregnancy rates as well as the cycle cancellation rates are not as satisfactory as with the other methods of stimulation. More recently, the majority of the Australian teams, as well as those in Europe and the United States, have used clomiphene citrate plus hMG plus hCG (Vargyas *et al.*, 1984; Wentz *et al.*, 1983; Testart *et al.*, 1982). Here at EVMS hMG plus hCG stimulation has been used almost from the beginning.

1. *Clomiphene Citrate plus hCG*

Monitoring for clomiphene citrate plus hCG-stimulated cycles was reported early on by Trounson and Wood (1981). These investigators relied upon ultrasound as the major method of monitoring, although urinary estrogen and luteinizing hormone (LH) assays were also performed. Thus, 50–150 mg clomiphene citrate was administered daily beginning on day 3–5 of the cycle, and hCG was administered when the ultrasound indicated the largest follicular diameter was 20 mm or above. If the LH surge was detected, the cycle was usually canceled. Estrogen assays in serum were estimated to be 400 pg/ml times the number of the follicules visualized on ultrasound; thus, if three follicles were visualized, the serum estrogen should be approximately 1200 pg/ml.

2. *Clomiphene Citrate plus hMG plus hCG*

Clomiphene citrate is given at 50–150 mg/day beginning about day 5 of the cycle. Two ampules of hMG [75 IU each of follicle-stimulating hormone (FSH) and LH] are given on days 6, 8, and 10 of the cycle. Follicular ultrasound and serum estrogens are the major methods used for monitoring; typically, hCG is given when two 15-mm follicles are seen. The Women's Hospital group in Melbourne, Australia has individualized cases by using serum estradiol and biological parameters to determine when to give hCG. It is important to realize that each *in vitro* fertilization team may favor minor variations in these generic protocols.

3. *hMG plus hCG*

At EVMS, hMG (75 IU each of FSH and LH) was given at the rate of two ampules of Pergonal (Serono Labs, Randolph, MA) daily, beginning on cycle day 3 in patients having a cycle of 28 ± 3 days. The hMG was administered as needed im at 4 PM after the estradiol values were reported at 3 PM. HMG was discontinued or decreased as determined by monitoring (Jones *et al.,* 1982). This protocol produced good responses in many patients, but was not optimal for several subgroups. Accordingly, in recent months we have intensified evaluations of FSH-rich stimulation protocols.

4. *"Pure" FSH plus hMG plus hCG*

Preliminary findings indicate that many patients treated with greater relative amounts of FSH to LH, especially early in the stimulation protocol, became pregnant in the EVMS *in vitro* fertilization program (Jones *et al.,* 1984). Current results favor the "pure" FSH plus hMG plus hCG over all other regimens tested. Whether "pure" FSH (Metrodin, Serono Labs, Randolph, MA) alone, or in combination with hMG and/or hCG (by a protocol yet to be evaluated), will ultimately prove superior for certain patients to previous regimens, is being tested (Schenken *et al.,* 1984).

B. Rationale for the Treatment Regimen

Days 3 to 5 were chosen for beginning most regimens because typically the dominant follicle is not selected before about day 6 (Goodman and Hodgen, 1983). Thus, cycle days 3 to 5 will usually accommodate two or three additional follicles from the maturing cohort of follicles developing concurrently. Two ampules of hMG per day were given because, in the prior experience with ovulation induction, this amount stimulated patients with minimal hypothalamic–pituitary function within an 8- to 10-day period. Importantly, by starting with the highest amount of hMG thought required and then reducing dosage if indicated, the stimulation is more manageable than starting with a low dosage and increasing.

Cycles are monitored by all available parameters of follicular growth and development which should, theoretically, parallel maturation of the oocytes: serum estradiol; the biological response to estradiol, measured by the peripheral end-organ responses, such as maturation of the vaginal cells and cervical mucus changes; and the numbers of follicles and their anatomic growth as measured by daily ultrasound.

C. Follicular Ultrasound Measurements

The diameter of the hMG-stimulated follicles was found by ultrasound to be smaller than anticipated from the size of the dominant follicle in the natural cycle (Mantzavinos *et al.*, 1983; Quinn *et al.*, 1984; Hackeloer *et al.*, 1979). The average diameter of the largest follicles when hMG was discontinued was 13.7 ± 1.4 mm and 15.1 ± 1.5 mm when hCG was given, as compared to 15 and 21 mm in the natural cycle. The clarity of the follicular borders is also somewhat obscured by the edema which develops in the hMG/hCG-stimulated ovary. Although the ultrasound is invaluable in determining the side in which the largest follicles occur, and the location as well as the number of follicles, it has not been used at EVMS as a primary monitoring method. Here, it may influence the discontinuation of the hMG by ± 1 day. However, other *in vitro* fertilization teams utilize quite nicely ultrasound as the principal tool for patient monitoring (Quigley *et al.*, 1984).

D. Monitoring Patient Response

The ideal time for discontinuing hMG depends on individual patient responses. Three patient response categories were identified and arbitrarily classified as low, intermediate, or high in relation to the effect of serum estradiol on peripheral estrogen. It was determined that hMG should be discontinued in the majority of patients when the estradiol, E_2, was 300 pg/ml or above, if the peripheral biological estrogen responses (vaginal and cervical) were evident. The intermediate group comprised the largest number of patients. HMG should be discontinued in patients designated as the high-responder group when estradiol concentrations >600 pg/ml were reached, without regard for biological response (Fig. 3). HMG should be discontinued in the low-responder group if the biological response can be detected up to 3 days in advance, even if serum estradiol concentrations are below 300 pg/ml (Fig. 4).

The etiology of the characteristic high, intermediate, or low patient response to hMG resides in the complex physiology of the hypothalamic–pituitary–ovarian (HPO) axis. It is not due to a higher total

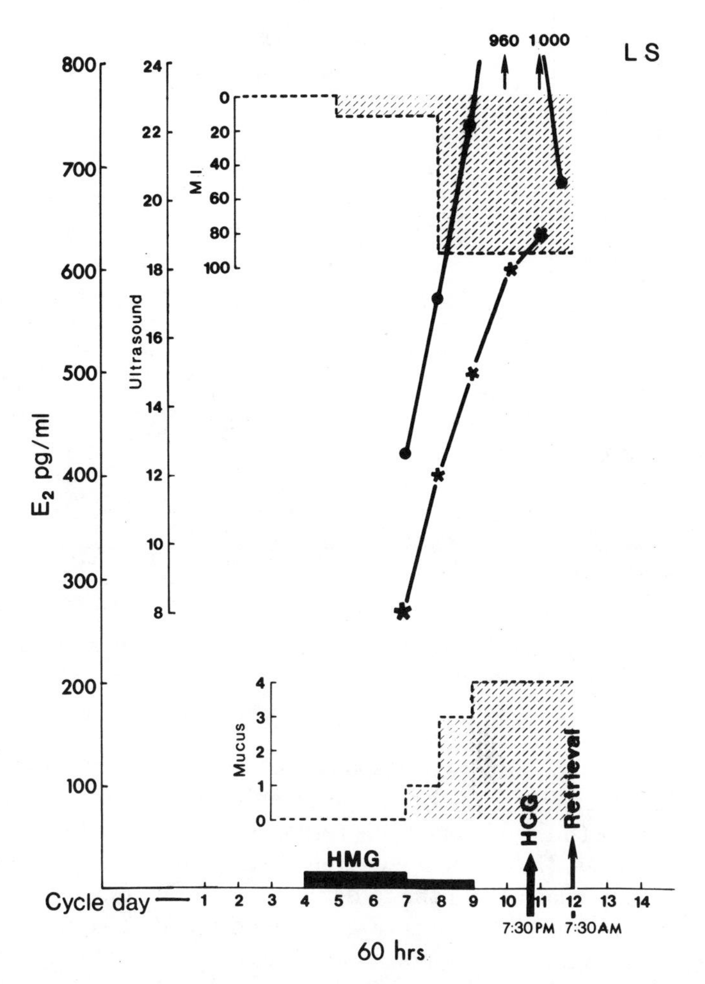

FIG. 3. A high responder to estradiol, E_2. The patient does not show an estrogen shift in the peripheral response until the serum E_2 is above 600 pg/ml. From G. S. Jones (1984).

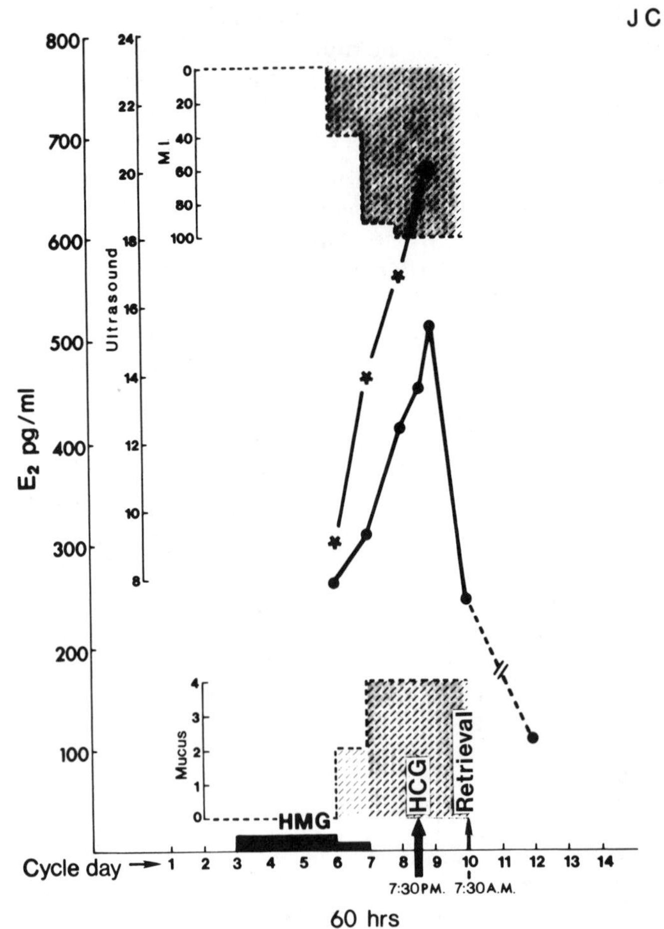

FIG. 4. A low responder. The patient has had an estrogen shift in the peripheral response for 48 hours but the serum E_2 has not reached 300 pg/ml. From G. S. Jones (1984).

hMG dosage given to the high responders, because the high responders require less dosage over a shorter period of time to induce a comparable effect on both the biological E_2 response and estradiol and progesterone synthesis. Note that the degree of steroidogenesis in the luteal phase reflects responses in the follicular phase (Fig. 5).

Importantly, recent findings (Fig. 6) suggest that co-administration of a gonadotropin releasing hormone (GnRH) antagonist with gonadotropin, to achieve a state approaching reversible "medical hypophysectomy," may markedly reduce the individual variability of response to FSH or FSH–LH mixtures (Kenigsberg *et al.*, 1984a,b).

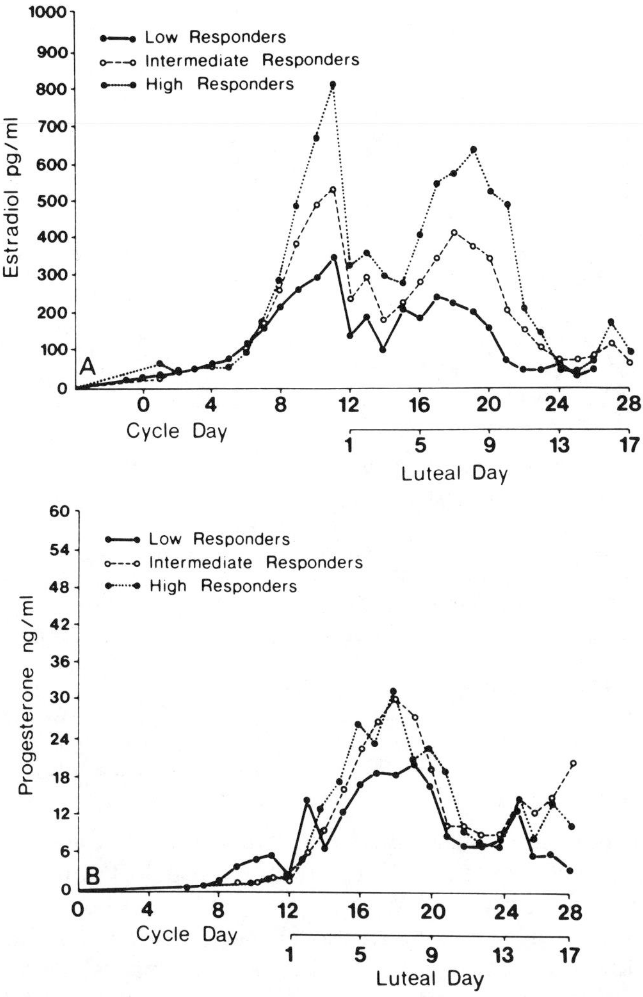

FIG. 5. Both the luteal E_2 (A) and progesterone (B) reflect the patterns of the steroidogenesis in the follicular phase of the cycle, indicating that the responses are dependent upon the initial response to the hMG stimulus, perhaps favoring a receptor theory. From G. S. Jones (1984).

E. IMPORTANCE OF THE FSH : LH RATIO

The importance or unimportance of the ratio of FSH to LH remains an unsettled issue. However, the trend of interpretation of recent data (Fig. 7) indicates that the amount of FSH is of much greater relative significance than is LH (Jones *et al.*, 1984; Schenken *et al.*, 1984; Kenigsberg *et al.*, 1984b). Thus, the ratio of FSH to LH per se may be a

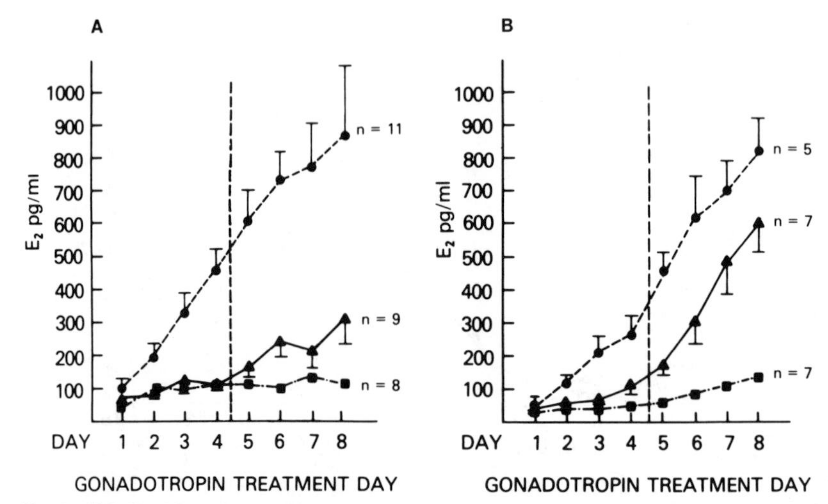

FIG. 6. "Medical hypophysectomy" in monkeys. (A) Groups I and II did not receive and (B) groups III and IV did receive pretreatment with gonadotropin and concurrent treatment with a GnRH antagonist. Among responders, area under the curve (AUC) computations for days 1–4 and days 5–8 (comparing fast and slow responders), analysis of variance, and Kramer's modification of Duncan's multiple range test showed a significant difference ($p > 0.05$) between responses during treatment with the GnRH antagonist. Note: n = the number of subjects for AUC analysis, whereas the number of subjects for daily mean E_2 values may be greater. Coefficients of variation among responders for total AUC in groups I–IV were 63.1, 70.5, 43.1, and 28.3, respectively. When grouped as in (A) and (B), the AUC coefficients of variation were 69.0 and 47.0, respectively. (●) Fast responder, (▲) slow responder, (■) nonresponder. From Kenigsberg *et al.* (1984b).

futile consideration. Rather, it is more important that adequate ovarian response requires more FSH in some patients than others. This much seems clear already. What is less obvious is how much LH is required to support optimal folliculogenesis for *in vitro* fertilization, or whether LH is needed at all. Ongoing studies may show that extra amounts of FSH will directly compensate for an overt LH deficiency.

One myth that deserves squelching is that a major variable in patient response is the FSH:LH ratio in commercial preparations of hMG. To the contrary, when one considers the enormous diversity in patient sensitivity to exogenous gonadotropins compared to as much as a 25% variation (usually about 10%) in FSH:LH biopotency among particular batches of hMG preparations, the former variable (patient response) is so overwhelming as to extinguish the minor impacts of differences in the medications themselves. Besides, patient monitoring is structured to accommodate the need for increasing or decreasing the stimulation regimen based on individualized responses. Thus, while

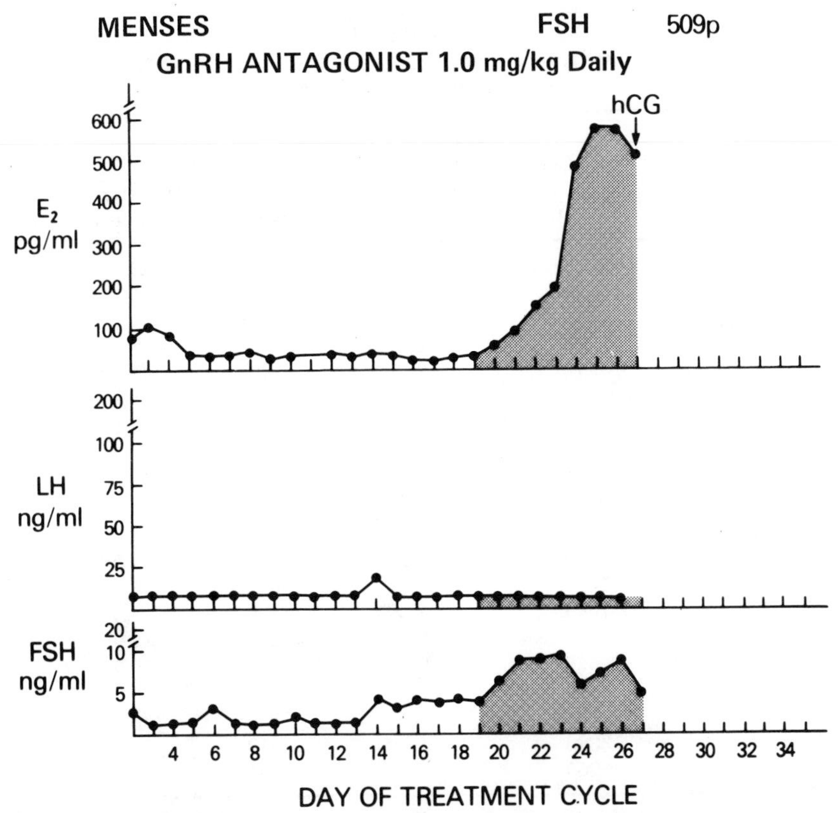

FIG. 7. Representative serum E_2, LH, and FSH values in a typical monkey treated with gonadotropin and GnRH antagonist. Plasma E_2 exceeded 300 pg/ml, qualifying the subject as a responder; but since the level of 300 pg/ml was not reached on or before gonadotropin treatment on day 5, this monkey was classified as a slow responder. The shaded area corresponds to gonadotropin treatment days 1–8. From Kenigsberg *et al.* (1984b).

some variation in the bioavailability of FSH and/or LH surely is inherent to all commercial hMG preparations, its contribution to overall results with *in vitro* fertilization is overshadowed by larger factors. Moreover, radioimmunoassay of FSH and LH in hMG preparations is irrelevant and is a valueless parameter of patient response, which depends strictly on the biologically active forms of FSH and LH contained in the preparation. Although certain patients do respond reproducibly in subsequent cycles (G. S. Jones, 1984), others depart radically, despite repeating the exact protocol in the same woman (J. Cohen, personal communication, 1985) (Table VI).

TABLE VI
RESPONSE OF INDIVIDUAL PATIENTS DURING TWO SEPARATE CYCLES TO IDENTICAL TREATMENT[a]

Case	Pre-hCG E_2 (pg/ml)	Number of mature follicles	Luteal phase	
			E_2 (pg/ml)	Progesterone (ng/ml)
1	1660	3	1100	21
	840	2	650	17
2	2390	5	1580	17
	3700	2	780	21
3	1310	3	400	12
	940	2	620	16.5
4	1280	2	435	1.2
	980	1	470	6
5	1810	6	1310	20
	3020	3	870	50
6	150	3	420	12
	1590	2	680	12.5
7	1420	5	630	14
	1000	3	530	
8	770	3	265	12
	520	6	520	15.5
9	800	2	680	5.5
	133	4	1040	30
10	3320	5	1010	31
	1260	?	35	38

[a] From Cohen (1985).

F. OOCYTE MATURATION IN CULTURE

With hMG stimulation, the cohort of follicles is seldom completely synchronized. One, therefore, may obtain a number of immature oocytes associated with the preovulatory oocytes. Although the fertilization rate of immature oocytes is not high (Table VII), by varying of the duration of time in culture before fertilization, the success rate can be improved. Those oocytes judged to be more mature (germinal vesicle breakdown), may require only 12 hours in culture for polar body extrusion. More immature oocytes (with germinal vesicles) may need up to 32 hours for polar body extrusion. Fertilization should not be attempted before polar body extrusion. Maturation of such oocytes allows an increased number of concepti to be transferred (Suzuki *et al.*, 1983); as previously reported, successful pregnancies from only immature oocytes matured *in vitro* have occurred but may be few in number (Veeck *et al.*, 1983).

TABLE VII

RESULTS OF ATTEMPTS TO MATURE AND FERTILIZE HUMAN OOCYTES *in Vitro* AS COMPARED TO ATTEMPTS TO FERTILIZE PREOVULATORY OOCYTES DURING THE SAME PERIOD, SEPTEMBER 1, 1983 TO JULY 31, 1982[a]

	Immature	Preovulatory
Total number oocytes	74	216
Failed maturation	10 (13.5%)	
Inseminated before completion of maturation	2 (2.7%)	
Failed fertilization after maturation	5 (6.8%)	27 (12.5%)
Fertilized with more than two pronuclei	6 (8.1%)	19 (8.8%)
Failed cleavage after apparently normal fertilization	7 (9.5%)	6 (2.8%)
Total number of concepti undergoing fertilization and transfer	44 (59.5%)	165 (76.4%)
Transferred with cleavage	35 (79.5%)	165 (100%)
Transferred at pronuclear or postpronuclear stage before cleavage	9 (20.5%)	0 (0%)

[a] From Veeck *et al.* (1983).

G. THE SURROGATE LH SURGE

Administration of hCG is usually required after hMG is discontinued (Collins *et al.*, 1984). In choosing the time for aspiration, ovulation will begin within approximately 36–40 hours after hCG administration. In the EVMS program, oocytes are aspirated at 7:50 AM; therefore, hCG is usually administered between 7 and 9 PM, 34–36 hours before the aspiration schedule. If ultrasound and other parameters indicate that follicle maturation is progressing normally, hCG is administered at 50 hours after the last hMG injection. If the ultrasound shows a rapidly increasing follicular size or the serum E_2 plateaus, hCG may be given between 30 and 32 hours after the last hMG injection. Timing of the hMG to hCG interval has been varied throughout several series. A study of results with shortened intervals suggested that, although the numbers of fertilizable eggs retrieved, as well as fertilization, cleavage, and transfer rates, were independent of interval, the pregnancy rate per cycle and per transfer was higher after a 50- or 60-hour interval. Therefore, the hMG to hCG interval should be shortened only by specific indications as stated above.

HCG, which substitutes for the LH surge in the natural cycle, initiates the resumption of oocyte meiosis, the nuclear change which signals oocyte maturation. This requires approximately 28 hours from the beginning of the LH surge and 36 hours from the administration of hCG. From this study, it seems that an interval of 50–60 hours from stopping hMG to giving of hCG may represent a necessary interval for cytoplasmic oocyte maturation to reach completion in the 36 hours after hCG administration. Recent work by Moor *et al.* (1983) in Cambridge would seem to substantiate this theory. The oocytes obtained after a shortened hMG/hCG interval did not seem to show a difference in nuclear maturation but only in the ability to induce a normal pregnancy. Thus it would seem that germinal vesicle breakdown and polar body extrusions representing nuclear maturation are not influenced by the hMG to hCG time interval.

The first 31 EVMS cycles were monitored by analyzing serum LH every 4 hours after the serum estradiol peak indicated an LH surge might be expected, and it was found that no LH surge developed (Fig. 8). LH has not been used, therefore, in monitoring patients in the subsequent series (Ferraretti *et al.*, 1983). Oocyte aspiration for *in vitro* fertilization has been performed in 207 cycles stimulated by hMG with this method and no spontaneous ovulation has occurred before the administration of hCG.

H. Blockade, Delay, or Attenuation of the LH Surge

The finding that hMG stimulation is associated with failure of the LH surge in response to normal or supranormal amounts of estradiol over a 48-hour period in women with normal feedback mechanisms is consistent with the findings of other investigators. Fowler and coworkers (1978) stated that the LH surge "seldom occurs after hMG stimulation of normally menstruating women." These are the only investigators having extensive experience with hMG stimulation in normally ovulating women. In normally ovulating women stimulated with varying gonadotropin protocols at different phases of the cycle, if even a single follicle is stimulated, or if estradiol reaches 2000 pg/ml, an LH surge may occur; otherwise, spontaneous LH surges are unlikely.

Although hCG administration is usually necessary among anovulatory women, it has long been recognized among anovulatory women, particularly those patients with polycystic ovarian disease, who frequently generate inappropriate LH surges, that ovulation can occasionally occur without administration of hCG. Schoemaker *et al.* (1978) demonstrated inhibition of LH secretion in anovulatory patients receiving "pure" pituitary FSH (National Pituitary Agency). The assumption is that LH suppression is mediated by the FSH content of the hMG and not by a direct LH inhibition of LH. The inhibition of the LH surge in hMG-stimulated cycles is apparently not an absolute one, but is related to the amount of stimulated estradiol balanced by the numbers of follicles which are stimulated.

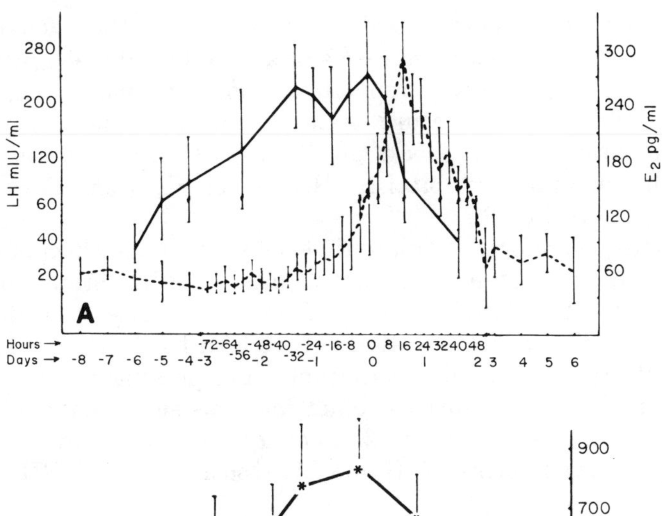

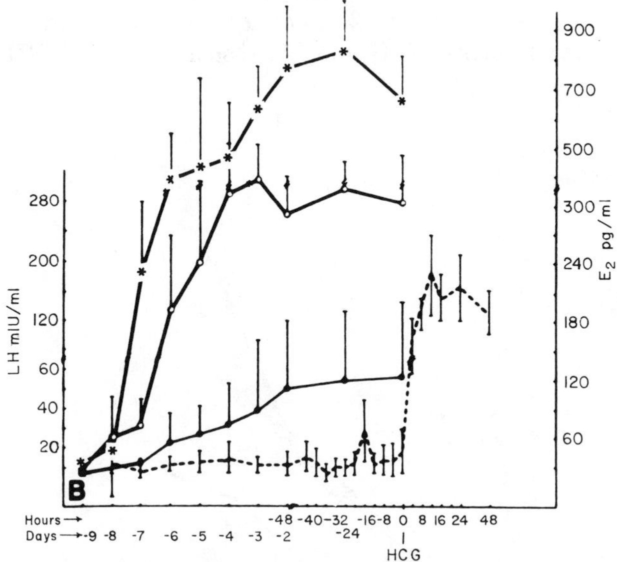

FIG. 8. (A) Serum LH (50 cycles) (- - -) and 17β-estradiol (E_2, 10 cycles) (——) in spontaneous cycles (control group) normalized to the time of initial LH rise (over 60 mIU/ml). Time 0 = time of initial LH rise. (B) Serum LH (16 cycles) (- - -) and 17β-estradiol (——) in hMG/hCG-stimulated cycles, normalized to the time of hCG administration (day 0). Three different E_2 responses are represented. $*$, High E_2 response (6 cycles); ○, normal E_2 response (5 cycles); ●, low E_2 response (5 cycles). All cycles resulted in aspiration of preovulatory oocytes. From Ferraretti *et al.* (1983).

In hMG-treated cycles, any preovulatory oocytes retrieved show decreased size, both by ultrasound and by amount of follicular fluid aspirated. Channing *et al.* (1983) analyzed follicular fluid from these preovulatory follicles and found decreased levels of steroids, estradiol, progesterone, and androstenedione, in relation to those found in the natural cycle, and increased levels of an inhibin-like activity (Channing *et al.*, 1984). This was from 3 to 10 times the amount found in the dominant follicle of the natural cycle. Although porcine follicular fluid "inhibin" preferentially blocks pituitary FSH release, it may also, in sufficient amounts, inhibit LH (Hodgen *et al.*, 1980; Sopelak and Hodgen, 1984) (Fig. 9).

One may, therefore, postulate that the suppressive effect of hMG on the LH surge is related to an increase in inhibin-like protein produced by the hMG-stimulated follicles. We have advanced this theory by determining that administration of pure FSH blocks the FSH and LH surge release in normally cycling monkeys presenting with ovarian hyperstimulation. We further found that this suppression originated at the ovarian level. In contrast, oophorectomized, hMG-stimulated monkeys showed normal FSH and LH responses to a GnRH or estra-

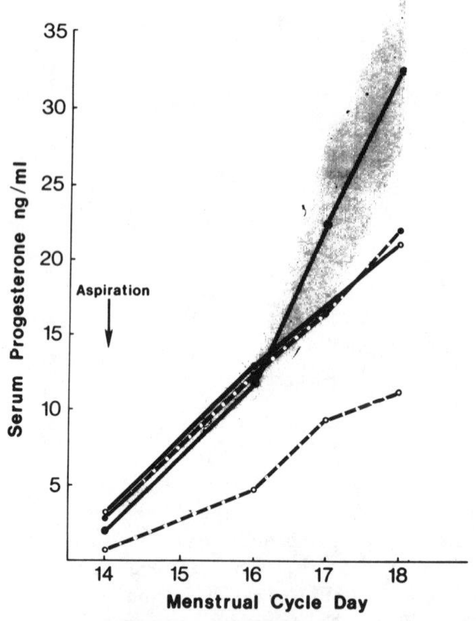

FIG. 9. The shadowed area represents progesterone levels, ± SE, of the pregnant* group (●—●) after hMG/hCG-stimulated cycles during early luteal phase. Notice how progesterone levels of the nonpregnant* (● - - ●) and "advanced" endometrial biopsy (○—○) groups were within the same range of the pregnant group on days 14 and 16 of the menstrual cycle. By day 17, progesterone levels were lower in the nonpregnant and advanced endometrial biopsy groups, but were still within the 1 SE. All progesterone levels on day 18 are significantly lower than the pregnancy levels. (○ - - ○), "In phase" endometrial biopsy group; *progesterone 12.5 mg everyday after day 16. From Garcia *et al.* (1984).

diol stimulation. Blockade of pituitary LH secretion during hMG-induced hyperstimulation is highly transient after ovariectomy (Littman and Hodgen, 1984). The proof of this hypothesis awaits purification and identification of this follicular factor(s).

I. Endometrial Development in a Pharmacological Milieu

The greatest inefficiency in the program for *in vitro* fertilization is found in the step beyond transfer. Why does implantation fail in 75% of cycles? The two obvious considerations are that (1) the endometrium is defective and unable to receive an implantation signal, or (2) the oocyte is defective and unable to signal the endometrium.

It was initially assumed that there was no problem with the endometrium in the hMG-stimulated cycle, as the majority show progesterone serum values in excess of those found in the natural cycle. Nevertheless, in cycles in which estradiol is significantly above that seen in the natural cycle, it is possible that there could be a physiological imbalance in the stimulation of the endometrium. Endometrial biopsies were, therefore, performed on 22 patients who for one reason or another did not receive a conceptus transfer. These biopsies were dated according to the Noyes criteria by three separate pathologists who had no knowledge of the history of the patients. The day of follicular aspiration was arbitrarily designated as cycle day 14 to correspond with the presumed ovulation date in the natural cycle. One biopsy was taken on day 14, one on day 15, and the other 20 biopsies were taken on day 16, the day on which transfer would have occurred. Biopsies obtained on days 14 and 15 were reported as proliferative endometrium, as was one biopsy taken on day 16. Five of the biopsies taken on day 16 were "in phase" by histological dating, in contrast to 11 which were dated 1, 2, or 3 days in advance of normal (Garcia *et al.*, 1984).

The biopsy dates were then compared to serum progesterone results and a good correlation between the dating and the serum progesterone was found (Table VIII). Therefore, serum progesterone at the time of transfer might be used to estimate whether the endometrium into which the conceptus was transferred was advanced or in phase at the time of transfer. Those cycles in which pregnancy occurred were associated with the high progesterone values, similar to values seen in the cycles in the advanced endometrial patterns.

It must be recalled that after *in vitro* fertilization, typically a four-cell conceptus is transferred on day 16 of the cycle, while in the natural cycle a blastocyst arrives in the uterus on day 17 and 18 of the cycle. Therefore, during *in vitro* fertilization with hMG stimulation, a con-

TABLE VIII
SERUM PROGESTERONE LEVELS AT THE TIME OF THE ENDOMETRIAL BIOPSY[a]

Number of cycles	Day of endometrial biopsy			Progesterone (ng/ml) (mean)
	14[b]	15	16	
2	Proliferative			1.3
3		Proliferative		2.2
1			Proliferative	1.3
4			Secretory 16	5.2
5			Secretory 17	8.3
3			Secretory 17–18	16.2
2			Secretory 18	14.7
1			Secretory 19–20	20.8

[a] From Garcia *et al.* (1984)
[b] Follicular aspiration day.

ceptus is being transferred into a uterine endometrium which may be 1–3 days advanced (Fig. 1) in relation to conceptus development.

J. PREIMPLANTATION EMBRYO–ENDOMETRIAL–LUTEAL INTERACTIONS

A study of the luteal progesterone values indicates that progesterone values on the day of aspiration, day 14, and through day 17 are similar in the pregnant, nonpregnant, and advanced endometrial biopsy group of patients. However, by day 18, 1 day after conceptus transfer, there is a statistically significant increase in progesterone values in those patients who become pregnant (Fig. 9). The finding that serum progesterone is significantly elevated in the fertile cycles by even 1 day after transfer needs further study. If this can be substantiated it is hard to escape the conclusion that the embryo, even at this early state, is signaling to reinforce the function of the corpus luteum and to prevent luteolysis.

K. PREGNANCY RATES

The ultimate success of *in vitro* fertilization and embryo transfer therapy can be judged only by the take-home rate of normal healthy babies. In order to evaluate the efficacy of these pregnancy statistics, it is necessary to compare the pregnancy rates in the *in vitro* fertilization program to the expectancy of pregnancy and abortion in any one normal cycle of pregnancy exposure. (Fig. 10). Studies of the literature show that the *in vitro* results are approaching those of normal repro-

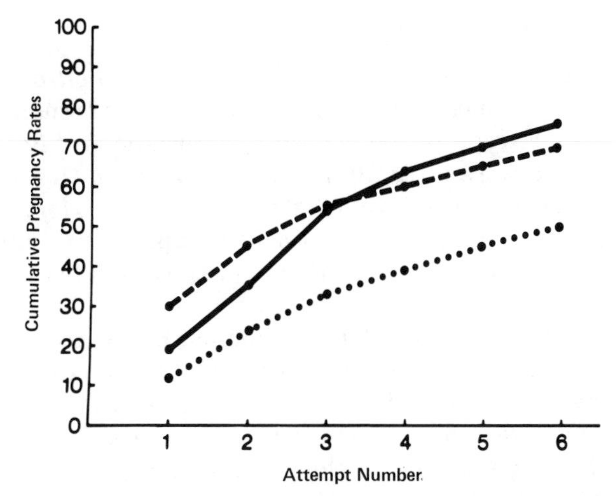

FIG. 10. Cumulative pregnancy rate of *in vitro* fertilization rivals *in vivo* conceptions. Data from the Norfolk *in vitro* fertilization program, 1981–1984. (——) *In vitro* fertilization, 509 patients, 932 cycles. (---) Natural conception, 2900 patients. (···) Artificial insemination of donor (AID), 259 patients, 1273 cycles. From H. W. Jones, Jr. (1985).

duction (Lutjen *et al.,* 1984). With the ability to transfer more than one conceptus, it is theoretically possible that when optimum conditions are known and achieved, the normal pregnancy rate of 25% may be exceeded by *in vitro* fertilization.

Although the pregnancy rate for *in vitro* fertilization is beginning to approach the normal expectancy for any given exposure cycle, many unknown technical and theoretical problems remain to be solved. Major among these are determining the best method to stimulate multiple follicle maturation for oocyte retrieval and improving the monitoring to ensure retrieval of the most mature oocyte. In addition to improving current methods of stimulation and monitoring, it is important to make an effort to improve the culture media for better oocyte cytoplasmic maturation.

The state of the art for *in vitro* fertilization today is aiming toward the induction of a more predictable stimulation pattern. Recognition of the high, intermediate, or low response patterns of individual patients to hMG stimulation, and perhaps also to clomiphene citrate, may be crucial. Patient individualization should allow increased pregnancy rates and fewer miscarriages, which now comprise up to 30% of all confirmed pregnancies. The problems associated with failure of implantation after transfer seem to reflect normalcy and stage of maturation of the oocyte itself, rather than the endometrium.

L. Unique Research Opportunities

We might note that until the era of successful *in vitro* fertilization, perhaps less than 10 persons had ever seen a living human preimplantation embryo. Except for the few early observations of Rock and Hertig (1942), there were virtually no direct studies on the early human conceptus. Indeed, it was the clinical utility of *in vitro* fertilization and embryo transfer for infertility treatment that provided simultaneously the professional impetus and ethical justification for crossing this threshold.

With the advent of *in vitro* fertilization has come access, for the first time, to the "substrates" requisite for renewal of human life. From this milieu, research opportunities emerge at two levels: (1) clinical investigation to improve and extend therapeutic success of *in vitro* fertilization; and (2) basic research on the fundamental processes controlling development, differentiation of the embryo, maternal immune tolerance, and response to the genomic signals that orchestrate timely gene expression and repression. Improvements in ovarian stimulation protocols, egg or embryo donation (Table IX and Fig. 11), cryopreservation of embryos, and oocyte maturation *in vitro* (Fig. 12) are immediate goals; such research holds potential significance beyond the brink of our current scientific anticipation. Indeed, newly acquired access to human gametes and preimplantation embryos provides the basis for direct study of the human germ line, the origins of teratogenic and genetic defects (lethal and nonlethal), the process of oncogenesis, and even aging itself.

Development of somatic cell gene therapy is virtually upon us, and it is not unreasonable to project manipulation of human germinal material for disease diagnosis and prevention by the onset of the twenty-first century, barely more than a dozen years away. Through the confluence of molecular biology and reproductive medicine, these op-

TABLE IX
Clinical Indications for Egg or Embryo Donation

Inaccessible ovaries
Genetic disease
Contraindications for *in vitro* fertilization
Ovarian dysgenesis
Premature menopause
Surgical castration
Failed *in vitro* fertilization

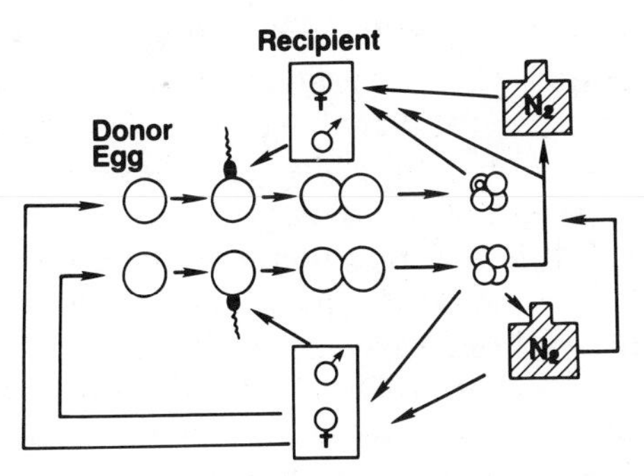

FIG. 11. A series of scenarios for egg or embryo donation. N_2, liquid nitrogen storage.

portunities surely rival the most monumental achievements of medical science from Pasteur to the present. A few examples will make my point. Cancer biologists are forging a persuasive theme that 20–30 oncogenes may spawn the aggressive behavior of virulent tumor cells; often these malignant tissues are able to preferentially sequester a vast blood supply, avoid immune rejection by the host, and elaborate unique gene products such as chorionic gonadotropin and α-fetoprotein (AFP) that reflect reactivation of embryonic genes, long dormant after completion of intrauterine life. The parallelisms of oncogenesis with embryogenesis and fetal development are extensive, including angiogenic expressions of the implanting blastocyst, the immune privilege of gestation, the copresence of unique trophoblastic hormones (hCG)

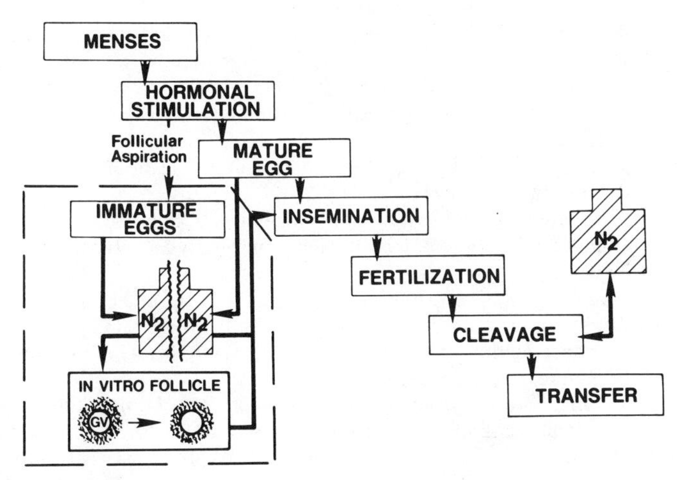

FIG. 12. A high scientific priority is the technology permitting *in vitro* maturation of the immature oocyte.

with fetal hepatic proteins (AFP), and finally, persistence of an accelerated mitogenic status. It is imperative to learn whether viral vectors are passed between generations along the human germinal line itself.

We have only begun to appreciate how these new investigative endeavors radiate outward from current *in vitro* fertilization and embryo transfer therapy. While the treatment of human infertility remains at the epicenter of these activities, past and current achievements may pale beside the nascent realities previously trapped within the inaccessible human embryo. That profound ethical, social, and legal concerns are raised by human embryo research is obvious. This, too, is a unique and special challenge to mankind, because the preservation and protection of what is human can be described and regarded in so many ways.

REFERENCES

Chang, M. C. (1971). Second Annual Carl G. Hartman Lecture. Experimental studies of mammalian spermatozoa and eggs. *Biol. Reprod.* **4,** 3.

Channing, C. P., Liu, C. Q., Evans, V., Gabliano, P., Jones, G. S., Veeck, L. L., and Jones, H. W., Jr. (1983). Decline of follicular oocyte maturation inhibitor coincident with maturation achievement of fertilizability of oocytes recovered at midcycle of gonadotropin-treated women. *Proc. Natl. Acad. Sci. U.S.A.* **80,** 4184.

Channing, C. P., Tanabe, K., Jones, G. S., Jones, H. W., Jr., and Lebech, P. (1984). Inhibin activity of preovulatory follicles of gonadotropin-treated and untreated women. *Fertil. Steril.* **42,** 243.

Chillik, C. F., Acosta, A. A., Garcia, J. E., Perera, S., van Uem, J. F. H. M., Rosenwaks, Z., and Jones, H. W., Jr. (1985). The role of *in vitro* fertilization in infertile patients with endometriosis. *Fertil. Steril.* **44,** 56.

Collins, R. L., Williams, R. F., and Hodgen, G. D. (1984). Endocrine consequences of prolonged ovarian hyperstimulation: Hyperprolactinemia, follicular atresia, and premature luteinization. *Fertil. Steril.* **42,** 436.

Edwards, R. G., and Purdy, J. M., eds. (1982). "Human Conception in Vitro." Academic Press, London.

Edwards, R. G., and Steptoe, P. C. (1983). Current status of *in vitro* fertilization and implantation of human embryos. *Lancet* **2,** 1265.

Ferraretti, A. P., Garcia, J. E., Acosta, A. A., and Jones, G. S. (1983). Serum LH during ovulation induction for *in vitro* fertilization in normally menstruating women. *Fertil. Steril.* **40,** 742.

Fowler, R. E., Edwards, R. G., Walters, D. E., Chan, S. T. H., and Steptoe, P. C. (1978). Steroidogenesis in preovulatory follicles of patients given human menopausal and chorionic gonadotrophins as judged by the radioimmunoassay of steroids in follicular fluid. *J. Endocrinol.* **77,** 161.

Garcia, J. E., Jones, G. S., Acosta, A. A., and Wright, G. L., Jr. (1983). HMG/hCG follicular maturation of oocyte aspiration. Phase I, 1981. *Fertil. Steril.* **39,** 167.

Garcia, J. E., Acosta, A. A., Hsiu, J.-G., and Jones, H. W., Jr. (1984). Advanced endometrial maturation after ovulation induction with human menopausal gonadotropin/human chorionic gonadotropin for *in vitro* fertilization. *Fertil. Steril.* **41,** 31.

Garcia, J. E., Jones, H. W., Jr., Acosta, A. A., and Andrews, M. C. (1985). Reconstructive pelvic surgery for *in vitro* fertilization. *J. In Vitro Fertil.*, in press.

Goodman, A. L., and Hodgen, G. D. (1983). The ovarian triad of the primate menstrual cycle. *Recent Prog. Horm. Res.* **39,** 1.

Guttmacher, A. F. (1952). Fertility of man. *Fertil. Steril.* **3,** 281.

Hackeloer, B. J., Fleming, R., Robinson, H. P., Adam, A. H., Coutts, J. R. (1979). Correlation of ultrasonic and endocrinologic assessment of human follicular development. *Am. J. Obstet. Gynecol.* **135,** 122.

HEW Ethics Advisory Board (1979). Report and conclusions: HEW support of research involving human *in vitro* fertilization and embryo transfer, May 4. Submitted to HEW Secretary Joseph Califano.

Hodgen, G. D. (1983). Surrogate embryo transfer combined with estrogen–progesterone therapy in ovariectomized monkeys: Implantation, gestation, and delivery without ovaries. *J. Am. Med. Asso.* **250,** 2167.

Hodgen, G. D. (1984). Testimony at Hearings of the Subcommittee on Investigations and Oversight, August 8, 9.

Hodgen, G. D., Channing, C., Anderson, L., Gagliano, P., Turner, C., and Stouffer, R. (1980). On the regulation of FSH secretion in the primate hypothalamic–pituitary–ovarian axis. *In* "Endocrinology 1980" (I. A. Cumming, J. W. Funder, and F. A. O. Mendelson, eds.), p. 263. Elsevier, New York.

Jones, G. S. (1984). Update on *in vitro* fertilization. *Endocr. Rev.* **5,** 62.

Jones, G. S., Garcia, J. E., and Acosta, A. A. (1982). Luteal phase evaluation in *in vitro* fertilization. *In* "Human Conception *In Vitro*" (R. G. Edwards and J. M. Purdy, eds.), p. 293. Academic Press, London.

Jones, G. S., Garcia, J. E., and Rosenwaks, Z. (1984). The role of pituitary gonadotropins in follicular stimulation and oocyte maturation in the human. *J. Clin. Endocrinol. Metab.* **59,** 178.

Jones, H. W., Jr. (1985). Indications for *in vitro* fertilization. "In Vitro Fertilization at Norfolk," Chap. 1. Williams & Wilkins, Baltimore.

Kenigsberg, D., Littman, B. A., and Hodgen, G. D. (1984a). Medical hypophysectomy. I: Dose-response using a GnRH antagonist. *Fertil. Steril.* **42,** 112.

Kenigsberg, D., Littman, B. A., and Hodgen, G. D. (1984b). Medical hypophysectomy. II: Variability of ovarian response to gonadotropin therapy. *Fertil. Steril.* **42,** 116.

Laufer, N., DeCherney, A. H., Haseltine, F. P., Polan, M. L., Mezer, H. C., Dlugi, A. M., Sweeney, D., Nero, F., and Naftolin, F. (1983). The use of high-dose human menopausal gonadotropin in an *in vitro* fertilization program. *Fertil. Steril.* **40,** 734.

Leung, P. C. S., Lopata, A., Kellow, G. N., Johnston, W. I. H., and Gronow, M. J. (1983). A histochemical study of cumulus cells for assessing the quality of preovulatory oocytes. *Fertil Steril.* **39,** 853.

Littman, B. A., and Hodgen, G. D. (1984). Human menopausal gonadotropin stimulation in monkeys: Blockade of the luteinizing hormone surge by a highly transient ovarian factor. *Fertil. Steril.,* **41,** 440.

Lutjen, P., Trounson, A., Leeton, J., Findlay, J., Wood, C., and Renou, P. (1984). The establishment and maintenance of pregnancy using *in vitro* fertilization and embryo donation in a patient with primary ovarian failure. *Nature* (*London*) **307,** 174.

Mantzavinos, T., Garcia, J. E., and Jones, H. W., Jr. (1983). Ultrasound measurement of ovarian follicles stimulated by human gonadotropins for oocyte recovery and *in vitro* fertilization. *Fertil. Steril.* **40,** 461.

Moor, R. M., Crosby, I. M., and Osborn, J. C. (1983). Growth and maturation of mammalian oocytes. *In* "*In Vitro* Fertilization and Embryo Transfer" (P. G. Crosignai and B.

L. Rubin, eds.), p. 39. Serono Clinical Colloquia on Reproduction 4. Academic Press, London.

Muasher, S., Garcia, J. E., and Jones, H. W., Jr. (1984). *Fertil. Steril.* **42,** 20.

Quigley, M. M., Berkowitz, A. S., Gilbert, S. A., and Wolf, D. P. (1984). Clomiphene citrate in an *in vitro* fertilization program: Hormonal comparisons between 50- and 150-mg daily dosages. *Fertil. Steril.* **41,** 809.

Quinn, P., Warnes, G., Kerin, J., and Kirby, C. (1984). Culture factors in relation to the success of human *in vitro* fertilization and embryo transfer. *Fertil. Steril.* **41,** 202.

Rock, J., and Hertig, A. T. (1942). Some aspects of early human development. *Am. J. Obstet. Gynecol.* **44,** 973.

Schenken, R. S., Williams, R. F., and Hodgen, G. D. (1984). Ovulation induction using "pure" follicle stimulating hormone in monkeys. *Fertil. Steril.* **41,** 629.

Schoemaker, J., Wentz, A. C., Jones, G. E., Dubin, N. H., and Sapp, K. C. (1978). Stimulation of follicular growth with "pure" FSH in patients with anovulation and elevated LH levels. *Obstet. Gynecol.* **51,** 270.

Sopelak, V. M., and Hodgen, G. D. (1984). Blockade of estrogen-induced LH surges in monkeys: A non-steroidal antigenic factor in porcine follicular fluid. *Fertil. Steril.* **41,** 108.

Suzuki, S., Endo, Y., Fujiwara, T., Tanaka, S., and Iizuka, R. (1983). Cytochemical study of steroid-producing activities of human oocytes. *Fertil. Steril.* **39,** 683.

Testart, J., Lassalle, B., and Frydman, R. (1982). Apparatus for the *in vitro* fertilization and culture of human oocytes. *Fertil. Steril.* **38,** 372.

Trounson, A., and Wood, C. (1981). Extracorporeal fertilization and embryo transfer. *Clin. Obstet. Gynecol.* **8,** 681.

Van Uem, J. F. H. M., Acosta, A. A., Swanson, R. J., Mayer, J., Ackerman, S., Burkman, L. J., Veeck, L., McDowell, J. S., Bernardus, R. E., and Jones, H. W., Jr. (1985). Male factor evaluation *in vitro* fertilization. Norfolk experience, in press.

Vargyas, J. M., Morente, C., Shangold, G., and Marrs, R. P. (1984). The effect of different methods of ovarian stimulation for human *in vitro* fertilization and embryo replacement. *Fertil. Steril.* **42,** 745.

Veeck, L. L., Wortham, J. W., Witmyer, J., Sandow, B. A., Acosta, A. A., Garcia, J. E., Jones, G. S., and Jones, H. W., Jr. (1983). Maturation and fertilization of morphologically immature human oocytes in a program of *in vitro* fertilization. *Fertil. Steril.* **39,** 594.

Wentz, A. C., Repp, J. E., Maxson, W. S., Pittaway, D. E., and Torbit, C. A. (1983). The problem of polyspermy in *in vitro* fertilization. *Fertil. Steril.* **40,** 748.

VITAMINS AND HORMONES, VOL. 43

Intracellular Processing and Secretion of Parathyroid Gland Proteins

DAVID V. COHN, RAMASAMY KUMARASAMY, AND WARREN K. RAMP

Departments of Oral Biology and Biochemistry,
Health Sciences Center,
University of Louisville,
Louisville, Kentucky 40292

I. Introduction

The parathyroid gland is of paramount interest to workers in fields related to calcium metabolism because of the important role its hormone PTH (parathormone, parathyroid hormone, parathyrin) plays in the regulation of body calcium. Additional attention has recently been focused on the gland because of the realization that it also synthesizes and secretes a major glycoprotein termed *secretory protein-I* (SP-I) that is similar, if not identical, to chromogranin A (CGA), a protein cosecreted with epinephrine by the adrenal. SP-I/CGA appears to be present in a large number of endocrine, but not exocrine, cells.

This review focuses on PTH, its synthesis, intracellular processing, and secretion, and provides current information on the chemistry and biology of SP-I and its possible relationship to PTH. Some recent reviews emphasizing different aspects of the subject that the reader might wish to consult include those by Cohn and MacGregor (1981), Potts *et al.* (1982), Cohn and Elting (1983, 1984), and Habener *et al.* (1984).

II. Calcium Homeostasis

The many functions of calcium in physiology are well known to readers of this review. Some that immediately come to mind include its role in muscular contraction, transmission of nerve impulses, coupled stimulus–secretion, and cell–cell interaction (Cheung, 1980, 1982). In addition, Ca^{2+} together with phosphate comprise the major components of the mineral hydroxyapatite that provides rigidity and structural strength to the skeleton (Glimcher, 1976). When the concentration of Ca^{2+} in the extracellular fluid moves out of the physiological range, those processes dependent upon Ca^{2+} are disrupted (Phang and Weiss, 1976; Neer, 1979). In rickets and osteomalacia, for example, lack of vitamin D limits Ca^{2+} absorption (DeLuca, 1983), and proper mineralization of the skeleton becomes impossible (Meunier, 1983). In hypoparathyroidism the concentration of extracellular Ca^{2+} declines and tetany may occur (Parfitt, 1979). When the concentration of Ca^{2+} in the extracellular fluid is too high, in hyperparathyroidism for example, nephrocalcinosis may result (Aurbach *et al.*, 1985).

Considering the many critical physiological processes dependent upon regulated Ca^{2+} concentration in intracellular fluids, it is not surprising that higher animals have developed a complex homeostatic system to maintain this concentration (Neer, 1979). The normal concentration of total extracellular calcium in man is about 2.5 m*M*, half of which is ionized. The nonionized fraction is bound primarily to serum proteins with smaller amounts associated with anions of blood serum such as phosphate, citrate, and carbonate.

A fall in serum Ca^{2+} concentration causes an increase in the rate of secretion of PTH (Mayer, 1979). The released hormone acts on bone cells to stimulate osteoclastic bone resorption, to increase osteoclastic Ca^{2+} release, and to limit new bone formation (Raisz, 1976; Ramp and McNeil, 1978; Cohn and Wong, 1979)—actions that bring skeletal Ca^{2+} into the extracellular fluid or limit its exit. It enhances renal Ca^{2+} retention and allows excess serum phosphate to be excreted by decreasing renal tubular reabsorption (Handler and Cohn, 1952; Pulman *et al.*, 1960). Finally PTH stimulates 1-hydroxylation of 25-hydroxycholecalciferol (Garabedian *et al.*, 1972; Fraser and Kodicek, 1973), enhancing the synthesis of 1,25-dihydroxycholecalciferol, the most active metabolite of vitamin D (DeLuca, 1983), which in turn increases the intestinal absorption of Ca^{2+}. Each of these actions leads to an increase in Ca^{2+} in the extracellular fluid which eliminates the secretory stimulus to the parathyroid through negative feedback.

When Ca^{2+} concentration rises above the normal level, the C cells of the thyroid secrete calcitonin, a peptide hormone that inhibits osteoclastic bone resorption (Luben *et al.*, 1976, 1977) and decreases the efflux of Ca^{2+} from the skeleton (Talmage *et al.*, 1983). In some animals calcitonin enhances renal excretion of Ca^{2+}. These actions all tend to lower the Ca^{2+} concentration of the extracellular fluid.

In this complex homeostatic scheme, PTH is considered responsible for the moment-to-moment regulation of the circulating Ca^{2+} concentration. Vitamin D metabolites modulate calcium balance over the longer term through relatively slowly developing effects on intestinal calcium absorption and parathyroid gland metabolism. Calcitonin modulates postprandial hypercalcemia in some species but there is no known function of calcitonin in adult man.

III. Biochemistry and Physiology of Parathyroid Hormone

A. Chemistry of PTH

The amino acid sequences of PTH have been completely defined for man (Keutmann *et al.*, 1978; Hendy *et al.*, 1981; Vasicek *et al.*, 1983), cow (Brewer and Ronan, 1970; Niall *et al.*, 1970), pig (Sauer *et al.*, 1974), and rat (Heinrich *et al.*, 1984), and partially determined for chicken (MacGregor *et al.*, 1976b) and dog (Cohn and Hamilton, 1976). In each species the hormone consists of 84 amino acids in a single chain with a molecular weight of about 9600 (Fig. 1). There is a high degree

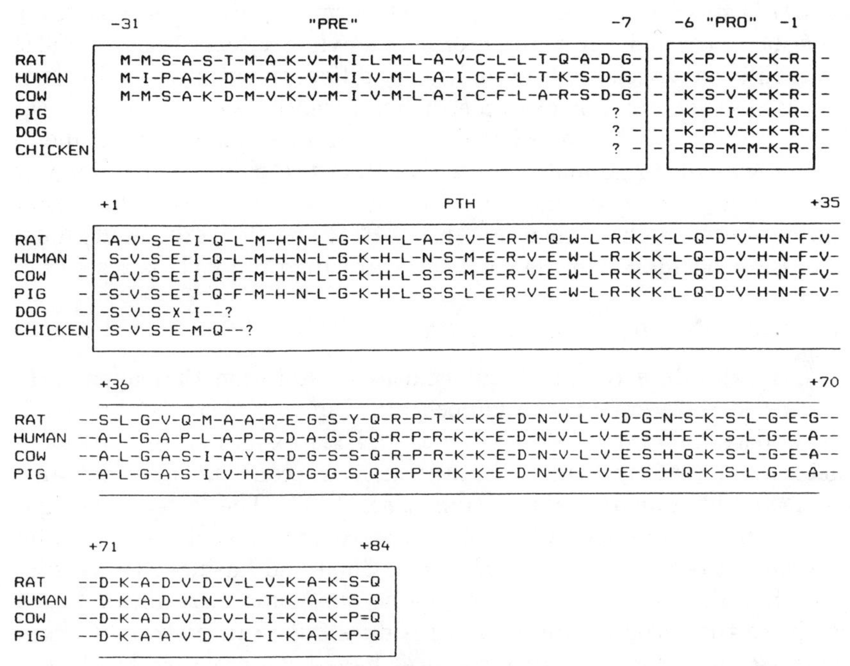

Fig. 1. Amino acid sequences of PTH peptides from different species. "PRE" represents the segment of the molecule denoted the "signal sequence"; "PRO," the prohormone hexapeptide; and PTH, the hormone sequence. Blank spaces and ? indicate that that portion of the molecule has not been sequenced. The one-letter code for amino acids is used as follows: A, Ala; C, Cys; D, Asp; E, Glu; F, Phe; G, Gly; H, His; I, Ile; K, Lys; L, Leu; M, Met; N, Asn; P, Pro; Q, Gln; R, Arg; S, Ser; T, Thr; V, Val; W, Trp; X, unknown; Y, Tyr.

of homology among the PTHs of different species, particularly in the amino terminal region that carries the biological activity (see below).

PTH is unglycosylated (Morrissey *et al.,* 1978) and generally does not contain modified amino acids. A recent report, however, suggests that a phosphorylated form of the hormone exists (Rabbani *et al.,* 1984). Phosphorylation developed during a 4-hour incubation of parathyroid tissue *in vitro* and it is not clear that it is physiological, particularly since the parathyroid cell contains protein kinase (Lasker and Spiegel, 1982; Brown and Thatcher, 1982) and PTH (residues 1–34) has been shown to be a general substrate for protein kinases of the brain (Raese *et al.,* 1980).

An extensive series of structure–function analyses (Rosenblatt, 1982; Potts *et al.,* 1982) show that the biological activity of PTH resides in the first third of the amino-terminal portion of the molecule, with the minimum molecule represented by residues 1–27. Generally, PTH (1–34) is fully as active as the intact hormone, although most tests have been carried out with *in vitro* adenylate cyclase assays. PTHs from different species exhibit markedly different activities in the various assay systems. For example, it has recently been found that rat PTH fragment 1–34 tested with rat or canine renal cortical membranes was up to 10-fold more active than the equivalent human or bovine hormone fragments (Keutmann *et al.,* 1985). It follows that evaluation of the biological activity of PTH and PTH fragments must take into consideration the conditions in which the PTH is tested.

B. Secondary and Tertiary Structure of PTH

PTH exhibits a complex conformation in solution that appears to reorder at different pHs (Edelhoch and Lippoldt, 1969; Cohn *et al.,* 1974c; Brewer *et al.,* 1975). Images of PTH examined by dark-field electron microscopy suggest that the molecule consists of two domains connected by a short stalk (Fiskin *et al.,* 1977). The latter investigators, using the predictive formulas for secondary structure (Chou and Fasman, 1974a,b; Fasman *et al.,* 1976; Chou and Fasman, 1977), suggest that PTH residues 1–29 comprise one domain, residues 43–84 comprise the second domain, and residues 30–42 in a straight chain comprise the stalk. Similar structures have been proposed by Geisow (1978) and by Zull and Lev (1980). Additional aspects of PTH conformation were considered by Cohn and Elting (1984).

C. The Physiological Precursors of PTH

Two biological precursors of PTH have been described. The immediate precursor is proparathormone (proPTH) (Hamilton *et al.,* 1971a;

Cohn *et al.*, 1972a,b; Kemper *et al.*, 1972). It represents PTH plus an additional hexapeptide segment, highly basic, at the amino terminus (Fig. 1). ProPTHs from cow (Hamilton *et al.*, 1974), human (Chu *et al.*, 1973b; Cohn *et al.*, 1974b; Jacobs *et al.*, 1974; Huang *et al.*, 1975), pig (Chu *et al.*, 1975), dog (Cohn and Hamilton, 1976), chicken (MacGregor *et al.*, 1976b), and rat (Heinrich *et al.*, 1984) have been studied thus far (Fig. 1). Only slight differences exist among the "pro" sequences in the proPTHs from the different species. In each instance, a Lys–Arg pair precedes the PTH sequence. This amino acid pair or the equally basic pair Arg–Arg is also found in other peptides that are cleaved to yield the secreted form of the protein from, for example, proinsulin, proglucagon, or proalbumin (Steiner *et al.*, 1984). ProPTH exhibits less immunoactivity and less biological activity than does PTH (Hamilton *et al.*, 1971a), suggesting that removal of its hexapeptide terminus to produce PTH yields a significant change in conformation of the molecule released to react in the periphery with target cell receptors.

The immediate precursor of proPTH, and the actual gene product, is preproPTH (Kemper *et al.*, 1976a, 1974b; Habner *et al.*, 1975b). As portrayed in Fig. 1, this molecule contains a 25 amino acid extension at the amino-terminal end of proPTH (Kemper *et al.*, 1976a; Habener *et al.*, 1978). This portion of the molecule is exceedingly hydrophobic and is typical of the so-called "signal" or "leader" sequence common for almost all proteins that are destined for export (Kreibich *et al.*, 1980; Blobel, 1983).

An analysis of the internal homology of preproPTH (Cohn *et al.*, 1979) using a mutation matrix designed to detect distant protein relationships (Barker and Dayhoff, 1972; Dayhoff *et al.*, 1972) and the Chou–Fasman technique for predicting secondary structure (Chou and Fasman, 1974a,b, 1977; Fasman *et al.*, 1976) indicates that the molecule was generated by gene duplication with the result that residues −23 to +29 match residues +30 to +81. A recent extension of this work suggests that each half of the molecule is itself the product of an earlier gene duplication (Mallette *et al.*, 1985). It was estimated by Cohn *et al.* (1979a) that the most recent gene duplication occurred about 150 million years ago, the time in evolution at which amphibia first appeared. Since more primitive animals of earlier evolutionary age than amphibia lack parathyroid glands, it had been assumed that the hormone did not circulate in such species. The reports of a hypercalcemic factor in fish pituitary (Parsons *et al.*, 1978) and in eel corpuscles of Stannius (Lopez *et al.*, 1984), the latter containing factor(s) chemically and immunologically similar to mammalian PTH, suggest that a primitive PTH partially homologous to today's molecule exists in pre-amphibians (Cohn *et al.*, 1979a).

D. The PTH Gene

Chromosome mapping studies have localized the human PTH gene to the short arm of chromosome 11 (11p) (Antonarakis *et al.,* 1983; Kittur *et al.,* 1985). Relatively close are the genes for calcitonin, β-globin, the oncogene HRAS1, IGF-2, and insulin. It is not known whether the proximity of the PTH gene to the other endocrine factors is of biological significance.

The genes coding for bovine, human, and rat PTH are not continuous (Hendy *et al.,* 1981; Kemper *et al.,* 1981; Weaver *et al.,* 1982; Vasicek *et al.,* 1983; Heinrich *et al.,* 1984). There are two intervening sequences that separate the gene into a 5′ noncoding domain, a pre sequence and a partial pro sequence domain (to residue −3) and a domain containing the remainder of the pro sequence, the entire PTH sequence, and the 3′ noncoding region. The location of the introns are identical in the bovine, human, and rat genes but their sizes differ. The flanking sequences are about 80% homologous.

E. Intracellular Traffic Patterns of Proteins

The biosynthesis, processing, and directing of proteins to their appropriate locales within the cell are each specific phases of a complex and varied intracellular traffic program (Kreil, 1981; Blobel, 1983; Steiner *et al.,* 1984). One class of protein after synthesis (e.g., a cytosolic protein) remains in the cytoplasm. Another enters and becomes part of a membrane, in which, depending upon function, it may be totally enclosed (e.g., a structural protein) or partially enclosed (e.g., a hormone receptor). A third, including proteins destined for export (e.g., hormones, digestive enzymes, or lysosomal enzymes) pass through a membrane to be encased within a vesicle. The fate of these latter proteins then depends upon the fate of the vesicle, which may undergo exocytosis or fusion with other intracellular vesicles.

The chemical basis explaining why some proteins are exported and others are retained within the cell is now becoming evident. Regardless of destination, all proteins are synthesized in the same way. The fundamental process involves translation of the mRNA by the ribosomal complex and discharge from the mRNA–ribosomal complex of the still-growing nascent chain (Blobel, 1983). The routing of a protein to the cytoplasm or a particular intracellular membrane is governed by the primary amino acid sequence of the protein. Almost without exception those proteins destined for export are synthesized as a larger precursor molecule containing at its amino-terminal end a hydrophobic leader sequence, the so-called signal sequence (Milstein *et al.*, 1972; Blobel and Dobberstein, 1975). This sequence, as it is spun out of the ribosome, permits the nascent protein–ribosome–mRNA complex to bind to a so-called signal recognition particle (SRP) consisting of six nonidentical polypeptides and a 7 S RNA (Walter and Blobel, 1980, 1981a,b, 1982; Walter *et al.*, 1981). This complex then binds to an endoplasmic reticulum "docking protein," an interaction that allows the nascent protein chain to pass through the membrane and enter the cisternal space. The signal sequence is then removed by peptidase, a cleavage required for the protein to move from the membrane (Dalbey and Wickner, 1985).

In their classic studies, Palade and associates (see Palade, 1975) elucidated the traffic pattern of exportable proteins: transport from site of synthesis to the cisternal space of the rough endoplasmic reticulum (RER), RER to Golgi, Golgi to secretory vesicles, secretory vesicles to extracellular site via exocytosis.

Those proteins that are integrated into a membrane rather than passing totally through it contain amino acid sequences downstream of the signal sequence that act as a "stop" message. In addition to conveying information as to where the protein should be directed, the primary amino acid sequence carries information relative to co- and posttranslational modification including glycosylation, phosphorylation, and proteolytic cleavage.

F. Biosynthesis and Processing of PTH

The biosynthesis and processing of PTH are not exceptions to the considerations just mentioned for exportable proteins. In addition to directed transport, however, PTH is subject to substantial posttranslational proteolytic degradation that plays an important physiological role in its formation and secretion.

Supporting the general description of the intracellular flow of PTH-related peptides are data from autoradiographic examination of the parathyroids after injection of radiolabeled amino acids or carbohydrates into rats (Nakagami *et al.*, 1971; Habener *et al.*, 1979) or after incubation of the gland with radioactive amino acids (Habener *et al.*, 1981). As early as 2 minutes after labeling of the tissue, autoradiographic grains were located over the RER. Most of the label was over the Golgi by 10 minutes, and over secretory vesicles by 20–30 minutes. These data, by themselves, are equivocal since specific identification of the radioactive proteins giving rise to autoradiographic grains was not possible. Indeed, it is likely that the majority of the grains attributed to PTH were caused by SP-I since per unit of time about sevenfold more radioactivity is incorporated into the latter protein than into PTH (Cohn and Elting, 1984). Nonetheless, the projected intracellular flow described for the PTH peptides is substantiated directly by several *in vitro* studies.

G. Synthesis and Vectorial Transport of preproPTH and proPTH

The synthesis of preproPTH is readily apparent in cell-free translation systems using PTH mRNA (Kemper *et al.,* 1974a, 1976b; Habener *et al.,* 1975b). Addition of pancreatic membranes (containing endoplasmic reticulum) to the incubation system yields proPTH, not preproPTH, as the product and it becomes segregated within the membranes (Dorner and Kemper, 1978). The signal sequence is likely degraded or left within the membranes since it has never been detected. Recently it was shown that cloned DNA encoding human preproPTH can be expressed by rat pituitary cells (Hellerman *et al.,* 1984). Modifications proposed to be made by these investigators in the DNA sequences coding for the pre sequence might provide specific details on how the signal sequence participates in the transport of the PTH molecule.

Intact parathyroid tissue, tissue slices, or dispersed cells incubated with radioactive amino acids give rise to proPTH in 2 minutes or less (Cohn *et al.,* 1972b; Chu *et al.,* 1975; Morrissey *et al.,* 1980b) and PTH in about 15 minutes (Hamilton and Cohn, 1969; Hamilton *et al.,* 1971b). In only one study was a trace of preproPTH detected and the investigators suggest that this might have been an artifact of the system (Habener and Potts, 1979). Examination of the parathyroid tissue after incubation *in vitro* with radioactive amino acids shows that the bulk of the newly synthesized PTH peptides is associated with those particulate fractions rich in membranes and secretory granules (MacGregor *et al.,* 1973, 1978a; MacGregor and Cohn, 1978; Habener and Potts, 1979a; Morrissey *et al.,* 1980b).

H. Transfer of proPTH to the Golgi and Its Conversion to PTH

The newly formed proPTH moves to the Golgi zone where it is enzymatically converted to PTH. This process requires 10–15 minutes as determined by the delay between appearance of radioactive proPTH and PTH in *in vitro* pulse–chase studies and on the information from the aforementioned autoradiographic studies (MacGregor *et al.,* 1973). By measuring delay times under different conditions, Chu *et al.* (1977) determined that the transport of the proPTH to the Golgi required energy and was independent of the rate of formation of proPTH or the subsequent utilization of PTH. They also showed that inhibitors of microtubulular function, such as colchicine, slowed transport (increased delay), suggesting that microtubules were involved in this process.

Direct support for Golgi involvement in the conversion process comes from studies with nonamphoteric amines such as diethylamine and Tris buffer [tris(hydroxymethyl)aminomethane]. Incubation of parathyroid tissue in physiological buffers containing these reagents causes the Golgi sacules to swell, the amount of proPTH to increase, and the amount of PTH to decrease in equivalent amounts (Chu *et al.*, 1974; MacGregor *et al.*, 1977). Moreover, the swelling action of one of these reagents, diethylamine, was reversible. When the tissue was placed in normal buffer, the Golgi saccules reverted to normal morphology and conversion of proPTH to PTH resumed (Cohn *et al.*, 1974a).

Trypsin readily cleaves the pro hexapeptide from proPTH (Cohn *et al.*, 1972b; Goltzman *et al.*, 1976). *In vivo*, however, the formation of PTH from proPTH appears to be catalyzed by an enzyme or enzymes associated with the Golgi membranes (MacGregor *et al.*, 1976a; Habener *et al.*, 1977). This membrane-associated convertase was tested *in vitro* (MacGregor *et al.*, 1976a, 1978b). It removed the pro hexapeptide as an intact unit from proPTH, yielding native PTH. The hexapeptide was then reduced to free amino acids by an amino- and carboxypeptidase attack, but the native PTH was not further affected.

I. Packaging and Storage of PTH

After synthesis, PTH is packaged in secretory vesicles and may either be secreted, stored, or degraded intracellularly. Examination of adenomatous parathyroids (Capen and Roth, 1973; Roth and Capen, 1974; Shannon and Roth, 1974) or of normal glands that have been activated or repressed *in vitro* by Ca^{2+} (Roth and Raisz, 1964, 1966; Roth *et al.*, 1968) suggests that parathyroid cells exist in different states of synthetic activity. Those cells that contained an abundance of secretory granules and rough endoplasmic reticulum were judged to be the most active. It should be noted, however, that a good correlation does not exist between glandular content of PTH and the number of secretory vesicles (Altenahr, 1970; Altenahr and Seifert, 1971; Setoguti *et al.*, 1981), in part because of the problems of identifying the vesicles which exist in an assortment of sizes, shapes, and states of condensation (Setoguti *et al.*, 1981).

Evaluation of the heterogeneity of parathyroid gland secretory vesicles is made more complex because at least two discrete pools of PTH-containing vesicles, each available for secretion, may exist within the gland. MacGregor *et al.* (1975) found that the secreted PTH from bovine parathyroid slices that had been incubated with radioactive amino acids showed a specific radioactivity severalfold higher than that of the tissue PTH. They suggested that newly synthesized PTH could "by-pass" existing stores during exocytosis. Dietel and Dorn-Quint (1980) with adenomatous human glands and Setogouti *et al.* (1981) studying rat glands by electron microscopy agreed that a by-pass route occurs in the gland. The latter workers concluded that the conventional storage granules serve only as an emergency supply of PTH.

Additional substantive data supporting the existence of multiple hormone pools has come from experiments in which the secretion of "old" PTH (that synthesized at least 60 minutes previously) and "new" PTH (that synthesized less than 60 minutes previously) were compared (Morrissey and Cohn, 1979a,b). Porcine parathyroid cells were pulse-labeled with ^{3}H- or ^{14}C-amino acids in order to produce intracellular PTH of different ages. Whereas hypocalcemia elicited the secretion of both "old" and "new" PTH to the same degree, dibutryl cAMP and the β-agonists L-isoproterenol and epinephrine preferentially elicited secretion from the pool of the older hormone. Kinetic studies indicated that the half-time for PTH to move from the "new" to "old" pool is about 3 hours.

What fraction of PTH normally secreted is derived from newly synthesized hormone and what fraction comes from the older stored hormone? Chu *et al.* (1983) measured the secretory rates of radiolabeled PTH from stimulated bovine parathyroid tissue incubated with cycloheximide to inhibit synthesis of PTH. The degree of inhibition of radioactive PTH produced by cycloheximide suggested that the major portion of the total hormone secreted by the tissue came from the newly synthesized hormone, a conclusion supporting the proposal of Setoguti *et al.* (1981) that stored PTH is generally not secreted.

It has yet to be determined if the two pools of PTH exist within the same cell, or in cells of different activity within the gland. Moreover, Chu *et al.* (1983) reported that in bovine tissue slices and dispersed cells isoproterenol stimulated secretion of both new *and* old PTH, in contrast to the results with porcine cells (Morrissey and Cohn, 1979a,b). These results could be explained by a more rapid transit in bovine than in porcine parathyroids of new PTH into the old pool, but might also signify that the multiple pools of PTH exist to quite different extents in glands from different animal species. Alternatively, the parathyroids of different species might respond differently to a specific secretogogue.

J. Intracellular Degradation of PTH

As much as 90% of the newly generated PTH is neither secreted nor stored, but proteolytically degraded within the cell (Chu *et al.,* 1973a; Habener *et al.,* 1975a; Morrissey and Cohn, 1979b). The amount degraded depends upon the secretory activity of the gland. For example, in parathyroids from rats fed low-calcium diets to elicit maximum PTH secretion, 86% of newly made hormone was degraded, compared to 68% in glands from rats fed a diet normal in calcium (Chu *et al.,* 1973a). Parathyroid cells cultured in medium containing 3.0 mM Ca^{2+} degraded 74% of the newly synthesized hormone, compared to 40% for cells kept in a medium containing 0.5 mM Ca^{2+} (Morrissey and Cohn, 1979b). In both studies, the amount of PTH secreted at the low calcium concentration was at least twice that under normal or high calcium conditions. In these studies the rate of synthesis of proPTH was the same regardless of the secretory activity of the glands. This observation has received independent support by the finding that the amount of preproPTH mRNA does not change when the glandular secretion is stimulated by incubating it for short periods in hypocalcemic medium (Heinrich *et al.,* 1983).

Balance studies reveal that loss of hormonal molecules (proPTH, cell + PTH, cell + PTH, medium) commenced 20 minutes after synthesis of proPTH (Morrissey and Cohn, 1979b). Since at this time most, if not all, of the newly synthesized proPTH had been converted to PTH, it was reasoned that PTH rather than proPTH was the species degraded. Moreover, since at 20 minutes the PTH had left the Golgi and PTH secreted to the medium was not noticeably degraded, the loss of PTH occurred within the cell.

This degradation of PTH has been interpreted as a manifestation of a physiological mechanism for allowing rapid response of the gland to hypocalcemic stress and, *pari passu,* controlling tissue stores of the hormone (Chu *et al.*, 1973a; Morrissey and Cohn, 1979b). Since the rate of synthesis of proPTH does not increase during acute hypocalcemia, the gland must produce more PTH than is normally needed and consequently have it readily available to meet acute secretory demands. The bulk of the hormone not secreted is degraded proteolytically. Proteolysis as a mechanism to control the amount of newly formed protein has been specifically invoked in other systems, such as the synthesis of collagen by fibroblasts (Baum *et al.*, 1980) and of tryptophan pyrrolase (Schimke *et al.*, 1965) and catalase (Recheigl and Heston, 1967) by the liver. Such may represent a general regulatory process whereby the type and tissue content of protein can be controlled (Mortimore, 1984).

Obviously, the degradative mechanism just described can only be physiologically effective as long as the need for PTH in the periphery does not exceed the gland's normal synthetic rate. How does the gland deal with a situation in which it faces a chronic hypocalcemic stimulus such as occurs in renal osteodystrophy? In this case, the gland becomes hyperplastic and hypertrophic (Aurbach *et al.* 1985) and in so becoming increases its capacity to synthesize PTH. The increase of PTH mRNA observed after several hours' incubation of parathyroid tissue with low-calcium media likely is a part of this phenomenon (Russell *et al.,* 1983).

The specific mechanism for triggering hypertrophy and hyperplasia is not understood. One intriguing possibility is that a feedback mechanism exists between vitamin D metabolites and the gland. Henry *et al.* (1977) reported that 1,25-dihydroxycholecalciferol and 24,25-dihydroxycholecalciferol, working in concert, reversed parathyroid gland hypertrophy in chicks fed a diet low in clacium. Recently, Silver *et al.* (1985) found that in parathyroid cells 1,25-dihydroxycholecalciferol caused a decrease in PTH mRNA upon incubation with the metabolite for several hours.

As might be expected for a tissue in which intracellular degradation is a major event, large amounts of carboxyl-terminal PTH fragments are present in and secreted from parathyroid tissue (Flueck *et al.,* 1977; Dibella *et al.,* 1978; Mayer *et al.,* 1979; Morrissey *et al.,* 1980a; MacGregor *et al.,* 1983). Cultured parathyroid cells secreted up to 1.5 mol of carboxyl-terminal fragments (PTH 34–84 and PTH 37–84) for each mole of intact PTH released (Morrissey *et al.,* 1980a). Mayer *et al.* (1979) assayed blood draining the parathyroids of calves and found that the amount of PTH fragment generally exceeded that of intact hormone. The ratio of carboxyl-terminal PTH fragments to intact PTH varied directly with the concentration of Ca^{2+} perfusing the parathyroids. In the *in vivo* and in separate *in vitro* studies, the ratio of fragment to intact PTH was greater the lower the rate of secretion (Hanley *et al.,* 1978; Morrissey *et al.,* 1980a; MacGregor *et al.,* 1983). These data also make clear that a significant fraction of the circulating PTH fragments of the blood (Berson and Yalow, 1968; Habener *et al.,* 1972; Silverman and Yalow, 1973; Benson *et al.,* 1974; Segre, 1979) are normally of glandular origin. A smaller proportion, accordingly, can be accounted for by peripheral degradation of secreted hormone (Habener *et al.*, 1972; Segre *et al.*, 1976; Hruska *et al.*, 1978; Barrett *et al.*, 1978a,b; D'Amour *et al.*, 1979; Martin *et al.*, 1979).

The kinetic studies of Morrissey and Cohn (1979b) with high and low Ca^{2+} concentrations indicate that there are two stages of PTH degradation within the gland: a calcium-independent stage that begins 20 minutes after prohormone synthesis, and a calcium-related stage that manifests itself after 40 minutes. In both instances the hormone is presumed to be in intracellular vesicles and/or secretory granules. Two enzymes implicated in the degradative process are cathepsin D (Hamilton *et al.*, 1983; Zull and Chuang, 1985) and cathepsin B (MacGregor *et al.*, 1979a,b). Both enzymes cleave PTH centrally. Cathepsin D yields PTH (1–34), PTH (1–37), and the complementary carboxyl-terminal fragments PTH (35–84) and PTH (38–84). Cathepsin B gives initially PTH (37–84) and a large amino-terminal fragment, presumably PTH (1–36). The enzyme does not act further on the carboxyl fragment but degrades the still bioactive amino-terminal piece to smaller, and now inactive, fragments by successive removal of residues from the carboxyl terminus. These modes of cleavage can account not only for the type of PTH fragments found in the circulation but also can explain the low abundance of amino-terminal fragments in tissue or in secreted material.

Fusion of PTH-containing secretion vesicles with lysosomes might permit proteolysis of the hormone by lysosomal enzymes, as proposed for the intracellular degradation of proalbumin in the liver (Quinn and Judah, 1978), proinsulin in the pancreas (Smith and Van Frank, 1975), and prolactin in the anterior pituitary (Smith and Farquar, 1966). Alternatively, nascent proteases might exist and become activated within the secretory granules. Either event would require substantial physical change in the degradation container, since MacGregor *et al.* (1983) reported that PTH fragments are found in membrane-associated compartments that differ from those containing the bulk of the cell's PTH.

It is not yet clear whether Ca^{2+} directly controls degradative events. It might directly activate proteolytic enzymes (Fischer *et al.*, 1972) or promote fusion of secretory vesicles with lysosomes, as it appears to do in the fusion of chromaffin granules with synexin (Pollard *et al.*, 1981). On the other hand, an indirect effect is possible. Since the majority of secreted PTH is that most recently synthesized (Chu *et al.*, 1983), and since intracellular degradation does not commence until or after the gland begins to secrete, calcium, by inhibiting secretion, may indirectly cause retention of the hormone within the gland, where it is more available for proteolysis.

K. Regulation of PTH Secretion

The fundamental mechanisms responsible for secretory control are at least as complex as those regulating intracellular formation and processing of the hormone. It is widely accepted that the primary regulator of secretion is Ca^{2+} (Cooper *et al.,* 1978; Mayer, 1979; Cohn and MacGregor, 1981; Potts *et al.,* 1982). As the Ca^{2+} concentration drops there are disproportionately large increments in secreted hormone. This "proportional" type of response provides the gland with a mechanism for more effectively responding to small changes in the Ca^{2+} signal (Sherwood *et al.,* 1968; Mayer and Hurst, 1978). Magnesium might modulate Ca^{2+}-regulated PTH secretion since in both *in vivo* and *in vitro* studies it is from one-third as active to equipotent with Ca^{2+} in inhibiting secretion of the hormone (Sherwood *et al.,* 1968; Buckle *et al.,* 1968; Targovnik *et al.,* 1971; Habener and Potts, 1976; Mayer, 1975; Morrissey and Cohn, 1978; Mahaffee *et al.,* 1982).

There is only limited speculation on how the parathyroid cell senses a change in Ca^{2+}. It is not known whether the gland contains specific surface receptors for Ca^{2+} or if, instead, Ca^{2+} acts internally. In addition, the mechanism by which the change in Ca^{2+} is translated into altered hormone secretion is unknown. Ca^{2+} markedly changes the parathyroid cell membrane potential (Bruce and Anderson, 1979; Sand *et al.,* 1981) and this might alter transmembrane ion fluxes (Hove and Sand, 1981; Wallfelt *et al.,* 1985). Changes in extracellular Ca^{2+} concentration also produce parallel changes in cytosolic Ca^{2+} (Shoback *et al.,* 1983, 1984). But whether such changes are directly related to secretory events, or are secondary phenomena, or are merely fortuitous is unclear.

The effect of Ca^{2+} on parathyroid secretion has been considered to be the reverse of its action on other secretory cells. In other cells secretion is related to an increase in cytosolic Ca^{2+}, so-called secretion-coupling (Douglas and Rubin, 1961; Douglas, 1974, 1981). In the parathyroid, in contrast, secretion has been correlated with a decrease in the concentration of cytosolic Ca^{2+} (Shoback *et al.,* 1984). Recent studies, however, suggest that the parathyroids handle intracellular Ca^{2+} in a manner similar to other secretory cells. Thus, parathyroid membranes contain an active Ca^{2+}-dependent ATPase (Dawson-Hughes *et al.,* 1983) and accumulate Ca^{2+} at about the same rate as other cell membranes (Dean *et al.,* 1986). Inositol trisphosphate, an agent believed to be an intracellular hormone messenger (Berridge and Irvine, 1984; Nishizuka, 1984), releases Ca^{2+} from these membranes (Dean *et al.,*

1986) and from permeabilized parathyroid cells (Epstein *et al.*, 1985) in a manner equivalent to other cell systems. Finally, as do other cells, the parathyroid contains calmodulin (Brown, 1980; Oldham *et al.*, 1982; Brown *et al.*, 1981). It may be that local rather than general changes in intracellular Ca^{2+} are responsible for the seemingly "backward" behavior of the parathyroid gland. If this is the case, more subtle measurements of cell Ca^{2+} and purified, rather than crude, membrane preparations will be required to obtain meaningful results.

Several PTH secretagogues that increase intracellular cAMP, such as L-isoproterenol, epinephrine, prostaglandin E_2, dopamine, cholera toxin, and dibutyryl cAMP, enhance secretion (Williams *et al.*, 1973; Blum *et al.*, 1974; Brown *et al.*, 1977a,b, 1979a,b; Ramp *et al.*, 1979; Gardner *et al.*, 1978, 1980, 1981a). Agents that decrease cAMP, such as α-adrenergic agents, prostaglandin $F_{2\alpha}$, and nitroprusside (Gardner *et al.*, 1979a,b, 1981b), inhibit secretion. An excellent correlation has been noted between PTH secretion and the cell level of cAMP generated by these agents, regardless of which one is used (Brown *et al.*, 1978a).

It seems likely that the secretagogues or inhibitors affecting cAMP act through a different mechanism than does Ca^{2+}; neither dopamine nor dibutyryl cAMP affect the concentration of cytosolic Ca^{2+} even though each strongly stimulates secretion (Shoback *et al.*, 1984). Furthermore, the agents that elevate cAMP activate protein kinase (Brown and Thatcher, 1982) and cause phosphorylation of specific parathyroid proteins (Lasker and Spiegel, 1982), whereas Ca^{2+} does not. A complicating factor in this interpretation, however, is that the level of cAMP changes in parallel with degree of secretion when extracellular Ca^{2+} or Mg^{2+} are varied (Morrissey and Cohn, 1979a). These results could represent a direct action of intracellular Ca^{2+} on phosphodiesterase via calmodulin or on adenylate cyclase, or both (Brown, 1980; Brown *et al.*, 1981; Oldham *et al.*, 1982).

A third class of substances, the vitamin D polar metabolites, are reported to either acutely enhance or inhibit secretion of PTH (see Cohn and Elting, 1983). Whether any of these metabolites other than Ca^{2+} is a true physiological regulator or merely pharmacological is not known. With epinephrine, however, clinical studies indicate that at normal circulating levels, this agent does not affect parathyroid secretory function (Body *et al.*, 1983; Heath *et al.*, 1980). That some of these agents, as mentioned earlier, elicit secretion from a unique intracellular hormone pool (Morrissey and Cohn, 1979a,b) makes interpretation of secretory events in the parathyroid all the more challenging.

IV. Parathyroid Secretory Protein-I (SP-I) and Adrenal Chromogranin A

A. Discovery of SP-I

The second major protein synthesized and secreted by the parathyroid cell is SP-I. Licata *et al.* (1972) were the first to note that Ca^{2+} inhibited the secretion of glycoproteins by rat parathyroid glands maintained in organ culture. Kemper *et al.* (1974b) independently noted that Ca^{2+} inhibited the secretion by bovine parathyroid slices of a rapidly synthesized protein they named parathyroid secretory protein. They pointed out that its secretion rate and that of PTH responded in parallel fashion to Ca^{2+}. It was subsequently reported that this same protein, called secretory protein-I (SP-I) by Morrissey *et al.* (1978) and Cohn *et al.* (1982b), was a glycoprotein and that both Ca^{2+} and Mg^{2+} inhibited its secretion in parallel with PTH. Ravazzola *et al.* (1978), using immunofluorescent probes, concluded that SP-I and PTH were in the same intracellular granules of the parathyroid cell. This colocalization is supported by the finding that newly synthesized SP-I, PTH, and proPTH were extracted in the same relative amounts from parathyroid membranes by dilute detergents (Morrissey *et al,* 1980b).

B. Biosynthesis and Secretion of SP-I

Translation of bovine mRNA for SP-I in wheat germ and reticulocyte lysate cell-free systems gave rise to four precursor species closely related to SP-I (preSP-I). The multiple species appeared to differ only in the lengths of the amino-terminal leader sequences, since addition of microsomes to the translation system led to the formation of a single protein of molecular weight of about 71,000 that lacked a leader sequence (Majzoub *et al.*, 1979, 1982). These workers noted that there did not appear to be an intermediate pro form of SP-I, a conclusion supported by Morrissey *et al.* (1980b), who did not detect a proSP-I during rapid pulse–chase experiments at a time when proPTH was readily observed.

Two major species of SP-I with apparent molecular weights of 72,000 and 64,000 are synthesized (among several other proteins) in and secreted from porcine parathyroid cells (Morrissey *et al.*, 1980b). The cellular forms are found mainly associated with membranes. Both the cellular and secreted forms of SP-I have almost identical peptide maps but differ slightly in isoelectric point. The particular apparent molecular weights of the pair of SP-I molecules depend upon the species from which they arise. Thus, from bovine parathyroid the molecular weights have been reported as 72,000 and 70,000 (Cohn *et al.*, 1981; Takatsuki *et al.*, 1981). Both nonglycosylated and glycosylated forms of SP-I are secreted (Majzoub *et al.*, 1982).

Tunicamycin, an antibiotic that blocks the synthesis of N-linked oligosaccharides (Struck and Lennarz, 1980), neither affected the incorporation of [^{3}H]GlcN into SP-I nor the secretion of SP-I into the medium (Majzoub *et al.*, 1982). It was concluded that SP-I was not glycosylated cotranslationally during synthesis at the RER, but rather acquired O-linked sugars at the Golgi. This conclusion is supported by the finding that [^{3}H]mannose, a sugar commonly found in N-linked oligosaccharides, was not incorporated into SP-I during *in vitro* incubation studies. Earlier, however, Morrissey *et al.* (1978) reported that SP-I could be metabolically labeled with [^{3}H]mannose as well as [^{3}H]GlcN and that SP-I secreted into the medium was bound to concanavalin A, a lectin with a high affinity for mannose. The reason for the differences observed in the metabolic labeling studies with the bovine and porcine tissues are not yet known.

C. Chemistry of SP-I

SP-I has been isolated and purified in bulk from bovine parathyroid glands (Cohn *et al.*, 1981; Takatsuki *et al.*, 1981) and partly characterized in porcine parathyroid cells (Morrissey *et al.*, 1980b). The best preparations contain two principal species, 70 and 72 kDa in bovine and 64 and 72 kDa in procine glands. In solution the purified bovine SP-I behaves as a tetramer during gel filtration (Cohn *et al.*, 1981) as do the secreted forms from porcine glands (R. Kumarasamy and D. V. Cohn, unpublished data).

Edman degradation of the two protein bands from porcine cells shows that they have identical amino-terminal regions (Morrissey *et al.*, 1980b). Bovine SP-I is high in proline content (about 9%) and highly acidic (isoelectric point about 4.5), containing 30% aspartic and glutamic acids. It is phosphorylated (Bhargava *et al.*, 1983) and sulfated (Cohn and Elting, 1983). Carbohydrate analysis reveals that the protein contains 10 μmol of neutral and amino sugars per 100 mg of protein. SP-I is resistant to enzymatic digestion with endo H and is not adsorbed to concanavalin A in serial lectin affinity chromatography according to the procedure of Kumarasamy and Blough (1985), a result indicating the lack of any "high mannose" or "complex" type asparagine-linked oligosaccharides. However, a significant amount of bovine SP-I binds strongly to wheat germ agglutinin–Sepharose and the glycoprotein possesses a large number of terminal sialic acid residues that can be readily removed by digestion with *Clostridium perfringens* neuraminidase (R. Kumarasamy and D. V. Cohn, unpublished data). On the basis of these results, it is likely that bovine SP-I contains mostly O-linked oligosaccharides with terminal sialic acid residues.

Takatsuki *et al.* (1981) reported a distinctly different composition for bovine SP-I. The protein they isolated contained only 1% proline and 36% acidic amino acid residues. Their preparation behaved as a dimer during gel filtration in contrast to the tetramer reported by Cohn *et al.* (1981). The reason for these sharp differences is not clear, but might relate to the existence of a family of SP-I-like proteins in the parathyroids, as is now being uncovered in other tissues for the related groups of chromogranins and secretogranins (Rosa *et al.*, 1985). Perhaps the different research groups have been examining different species of the same family of proteins.

D. Chromogranin A (CGA) of the Adrenal Medulla Chromaffin Cell

Investigators studying adrenal gland function have devoted much effort to characterizing the chemical and physical nature of the chromaffin granule and its contents (for example, see Winkler, 1976, 1977; Sage *et al.*, 1967; Winkler and Carmichael, 1982; Pollard *et al.*, 1985). These structures represent storage vesicles for the catecholamines, but contain, as well, an assortment of other constituents including dopamine, dopamine β-hydroxylase, Met- and Leu-enkephalins, ATP and other nucleotides, ascorbic acid, Ca^{2+}, Mg^{2+}, and other metallic ions, glycosaminoglycans, and a large amount of several acidic soluble proteins termed *chromogranins*. The major component of the protein fraction is CGA, comprising 40% of the soluble protein or about 30% of the total protein of the granule (membrane protein represents about 20% of the total protein). CGA has also been identified in sympathetic nerve endings (Banks *et al.*, 1969) in which it is associated with norepinephrine-containing vesicles.

Although the physiological function of CGA is not known, it is secreted along with the catecholamines and other granule contents upon nervous or chemical stimulation (Sage *et al.*, 1967; Kirschner *et al.*, 1967; Banks *et al.*, 1969; Winkler and Carmichael, 1982).

CGA, like SP-I, is a highly acidic glycoprotein containing over 30% aspartic and glutamic acid residues (Hogue-Angeletti, 1977; Winkler and Carmichael, 1982) and predominantly O-linked oligosaccharides (Kiang *et al.*, 1982). Both higher and lower molecular weight forms have been identified which range from 100,000 to 65,000 (Winkler, 1976; Hogue-Angeletti, 1977; O'Connor and Frigon, 1984; Settleman *et*

```
1                                                        10
Leu-Pro-Val-Asn-Ser-Pro-Met-Asn-Lys-Gly---

11                                                          20
---Asp-Thr-Glu-Val-Met-Lys-Xxx-Ile-Val-Glu-?
```

FIG. 2. Amino-terminal sequence of SP-I (Cohn *et al.*, 1981a). This sequence is identical to that of CGA (Kruggel *et al.*, 1985). Residue 17 of SP-I is unknown. Kruggel *et al.* (1985) did not detect a specific amino acid residue at this position and have assumed it to be cysteine.

al., 1985a). Amino-terminal sequence analysis of the multiple forms of CGA ranging from 65,000 to 100,000 in molecular weight reveals a high degree of homology and immunological cross-reactivity (Settleman *et al.*, 1985a).[1] In addition, CGA of apparent molecular weight of 75,000 also exhibits internal homology and contains repeat sequences, suggesting possible gene duplication in its evolutionary development. Even though the majority of CGA exists in soluble form (Winkler and Carmichael, 1982; O'Connor and Frigon, 1984), it has been reported that based on extraction studies, a significant proportion of the protein is tightly associated with the granule membrane and behaves as an integral membrane protein (Settleman *et al.*, 1985b).

E. CHEMICAL AND IMMUNOLOGICAL SIMILARITY OF SP-I AND CGA

A remarkable similarity, if not identity, of SP-I to CGA was demonstrated by comparing immunological cross-reactivities, amino acid and carbohydrate compositions, and amino-terminal sequences of the purified proteins (Cohn *et al.*, 1982a). Of the first 20 amino acid residues of SP-I, 18 were identical to those published earlier (Hogue-Angeletti, 1977) for CGA. More recent data show that human and bovine CGA and bovine SP-I possess *identical* amino-terminal sequences for at least the first 20 residues (Kruggel *et al.*, 1985). It appears, therefore, that the previously published sequence for CGA (Hogue-Angeletti, 1977) is incorrect at positions 2 and 19. The amino acid sequence for SP-I and bovine and human CGA is presented in Fig. 2. The cell-free synthesis of chromogranin A (Falkensammer *et al.*, 1985) closely resembles that of SP-I, providing further evidence for similarity of these proteins.

[1] The molecular weight of the unmodified amino acid chain appears to be substantially less than the apparent molecular weight determined by SDS-polyacrylamide electrophoresis. Benedum *et al.* (1986) have reported the primary structure of bovine chromogranin A as deduced from sequencing a cDNA clone containing the entire coding region of bovine CGA. The molecule contains 431 amino acid residues giving a calculated molecular weight of 48 kDa. The first 20 residues agree exactly with those directly determined by amino acid sequencing of bovine SP-I (see Fig. 2). Residue 17 is cysteine as assumed.

F. Distribution of SP-I/CGA in Endocrine and Neuronal Cells

Using an immunoassay developed for SP-I, Takatsuki *et al.* (1982) detected this protein in extracts of several tissues including pituitary, ovary, pancreas, and kidney (data presented in Cohn and Elting, 1983). Subsequently, CGA immunoreactivity was detected in extracts of a variety of endocrine tissue, serum, and brain homogenates (O'Connor, 1983; O'Connor *et al.*, 1983; O'Connor and Frigon, 1984). CGA was found in neural and endocrine secretory granules by means of a monoclonal antibody (Lloyd and Wilson, 1983; Wilson and Lloyd, 1984). Both SP-I and CGA were detected in cells of the thyroid that contained calcitonin, but not thyroglobulin, in cells of anterior pituitary staining for the α subunits of TSH/FSH/LH, but not in cells staining for growth hormone, prolactin, or ACTH (Cohn *et al.*, 1984). O'Connor *et al.* (1983), Lloyd and Wilson (1983), and Cohn *et al.* (1984) each detected immunoactive SP-I/CGA in the pancreatic islets, but reported different cellular locations in the insulin-producing beta cells, the glucagon-producing alpha cells, or the somatostatin and pancreatic polypeptide-containing gamma cells, respectively. Detecting these differences was possibly due to the unique specificities of the different antibodies used. Immunoreactivity has also been reported to be widely distributed in the brain and spinal cord in locales that overlapped partially those of neurotransmitters and neuroactive peptides (Somogyi *et al.*, 1984). Recently, another group of acidic proteins, termed *secretogranin I* and *II* of molecular weights of 113,000/105,000 and 86,000/84,000, respectively, and similar to CGA in many respects, has been found in several endocrine and neuronal cells (Rosa *et al.*, 1985).

G. Is There a Physiological Role for SP-I/CGA?

No physiological function has been established for the chromogranins, secretogranins, or SP-I, although several have been proposed (Winkler and Westhead, 1980; Phillips, 1982; Kemper *et al.* 1974a,b; Cohn *et al.*, 1982a). Among these are that SP-I/CGA species plays a general role in storage or release of bioactive substances in secretory granules of endocrine cells and synaptic veiscles of neurons; that it may exhibit bioactivity alone or in conjunction with the substances with which it is cosecreted, that the membrane-associated form plays a specific role in the fusion of the secretory granule membrane with the plasma membrane during exocytosis, and that it may participate actively or passively in the proteolytic processing of PTH. The steadily increasing number of reports on these proteins suggests that definitive information on this aspect of parathyroid physiology, in particular, and endocrine regulation in general, will soon be forthcoming.

REFERENCES

Abe, M., and Sherwood, L. M. (1972). Regulation of parathyroid hormone secretion by adenyl cyclase. *Biochem. Biophys. Res. Commun.* **48,** 396.

Altenahr, E. (1970). Ultrastructure of rat parathyroid glands in normo-, hyper-, and hypocalcemia. *Virchows Arch. Abt. A* **351,** 122.

Altenahr, E., and Seifert, G. (1971). Ultrastructural comparison of human parathyroid glands in secondary hyperparathyroidism and primary parathyroid adenoma. *Virchows Arch. Abt. A* **353,** 60.

Angeletti, R. H., and Hickey, W. F. (1985). A neuroendocrine marker in tissues of the immune system. *Science* **230,** 89.

Antonarakis, S. E., Phillips, J. A., III, Mallonee, R. L., Kazazian, H. H., Jr., Rearon, E. R., Waber, P. G., Kronenberg, H. M., Ullrich, A., and Meyers, D. A. (1983). β-Globin locus is linked to the parathyroid hormone (PTH) locus and lies between the insulin and PTH loci in man *Proc. Natl. Acad. Sci. U.S.A.* **80,** 6615–6619.

Aurbach, G. D., Marx, S., and Spiegel, A. M. (1985). Parathyroid hormone, calcitonin and the calciferols. *In* "Textbook of Endocrinology" (R. H. Williams, ed.), Chap. 29. Saunders, Philadelphia.

Banks, P., Helle, K. B., and Mayor, D. (1969). Evidence for the presence of a chromogranin-like protein in bovine splenic nerve granules. *Mol. Pharmacol.* **5,** 210.

Barker, W. C., and Dayhoff, M. O. (1972). Detecting distant relationships: Computer methods and results. *In* "Atlas of Protein Sequence and Structure" (M. O. Dayhoff, ed.), Vol. 5, p. 101. National Biomedical Research Foundation, Silver Spring, Maryland.

Barrett, P. Q., Teitelbaum, A. P., and Neuman, W. F. (1978a). The heterogeneity of radioiodinated parathyroid hormone in rat plasma. *Metabol. Bone Dis. Relat. Res.* **1,** 263.

Barrett, P. Q., Teitelbaum, A. P., Neuman, W. F., and Neuman, M. W. (1978b). The role of the liver in the peripheral metabolism of parathyroid hormone. *In* "Endocrinology of Calcium Metabolism" (D. H. Copp and R. V. Talmage, eds.), p. 324. Excerpta Medica, Amsterdam.

Baum, B. J., Moss, J., Breul, S. D, Berg, R. A., and Crystal, R. G. (1980). Effect of cyclic AMP on the intracellular degradation of newly synthesized collagen, *J. Biol. Chem.* **255,** 2843.

Benedum, V. M., Baeuerle, P. A., Kanecki, D. S., Rainer, F., Powell, J., Mallet, J., and Huttner, W. B. (1986). The primary structure of bovine chromogranin A: A representative of a class of acidic secretory proteins, common to a variety of peptidergic cells. *EMBO J.* **5,** 1495.

Benson, R. C., Jr., Riggs, G. L., Pickard, B. M., and Arnaud, C. D. (1974). Immunoreactive forms of circulating parathyroid hormone in primary and ectopic hyperparathyroidism. *J. Clin. Invest.* **54,** 175.

Berridge, M., and Irvine, R. R. (1984). Inositol trisphosphate, a novel second messenger in cellular signal transduction. *Nature (London)* **312,** 315–321.

Berson, S. A., and Yalow, R. S. (1968). Immunochemical heterogeneity of parathyroid hormone in plasma. *J. Clin. Endocrinol. Metab.* **28,** 1037.

Bhargava, F., Russell, J., and Sherwood, L. M. (1983). Phosphorylation of parathyroid secretory protein. *Proc. Natl. Acad. Sci. U.S.A.* **80,** 878.

Blobel, G. (1983). Control of intracellular protein traffic. *In* "Methods in Enzymology" (S. Fleischer and B. Fleischer, eds.), Vol. 96, p. 663, Academic Press, New York.

Blobel, G., and Dobberstein, B. (1975). Transfer of proteins across membranes. I. Presence of proteolytically processed and unprocessed nascent immunoglobulin light chains on membrane-bound ribosomes of murine myeloma. *J. Cell Biol.* **67,** 835.

Blum, J. W., Fischer, J. A., Schwoerer, D., Hunziker, W., and Binswanger, U. (1974). Acute parathyroid hormone response: Sensitivity, relationship to hypocalcemia and rapidity. *Endocrinology* **95,** 753.

Body, J., Cryer, P. E., Offord, K. P., and Heath, H., III (1983). Epinephrine is a hypophosphatemic hormone in man. Physiological effects of circulating epinephrine on plasma calcium, magnesium, phosphorus, parathyroid hormone and calcitonin. *J. Clin. Invest.* **71,** 572.

Brewer, H. B., and Ronan, R. (1970). Bovine parathyroid hormone: Amino acid sequence. *Proc. Natl. Acad. Sci. U.S.A.* **67,** 1862.

Brewer, H. B., Fairwell, T., Ronan, R., Rittel, W., and Arnaud, C. (1975). Human parathyroid hormone. *In* "Calcium-Regulating Hormones" (R. V. Talmage, M. Owen, and J. A. Parsons, eds.), p. 23. Excerpta Medica, Amsterdam.

Brown, E. M. (1980). Calcium regulated phosphodiesterase in bovine parathyroid cells. *Endocrinology* **107,** 1998.

Brown, E. M., and Thatcher, J. G. (1982). Adenosine 3′,5′-monophosphate (cAMP)-dependent protein kinase and the regulation of parathyroid hormone release by divalent cations and agents elevating cellular cAMP in dispersed bovine parathyroid cells. *Endocrinology* **110,** 1374.

Brown, E. M., Carroll, R., and Aurbach, G. D. (1977a). Dopaminergic stimulation of cyclic AMP accumulation and parathyroid hormone release from dispersed bovine parathyroid cells. *Proc. Natl. Acad. Sci. U.S.A.* **74,** 4210.

Brown, E. M., Hurwitz, S., and Aurbach, G. D. (1977b). Beta-adrenergic stimulation of cyclic AMP content and parathyroid hormone release from isolated bovine parathyroid cells. *Endocrinology* **100,** 1696.

Brown, E. M., Gardner, D. G., Windeck, R. A., and Aurbach, G. D. (1978a). Relationship of intracellular 3′,5′-adenosine monophosphate accumulation to parathyroid hormone release from dispersed bovine parathyroid cells. *Endocrinology* **103,** 2323.

Brown, E. M., Hurwitz, S., and Aurbach, G. D. (1978b). Alpha-adrenergic inhibition of adenosine 3′,5′-monophosphate accumulation and parathyroid hormone release from dispersed bovine parathyroid cells. *Endocrinology* **103,** 893.

Brown, E. M., Gardner, D. G., Windeck, R. A., and Aurbach, G. D. (1979a). Cholera toxin stimulates 3′,5′-adenosine monophosphate accumulation and parathyroid hormone release from dispersed bovine parathyroid cells. *Endocrinology* **104,** 218.

Brown, E. M., Gardner, D. G., Windeck, R. A., Hurwitz, S., Brennan, M. F., and Aurbach, G. D. (1979b). β-Adrenergically stimulated adenosine 3′5′-monophosphate accumulation in and parathyroid hormone release from dispersed human parathyroid cells. *J. Clin. Endocrinol. Metab.* **48,** 618.

Brown, E. M., Dawson-Hughes, B. F., Wilson, R. E., and Adragna, N. (1981). Calmodulin in dispersed human parathyroid cells. *J. Clin. Endocrinol. Metab.* **53,** 1064.

Bruce, B. R., and Anderson, N. C., Jr. (1979). Hyperpolarization in mouse parathyroid cells by low calcium. *Am. J. Physiol.* **236,** C15.

Buckle, R. M., Care, A. D., Cooper, C. W., and Gitelman, H. (1968). The influence of plasma magnesium concentration of parathyroid hormone secretion. *J. Endocrinol.* **42,** 529.

Capen, C. C., and Roth, S. I. (1973). Ultrastructural and functional relationships of normal and pathological parathyroid cells. *In* "Pathobiology Annual" (H. L. Ioachim, ed.), p. 129. Appleton, New York.

Cheung, W. Y. (1980). "Calcium and Cell Function," Vol. I. Academic Press, New York.

Cheung, W. Y. (1982). "Calcium and Cell Function," Vol. II. Academic Press, New York.

Chou, P. Y., and Fasman, G. D. (1974a). Conformational parameters for amino acids in helical, β-sheet and random coil regions calculated from proteins. *Biochemistry* **13,** 211.

Chou, P. Y., and Fasman, G. D. (1974b). Prediction of protein conformation. *Biochemistry* **13,** 222.

Chou, P. Y., and Fasman, G. D. (1977). β-Turns in proteins. *J. Mol. Biol.* **115,** 135.

Chu, L. L. H., MacGregor, R. R., Anast, C. S., Hamilton, J. W., and Cohn, D. V. (1973a). Studies on the biosynthesis of rat parathyroid hormone and proparathyroid hormone: Adaptation of the parathyroid gland to dietary restriction of calcium. *Endocrinology* **93,** 915.

Chu, L. L. H., MacGregor, R. R., Liu, P. I., Hamilton, J. W., and Cohn, D. V. (1973b). Biosynthesis of proparathyroid hormone and parathyroid hormone by human parathyroid glands. *J. Clin. Invest.* **52,** 3089.

Chu, L. L. H., MacGregor, R. R., Hamilton, J. W., and Cohn, D. V. (1974). Conversion of proparathyroid hormone to parathyroid hormone: The use of amines as specific inhibitors. *Endocrinology* **95,** 1431.

Chu, L. L. H., Huang, D. W. Y., Littledike, E. T., Hamilton, J. W., and Cohn, D. V. (1975). Porcine proparathyroid hormone: Identification, biosynthesis and partial amino acid sequence. *Biochemistry* **14,** 3631.

Chu, L. L. H., MacGregor, R. R., and Cohn, D. V. (1977). Energy-dependent intracellular translocation of proparathormone. *J. Cell Biol.* **72,** 1.

Chu, L. L. H., MacGregor, R. R., and Hamilton, J. W. (1983). Effects of isoproterenol and cycloheximide on parathyroid secretion. *Mol. Cell. Endocrinol.* **2–3,** 157–68.

Cohn, D. V., and Elting, (1983). Biosynthesis, processing and secretion of parathormone and secretory protein-I. *Recent Prog. Horm. Res.* **39,**

Cohn, D. V., and Elting, (1984). Synthesis and secretion of parathormone and secretory protein-I by the parathyroid gland. *In* "Bone and Mineral Research" (W. A. Peck, ed.), pp. 31–64. Elsevier, Amsterdam.

Cohn, D. V., and Hamilton, J. W. (1976). Newer aspects of parathyroid chemistry and physiology. *Cornell Vet.* **66,** 271.

Cohn, D. V., and MacGregor, R. R. (1981). The biosynthesis, intracellular processing and secretion of parathormone. *Endocr. Rev.* **2,** 1.

Cohn, D. V., and Wong, G. L. (1979). Isolated bone cells. *In* "Skeletal Research" (D. Simmons and A. Kunin, eds.), p. 3. Academic Press, New York.

Cohn, D. V., MacGregor, R. R., Chu, L. L. H., and Hamilton, J. W. (1972a). Studies on the biosynthesis *in vitro* of parathyroid hormone and other calcemic polypeptides of the parathyroid gland. *In* "Calcium, Parathyroid Hormone and Calcitonin" (R. V. Talmage and P. L. Munson, eds.), p. 173. Excerpta Medica, Amsterdam.

Cohn, D. V., MacGregor, R. R., Chu, L. L. H., Kimmel, J. R., and Hamilton J. W. (1972b). Calcemic fraction-A: Biosynthetic peptide precursor of parathyroid hormone. *Proc. Natl. Acad. Sci. U.S.A.* **69,** 1521.

Cohn, D. V., MacGregor, R. R., Chu, L. L. H., and Hamilton, J. W. (1974a). Structure–function relationships in the synthesis, packaging and secretion of parathyroid gland hormones. *In* "Calcium Regulating Hormones" (R. V. Talmage, M. Owen, and J. A. Parsons, eds.), p. 45. Excerpta Medica, Amsterdam.

Cohn, D. V., MacGregor, R. R., Chu, L. L. H., Huang, D. W. Y, Anast, C. S., and Hamilton, J. W. (1974b). Biosynthesis of proparathyroid hormone and parathyroid hormone. Chemistry, physiology, and role of calcium in regulation. *Am. J. Med.* **56,** 767.

Cohn, D. V., MacGregor, R. R., Sinha, D., Huang, D. W. Y., Edelhoch, H., and Hamilton,

J. W. (1974c). The migration behavior of proparathyroid hormone, parathyroid hormone, and their peptide fragments during gel filtration. *Arch. Biochem. Biophys.* **164,** 669.

Cohn, D. V., Morrissey, J. J., MacGregor, R. R., and Hamilton, J. W. (1978). The role of calcium in the biosynthesis and secretion of parathormone. *In* "Comparative Endocrinology" (P. Gaillard and H. H. Boer, eds.), p. 273. Elsevier, Amsterdam.

Cohn, D. V., Smardo, F. L., and Morrissey, J. (1979). Evidence for internal homology in bovine preproparathyroid hormone. *Proc. Nat. Acad. Sci. U.S.A.* **76,** 1469.

Cohn, D. V., Morrissey, J. J., Hamilton, J. W., Shofstall, R. E., Smardo, F. L., and Chu, L. L. H. (1981). Isolation and partial characterization of secretory protein-I from bovine parathyroid gland. *Biochemistry* **20,** 4135.

Cohn, D. V., Zangerle, R., Fischer-Colbrie, R., Chu, L. L. H., Elting, J. J., Hamilton, J. W., and Winkler, H. (1982a). Similarity of secretory protein-I from parathyroid gland to chromogranin A from adrenal medulla. *Proc. Natl. Acad. Sci. U.S.A.* **79,** 6056.

Cohn, D. V., Morrissey, J. J., Shofstall, R. E., and Chu, L. L. H. (1982b). Co-secretion of secretory protein-I and parathormone by dispersed bovine parathyroid cells. *Endocrinology* **110,** 625.

Cohn, D. V., Elting, J. J., Frick, M., and Elde, R. (1984). Selective localization of the parathyroid secretory protein-I/adrenal medulla chromogranin A protein family in a wide variety of endocrine cells of the rat. *Endocrinology* **114,** 1963.

Cooper, C. W., Ramp, W. K., Ross, A. J., III, and Wells, S. A., Jr. (1978). Concurrent secretion of calcitonin and parathyroid hormone *in vitro* from the rat thyroparathyroid complex *Proc. Soc. Exp. Biol. Med.* **158,** 299–303.

Dalbey, R. E., and Wickner, W. (1985). Leader peptidase catalyzes the release of exported proteins from the outer surface of the *Escherichia coli* plasma membrane. *J. Biol. Chem.* **260,** 15925.

D'Amour, P., Segre, G. V., Roth, S. I., and Potts, J. T., Jr. (1979). Analysis of parathyroid hormone and its fragments in rat tissues. Chemical identification and microscopical localization. *J. Clin. Invest.* **63,** 89.

Dawson-Hughes, B. F., Underwood, R. H., and Brown, E. M. (1983). Ca-ATPase activity in bovine parathyroid cells. *Metabolism* **32,** 874–880.

Dayhoff, M. O., Eck, R. V., and Park, C. M. (1972). A model of evolutionary change in proteins. *In* "Atlas of Protein Sequence and Structure" (M. O. Dayhoff, ed.), Vol. 5, p. 89. National Biomedical Research Foundation, Silver Spring, Maryland.

Dean, W. L., Adunyah, S., and Cohn, D. V. (1986). Calcium uptake and inositol trisphosphate-induced calcium release from parathyroid gland membranes. *Bone Mineral* **1,** 59.

DeLuca, H. F. (1983). Metabolism and mechanisms of action of vitamin D—1982. *In* "Bone and Mineral Research Annual I" (W. A. Peck, ed.), p. 7. Excerpta Medica, Amsterdam.

Dibella, F. P., Gilkenson, J. B., and Arnaud, C. D. (1978). Carboxyl-terminal fragments of human parathyroid hormone in parathyroid tumors: Unique new source of immunogens for the production of antisera potentially useful in the radioimmunoassay of parathyroid hormone in human serum. *J. Clin. Endocrinol. Metab.* **46,** 604.

Dietel, M., and Dorn-Quint, G. (1980). By-pass secretion of human parathyroid adenomas. *Lab. Invest.* **43,** 116.

Dorner, A., and Kemper, B. (1978). Conversion of pre-proparathyroid hormone to proparathyroid hormone by dog pancreatic microsomes. *Biochemistry* **17,** 5550.

Douglas, W. W. (1974). Involvement of calcium in exocytosis and the exocytosis–vesiculation sequence. *Biochem. Soc. Symp.,* **39,** 1.

Douglas, W. W. (1981). Aspects of the calcium hypothesis of stimulus–secretion coupling: Electrical activity in adenopophyseal cells, and membrane retrieval after exocytosis. *Methods Cell Biol.* **23,** 483–501.

Douglas, W. W., and Rubin, R. P. (1961). The role of calcium in the secretory response of the adrenal medulla to acetycholine. *J. Physiol. (London)* **159,** 40–57.

Edelhoch, H., and Lippoldt, R. E. (1969). Structural studies on polypeptide hormones. *J. Biol. Chem.* **244,** 3876.

Epstein, P. A., Prentki, M., and Attie, M. F. (1985). Modulation of intracellular Ca^{2+} in the parathyroid cell: Release of Ca^{2+} from non-mitochondrial pools by inositol trisphosphate. *FEBS Lett.* **188,** 141–144.

Falkensammer, G., Fischer-Colbrie, R., Richter, K., and Winkler, H. (1985). Cell-free and cellular synthesis of chromogranin A and B of bovine adrenal medulla. *Neuroscience* **14,** 735–746.

Fasman, G. D., Chou, P. Y., and Adler, A. (1976). Prediction of the conformation of the histones. *Biophys. J.* **16,** 1201.

Fischer, J. A., Oldham, S. B., Sizemore, G. W., and Arnaud, C. D. (1972). Calcium regulated parathyroid hormone peptidase. *Proc. Natl. Acad. Sci. U.S.A.* **69,** 2341.

Fiskin, A. M., Cohn, D. V., and Peterson, G. S. (1977). A model for the structure of bovine parathormone derived by dark field electron microscopy. *J. Biol. Chem.* **252,** 8261.

Flueck, J. A., Dibella, F. P., Edis, A. J., Kehrwald, J. M., and Arnaud, C. D. (1977). Immunoheterogeneity of parathyroid hormone in venous effluent serum from hyperfunctioning parathyroid glands. *J. Clin. Invest.* **60,** 1367.

Fraser, D. R., and Kodicek, E. (1973). Regulation of 25-hydroxycholecalciferol-1-hydroxylase activity in kidney by parathyroid hormone. *Nature (London) New Biol.* **241,** 163.

Garabedian, M., Holick, M. F., DeLuca, H. F., and Boyle, I. T. (1972). Control of 25-hydroxycholecalciferol metabolism by the parathyroid glands. *Proc. Natl. Acad. Sci. U.S.A.* **69,** 1673.

Gardner, D. G., Brown, E. M., Windeck, R., and Aurbach, G. D. (1978). Prostglandin E_2 stimulation of adenosine 3′,5′-monophosphate accumulation and parathyroid hormone release in dispersed bovine parathyroid cells. *Endocrinology* **103,** 577.

Gardner, D. G., Brown, E. M., and Aurbach, G. D. (1979a). Inhibition of adenosine 3′,5′-monophosphate accumulation and parathyroid hormone release by sodium nitroprusside. *Endocrinology* **105,** 360.

Gardner, D. G., Brown, E. M., Windeck, R., and Aurbach, G. D. (1979b). Prostaglandin F_{2a} inhibits 3′,5′-adenosine monophosphate accumulation and parathyroid hormone release from dispersed bovine parathyroid cells. *Endocrinology* **104,** 1.

Gardner, D. G., Brown, E. M., Attie, M. F., and Aurbach, G. D. (1980). Prostaglandin-mediated stimulation of adenosine 3′,5′-monophosphate accumulation and parathyroid hormone release in dispersed human parathyroid cells. *J. Clin. Endocrinol. Metab.* **51,** 20.

Gardner, D. G., Brown, E. M., Attie, M. F., and Aurbach, G. D. (1981a). Effects of prostaglandins on adenosine 3′,5′-monophosphate content and adenylate cyclase activity in dispersed bovine parathyroid cells. *Endocrinology* **109,** 1545.

Gardner, D. G., Brown, E. M., and Aurbach, G. D. (1981b). Sodium nitroprusside inhibition of parathyroid hormone release is not mediated through cyclic GMP. *Metabolism* **30,** 1179.

Geisow, M. (1978). Polypeptide secondary structure may direct the specificity of prohormone conversion. *FEBS Lett.* **87,** 111.

Glimcher, M. J. (1976). Composition, structure, and organization of bone and other mineralized tissues and the mechanism of calcification. *In* "Handbook of Physiology" (G. D. Aurbach, ed.), Sect. 7, Vol. 7, p. 25. Am. Physiological Soc., Washington, D.C.

Goltzman, D., Callahan, E. N., Tregear, G. W., and Potts, J. T., Jr. (1976). Conversion of proparathyroid hormone to parathyroid hormone: Studies *in vitro* with trypsin. *Biochemistry* **15,** 5076.

Habener, J. F., and Potts, J. T., Jr. (1976). Relative effectiveness of magnesium and calcium on the secretion and biosynthesis of parathyroid hormone *in vitro. Endocrinology* **98,** 197.

Habener, J. F., and Potts, J. T., Jr. (1979). Subcellular distributions of parathyroid hormone, hormonal precursors, and parathyroid secretory protein. *Endocrinology* **104,** 265.

Habener, J. F., Segre, G. V., Powell, D., Murray, T. M., and Potts, J. T., Jr. (1972). Immunoreactive parathyroid hormone in circulation of man. *Nature (London)* **238,** 152.

Habener, J. F., Kemper, B., and Potts, J. T., Jr. (1975a). Calcium-dependent intracellular degradation of parathyroid hormone: A possible mechanism for the regulation of hormone stores. *Endocrinology* **97,** 431.

Habener, J. F., Kemper, B., Potts, J. T., Jr., and Rich, A. (1975b). Parathyroid mRNA directs the synthesis of pre-proparathyroid hormone and proparathyroid hormone in the Krebs ascites cell-free system. *Biochem. Biophys. Res. Commun.* **67,** 1114.

Habener, J. F., Change, H. T., and Potts, J. T., Jr. (1977). Enzymic processing of proparathyroid hormone by cell-free extracts of parathyroid glands. *Biochemistry* **16,** 3910.

Habener, J. F., Rosenblatt, M., Kemper, B., Kronenberg, H. M., Rich, A., and Potts, J. T., Jr. (1978). Preproparathyroid hormone: Amino acid sequence, chemical synthesis and some biological studies of the precursor region. *Proc. Natl. Acad. Sci. U.S.A.* **75,** 2616.

Habener, J. F., Amherdt, M., Ravazzola, M., and Orci, L. (1979). Parathyroid hormone biosynthesis. Correlation of conversion of biosynthetic precursors with intracellular protein migration as determined by electron microscopy autoradiography. *J. Cell. Biol.* **80,** 715.

Habener, J. F., Kronenberg, H. M., and Potts, J. T., Jr. (1981). Biosynthesis of preproparathyroid hormone. *Methods Cell Biol.* **23,** 51.

Habener, J. F., Rosenblatt, M., and Potts, J. T., Jr. (1984). Parathyroid hormone: Biochemical aspects of biosynthesis, secretion, action and metabolism. *Physiol. Rev.* **64,** 985.

Hamilton, J. W., and Cohn, D. V. (1969). Studies on the biosynthesis *in vitro* of parathyroid hormone. I. Synthesis of parathyroid hormone by bovine parathyroid gland slices and its control by calcium. *J. Biol. Chem.* **244,** 5421.

Hamilton, J. W., MacGregor, R. R., Chu, L. L. H., and Cohn, D. V. (1971a). The isolation and partial purification of a nonparathyroid hormone calcemic fraction from bovine parathyroid glands. *Endocrinology* **89,** 1440.

Hamilton, J. W., Spierto, F. W., MacGregor, R. R., and Cohn, D. V. (1971b). Studies on the biosynthesis *in vitro* of parathyroid hormone. II. The effect of calcium and magnesium on synthesis of parathyroid hormone isolated from bovine parathyroid tissue and incubation medium. *J. Biol. Chem.* **245,** 3224.

Hamilton, J. W., Niall, H. D., Jacobs, J. W., Keutmann, H. T., Potts, J. T., Jr., and Cohn, D. V. (1974). The N-terminal amino acid sequence of bovine proparathyroid hormone. *Proc. Natl. Acad. Sci. U.S.A.* **71,** 653.

Hamilton, J. W., Jilka, R. L., and MacGregor, R. R. (1983). Cleavage of parathyroid hormone to the 1–34 and 35–84 fragments by cathepsin D-like activity in bovine parathyroid gland extracts. *Endocrinology* **113,** 285–292.

Handler, P., and Cohn, D. V. (1952). Effect of parathyroid extract on renal function. *Am. J. Physiol.* **169,** 188.

Hanley, D. A., Takatsuke, K., Sultan, J. M., Schneider, A. B., and Sherwood, L. M. (1978). Direct release of parathyroid hormone fragments from functioning bovine parathyroid glands *in vitro*. *J. Clin. Invest.* **62,** 1247.

Heath, H., III, Larson, J. M., and Laakso, K. (1980). Provocative tests of parathyroid and C cell function in adrenalectomized and chemically sympathectomized rats. *Endocrinology* **107,** 977.

Heinrich, G., Kronenberg, H. M., Potts, J. T., Jr., and Habener, J. F. (1983). Parathyroid hormone messenger ribonucleic acid: Effects of calcium on cellular regulation *in vitro*. *Endocrinology* **112,** 449.

Heinrich, G., Kronenberg, H. M., Potts, J. T., Jr., and Habener, J. F. (1984). Gene encoding parathyroid hormone: Nucleotide sequence of the rat gene and deduced amino acid sequence of rat preproparathyroid hormone. *J. Biol. Chem.* **259,** 3320.

Hellerman, J. G., Cone, R. C., Potts, J. T., Jr., Rich, A., Mulligan, R. C., and Kronenberg, H. M. (1984). Secretion of human parathyroid hormone from rat pituitary infected with a recombinant retrovirus encoding preproparathyroid hormone. *Proc. Natl. Acad. Sci. U.S.A.* **81,** 5340–5344.

Hendy, G. N., Kronenberg, H. M., Potts, J. T., Jr., and Rich, A. (1981). Nucleotide sequence of cloned cDNAs encoding human preproparathyroid hormone. *Proc. Natl. Acad. Sci. U.S.A.* **78,** 7365.

Henry, H. L., Taylor, A. N., and Norman, A. W. (1977). Effect of the vitamin D metabolites 1,25-dihydroxyvitamin D and 24,25-dihydroxyvitamin D on chick parathyroid gland size. *J. Nutr.* **107,** 1918.

Hogue-Angeletti, R. A. (1977). Nonidentity of chromogranin A and dopamine-β-monooxygenase. *Arch. Biochem. Biophys.* **184,** 364.

Hove, K., and Sand, O. (1981). Evidence for a function of calcium influx in the stimulation of hormone release from the parathyroid gland in the goat. *Acta Physiol. Scand.* **113,** 37.

Hruska, K., Marian, K., Greenwalt, A., Klahr, S., and Slatopolsky, E. (1978). Characterization of parathyroid hormone uptake, degradation and fragment production by liver and kidney. *In* "Endocrinology of Calcium Metabolism (D. H. Copp and R. V. Talmage, eds.), p. 313. Excerpta Medica, Amsterdam.

Huang, D. W. Y., Chu, L. L. H., Hamilton, J. W., MacGregor, D. H., and Cohn, D. V. (1975). The NH_2-terminal amino acid sequence of human proparathyroid hormone by radioisotope microanalysis. *Arch. Biochem. Biophys.* **166,** 67.

Jacobs, J. W., Kemper, B., Niall, H. D., Habener, J. F., and Potts, J. T., Jr. (1974). Structural analysis of human proparathyroid hormone by a new microsequencing approach. *Nature (London)* **249,** 155.

Kemper, B., Habener, J. F., Potts, J. T., Jr., and Rich, A. (1972). Proparathyroid hormone: Identification of a biosynthetic precursor to parathyroid hormone. *Proc. Natl. Acad. Sci. U.S.A.* **69,** 643.

Kemper, B., Habener, J. F., Mulligan, R. C., Potts, J. T., Jr. and Rich, A. (1974a). Preproparathyroid hormone: A direct translation product of parathyroid messenger RNA. *Proc. Natl. Acad. Sci. U.S.A.* **71,** 3731.

Kemper, B., Habener, J. F., Rich, A., and Potts, J. T., Jr. (1974b). Parathyroid secretion: Discovery of a major calcium-dependent protein. *Science* **184,** 167.

Kemper, B., Habener, J. F., Ernst, M. D., Potts, J. T., Jr., and Rich, A. (1976a). Preproparathyroid hormone: Analysis of radioactive tryptic peptides and amino acid sequence. *Biochemistry* **15,** 15.

Kemper, B., Habener, J. F., Potts, J. T., Jr., and Rich, A. (1976b). Preproparathyroid hormone: Fidelity of the translation of parathyroid messenger RNA by extracts of wheat germ. *Biochemistry* **15,** 20.

Kemper, B., Weaver, C. A., and Gordon, D. F. (1981). Structure and function of bovine parathyroid hormone messenger RNA. *In* "Hormonal Control of Calcium Metabolism" (D. V. Cohn, R. V. Talmage, and J. L. Matthews, eds.), p. 19. Excerpta Medica, Amsterdam.

Keutmann, H. T., Sauer, M. M, Hendy, G. N., O'Riordan, J. L. H., and Potts, J. T., Jr. (1978). Complete amino acid sequence of human parathyroid hormone. *Biochemistry* **17,** 5723.

Keutmann, H. T., Griscom, A. W., Nussbaum, S. R., Reiner, B. F., Goud, A. N., Potts, J. T., Jr., and Rosenblatt, M. (1985). Rat parathyroid hormone (1–34) fragment: Renal adenylate cyclase activity and receptor binding properties *in vitro*. *Endocrinology* **117,** 1230.

Kiang, W. L., Krusius, T., Finne, J., Margolis, R. U., and Margolis, R. K. (1982). Glycoproteins and proteoglycans of the chromaffin granule matrix. *J. Biol. Chem.* **257,** 1651–1659.

Kirschner, N., Sage, H., and Smith, W. (1967). Mechanism of secretion from the adrenal medulla. II. Release of catecholamines and storage vesical protein in response to chemical stimulation. *Mol. Pharmacol.* **3,** 254.

Kittur, S. D., Hoppener, J. W. M., Antonarakis, S. E., Daniels, J. D. J., Meyers, D. A., Maestri, N. E., Jansen, M., Korneluk, R. G., Nelkin, B. D., and Kazazian, H. H., Jr. (1985). Linkage map of the short arm of human chromosome 11: Location of the genes for catalase, calcitonin, and insulin-like growth factor II. *Proc. Natl. Acad. Sci. U.S.A.* **82,** 5064.

Kreibich, G., Czako-Graham, M., Grebenau, R. C., and Sabatini, D. D. (1980). Functional and structural characteristics of endoplasmic reticulum proteins associated with ribosome binding sites. *In* "Precursor Processing in the Biosynthesis of Proteins" (M. Zimmerman, R. A. Mumford, and D. F. Steiner, eds.), p. 17. New York Academy of Sciences, New York.

Kreil, G. (1981). Transfer of proteins across membranes. *Annu. Rev. Biochem.* **50,** 317.

Kruggel, W., O'Connor, D. T., and Lewis, R. V. (1985). The amino terminal sequences of bovine and human chromogranin A and secretory protein. *Biochem. Biophys. Res. Commun.* **127,** 380–383.

Kumarasamy, R., and Blough, H. A. (1985). Galactose-rich glycoproteins are on the cell surface of herpes virus-infected cells. 1. Surface labeling and serial lectin binding studies of Asn-linked oligosaccharides of glycoprotein gC. *Arch. Biochem. Biophy.* **236,** 593–602.

Lasker, R. D., and Spiegel, A. M. (1982). Endogenous substrates for cAMP-dependent phosphorylation in dispersed bovine parathyroid cells. *Endocrinology* **111,** 1412.

Licata, A. A., Au, W. Y. W., and Raisz, L. G. (1972). Secretion of glucosamine-containing macromolecules by rat parathyroid glands in tissue culture. *Biochim. Biophys. Acta* **261,** 143.

Lloyd, R. V., and Wilson, B. S. (1983). Specific endocrine tissue marker defined by a monoclonal antibody. *Science* **222,** 628–630.

Lopez, E., Tisserand-Jochem, E. M., Vidal, B., Milet, C., Lallier, F., and Mac Intyre, I. (1984). Are corpuscles of stannius the parathyroid glands in fish? Immunocytochemical and ultrastructural arguments. *In* "Endocrine Control of Bone and Calcium Metabolism" (D. V. Cohn, J. T. Potts, Jr., and T. Fujita, eds.), Vol. 88, Abstract. Excerpta Medica, Amsterdam.

Luben, R. A., Wong, G. L., and Cohn, D. V. (1976). Biochemical characterization with parathormone and calcitonin of isolated bone cells: Provisional identification of osteoclasts and osteoblasts. *Endocrinology* **99,** 526.

Luben, R. A., Wong, G. L., and Cohn, D. V. (1977). Parathormone-stimulated resportion of devitalised bone by cultured osteoclast-type bone cells. *Nature (London)* **265,** 629.

MacGregor, R. R., and Cohn, D. V. (1978). The intracellular pathway for parathormone biosynthesis and secretion. *Clin. Orthop., Rel. Res.* **137,** 244.

MacGregor, R. R., Chu, L. L. H., Hamilton, J. W., and Cohn, D. V. (1973). Studies on the subcellular localization of proparathyroid hormone and parathyroid hormone in the bovine parathyroid gland: Separation of newly synthesized from mature forms. *Endocrinology* **93,** 1387.

MacGregor, R. R., Hamilton, J. W., and Cohn, D. V. (1975). The bypass of tissue hormone stores during the secretion of newly synthesized parathyroid hormone. *Endocrinology* **97,** 178.

MacGregor, R. R., Chu, L. L. H., and Cohn, D. V. (1976a). Conversion of proparathyroid hormone to parathyroid hormone by a particulate enzyme of the parathyroid gland. *J. Biol. Chem.* **251,** 6711.

MacGregor, R. R., Huang, W. Y., and Cohn, D. V. (1976b). Identification of chicken proparathormone: Comparison of its amino acid sequence to that of chicken parathormone. *Fed. Proc., Fed. Am. Soc. Exp. Biol.* **35,** 1695 (abstract).

MacGregor, D. H., Chu, L. L. H., MacGregor, R. R., and Cohn, D. V. (1977). Disruption of the Golgi zone and inhibition of the conversion of proparathyroid hormone to parathyroid hormone in human parathyroid tissue by tris(hydroxymethyl)aminomethane. *Am. J. Pathol.* **87,** 553.

MacGregor, R. R., Chu, L. L. H., Hamilton, J. W., and Cohn, D. V. (1978a). The intracellular translocation and metabolism of bovine proparathyroid hormone. *In* "Endocrinology of Calcium Metabolism" (D. H. Copp and R. V. Talmage, eds.), p. 291. Excerpta Medica, Amsterdam.

MacGregor, R. R., Hamilton, J. W., and Cohn, D. V. (1978b). The mode of conversion of proparathormone to parathormone by a particulate converting enzymic activity of the parathyroid gland. *J. Biol. Chem.* **253,** 2012.

MacGregor, R. R., Hamilton, J. W., Kent, G. N., Shofstall, R. E., and Cohn, D. V. (1979a). The degradation of proparathormone and parathormone by parathyroid and liver cathepsin B. *J. Biol. Chem.* **254,** 4428.

MacGregor, R. R., Hamilton, J. W., Shofstall, R. E., and Cohn, D. V. (1979b). Isolation and characterization of porcine parathyroid cathepsin B. *J. Biol. Chem.* **254,** 4423.

MacGregor, R. R., Cohn, D. V., and Hamilton, J. W. (1983). The content of carboxyl-terminal fragments of parathormone in extracts of fresh bovine parathyroids. *Endocrinology* **112,** 1019.

Mahafee, D. D., Cooper, C. W., Ramp, W. K., and Ontjes, D. A. (1982). Magnesium promotes both parathyroid hormone secretion and adenosine 3′,5′-monophosphate production in rat parathyroid tissues and reverses the inhibitory effects of calcium on adenylate cyclase. *Endocrinology* **110,** 487–495.

Majzoub, J. A., Kronenberg, H. M., Potts, J. T., Jr., Rich, A., and Habener, J. F. (1979). Identification and cell-free translation of mRNA coding for a precursor of parathyroid secretory protein. *J. Biol. Chem.* **254,** 7449.
Majzoub, J. A., Dee, P. C., and Habener, J. F. (1982). Cellular and cell-free processing of parathyroid secretory proteins. *J. Biol. Chem.* **257,** 3581.
Mallette, L., Thornby, J., and Pretorius, H. T. (1985). Internal homology in prepro-parathyroid hormone: Four copies of a primitive gene. *Abstr. Annu. Meet. Am. Soc. Bone Mineral Res., 7th.*
Martin, K. F., Hruska, K. A., Freitag, J. J., Klahr, S., and Slatopolsky, E. (1979). The peripheral metabolism of parathyroid hormone. *N. Engl. J. Med.* **301,** 1092.
Mayer, G. P. (1975). Effect of calcium and magnesium on parathyroid hormone secretion rate in calves. *In* "Calcium Regulating Hormones" (R. V. Talmage, M. Owen, and J. A. Parsons, eds.), p. 122. Excerpta Medica, Amsterdam.
Mayer, G. P. (1979). Parathyroid hormone secretion. *In* "Endocrinology" (L. DeGroot et al., eds.), p. 607. Grune and Stratton, New York.
Mayer, G. P., and Hurst, J. G. (1978). Sigmoidal relationship between parathyroid hormone secretion rate and plasma calcium concentration in calves. *Endocrinology* **102,** 1036.
Mayer, G. P., Keaton, J. A., Hurst, J. G., and Habener, J. F. (1979). Effects of plasma calcium concentration on the relative proportion of hormone and carboxyl fragments in parathyroid venous blood. *Endocrinology* **104,** 1778.
Meunier, P. J. (1983). Histomorphometry of the skeleton. *In* "Bone and Mineral Research Annual 1" (William A. Peck, ed.), p. 191. Excerpta Medica, Amsterdam.
Milstein, C., Brownlee, G. G., Harrison, T. M., and Matthews, M. B. (1972). A possible precursor of immunoglobulin light chains. *Nature (London)* **239,** 117.
Morrissey, J., and Cohn, D. V. (1978). The effects of calcium and magnesium on the secretion of parathormone and parathyroid secretory protein by isolated porcine parathyroid cells. *Endocrinology* **103,** 2081.
Morrissey, J., and Cohn, D. V. (1979a). Regulation of secretion of parathormone and secretory protein-I from separate intracellular pools by calcium, dibutyryl cyclic AMP, and (1)-isoproterenol. *J. Biol. Cell.* **82,** 93.
Morrissey, J., and Cohn, D. V. (1979b). Secretion and degradation of parathormone as a function of intracellular maturation of hormone pools: Modulation by calcium and dibutyryl cyclic AMP. *J. Biol. Cell.* **83,** 521.
Morrissey, J. J., Hamilton, J. W., and Cohn, D. V. (1978). The secretion of parathormone and glycosylated proteins by parathyroid cells in culture. *Biochem. Biophys. Res. Commun.* **82,** 1279.
Morrissey, J. J., Hamilton, J. W., MacGregor, R. R., and Cohn, D. V. (1980a). The secretion of parathormone fragments 34–84 and 37–84 by dispersed porcine parathyroid cells. *Endocrinology* **107,** 164.
Morrissey, J. J., Shofstall, R. E., Hamilton, J. W., and Cohn, D. V. (1980b). Synthesis, intracellular distribution and secretion of multiple forms of parathyroid secretory protein I. *Proc. Natl. Acad. Sci. U.S.A.* **77,** 6406.
Mortimore, G. E. (1984). Regulation of intracellular proteolysis. *Fed. Proc., Fed. Am. Soc. Exp. Biol.* **43,** 1281.
Nakagami, K., Warsharsky, H., and LeBlond, C. P. (1971). The elaboration of protein and carbohydrate by rat parathyroid cells as revealed by electron microscope autoradiography. *J. Cell Biol.* **51,** 596.
Neer, R. M. (1979). Calcium and inorganic phosphate homeostasis. *In* "Endocrinology" (L. DeGroot *et al.,* eds.), p. 669. Grune & Stratton, New York.

Niall, H. D., Keutman, H. T., Sauer, R., Hogan, M., Dawson, B., Aurbach, G. D., and Potts, J. T., Jr. (1970). The amino acid sequence of bovine parathyroid hormone. *Hoppe-Seyler's Z. Physiol. Chem.* **351,** 1586.

Nishizuka, Y. (1984). Turnover of inositol phospholipids and signal transduction. *Science* **225,** 1365–1370.

O'Connor, D. T. (1983). Chromogranin: Widespread immunoreactivity in polypeptide hormone producing tissues and serum. *Regul. Peptides* **6,** 263–280.

O'Connor, D. T., and Frigon, R. P. (1984). Chromogranin A: The major catecholamine storage vesicle soluble protein. *J. Biol. Chem.* **259,** 3237–3247.

O'Connor, D. T., Burton, D., and Deftos, L. (1983). Chromogranin A: Immunohistology reveals its universal occurrence in normal polypeptide hormone producing endocrine glands. *Life Sci.* **33,** 1657–1663.

Oldham, S. B., Fischer, A. A., and Shen, L. H. (1974). Isolation and properties of a calcium binding protein from porcine parathyroid glands. *Biochemistry* **14,** 4790.

Oldham, S. B., Lipson, L. G., and Tietjen, G. E. (1982). Presence of calmodulin in parathyroid adenomas. *Mineral Electrolyte Met.* **7,** 273.

O'Riordan, J. L. H., and Potts, J. T., Jr. (1974). The amino acid sequence of porcine parathyroid hormone. *Biochemistry* **13,** 1994.

Palade, G. (1975). Intracellular aspects of the process of protein synthesis. *Science* **189,** 347.

Parfitt, M. A. (1979). Surgical, idiopathic, and other varieties of parathyroid hormone-deficient hypoparathyroidism. *In* "Endocrinology," (L. J. DeGroot, ed.), Vol. 2, p. 755. Grune & Stratton, New York.

Parsons, J. A., Gray, D., Rafferty, B., and Zanelli, J. M. (1978). Evidence for a hypercalcemic factor in the fish pituitary immunologically related to mammalian parathyroid hormone. *In* "Endocrinology of Calcium Metabolism" (D. H. Copp and R. V. Talmage, eds.), pp. 111. Excerpta Medica, Amsterdam.

Phang, J. M., and Weiss, I. W. (1976). Maintenance of calcium homeostasis in human beings. *In* "Handbook of Physiology" Section 7, Vol. 7, p. 157. Am. Physiological Society, Washington, D.C.

Phillips, J. H. (1982). Dynamic aspects of chromaffin granule structure. *Neuroscience* **7,** 1595–1610.

Pollard, H. B., Pazoles, C., and Creutz, C. E. (1981). Mechanism of calcium action and release of vesicle-bound hormones during exocytosis. *Recent Prog. Horm. Res.* **37,** 299.

Pollard, H., Ornberg, R., Levine, M., Kelner, K., Morita, K., Levine, R., Forsgerg, E., Brocklehurst, K. W., Duong, L., Lelkes, P. I., Heldman, E., and Youdim, M. (1985). Hormone secretion by exocytosis with emphasis on information from the chromaffin cell system. *Vitam. Horm.* **42,** 109–196.

Potts, J. T., Jr., Kronenberg, H. M., and Rosenblatt, M. (1982). Parathyroid hormone: Chemistry, biosynthesis and mode of action. *Adv. Protein Chem.* **35,** 323.

Pullman, T. N., Lavender, A. R., Aho, I., and Rasmussen, H. (1960). Direct renal action of a purified parathyroid extract. *Endocrinology* **67,** 570.

Quinn, P. S., and Judah, J. D. (1978). Calcium-dependent golgi-vesicle fusion and cathepsin B in the conversion of proalbumin into albumin in rat liver. *Biochem. J.* **172,** 301.

Rabbani, S. A., Kremer, R., Bennett, H. P., and Goltzman, D. (1984). Phosphorylation of parathyroid hormone by human and bovine parathyroid glands. *J. Biol. Chem.* **259,** 2949–55.

Raese, J. D., Boarder, M. R., Makk, G., and Barchas, J. D. (1980). Phosphorylation of β-

lipotropin, β-endorphin, corticotorpin and parathyroid hormone: A potential control for peptide processing. *In* "Neural Peptides and Neuronal Communication" (E. Costa and M. Trabucchi, eds.), p. 377. Raven, New York.

Raisz, L. G. (1976). Mechanisms of bone resorption. *In* "Handbook of Physiology" (G. D. Aurbach, ed.), Section 7, Vol. 7, p. 117, Am. Physiological Society, Washington D.C.

Ramp, W. K., and McNeil, R. W. (1978). Selective stimulation of net calcium efflux from chick embryo tibiae by parathyroid hormone *in vitro*. *Calcif. Tissue Res.* **25,** 227–232.

Ramp, W. K., Cooper, C. W., Ross, A. J., III, and Wells, S. A., Jr. (1979). Effects of calcium and cyclic nucleotides on rat calcitonin and parathyroid hormone secretion. *Mol. Cell. Endocrinol.* **14,** 205–215.

Ravazzola, M., Orci, L., Habener, J. F., and Potts, J. T., Jr. (1978). Parathyroid secretory protein: Immunocytochemical localization within cells that contain parathyroid hormone. *Lancet* **2,** 371.

Recheigl, M., Jr., and Heston, W. E. (1967). Genetic regulation of enzyme activity in mammalian system by the alteration of the rates of enzyme degradation. *Biochem. Biophys. Res. Commun.* **27,** 119.

Rosa, P., Hille, A., Lee, R. W. H., Zanini, A., Camilli, P. D., and Huttner, W. B. (1985). Secretogranins I and II: Two tyrosine-sulfated secretory proteins common to a variety of cells secreting peptides by the regulated pathway. *J. Cell Biol.* **101,** 1999.

Rosenblatt, M. (1982). Structure–activity relations in the calcium-regulating peptide hormones. *In* "Endocrinology of Calcium Metabolism" (J. A. Parsons, ed.), Raven, New York.

Roth, S. I., and Capen, C. C. (1974). Ultrastructural and functional correlations of the parathyroid gland. *Int. Rev. Exp. Pathol.* **13,** 161.

Roth, S. I., and Raisz, L. G. (1964). Effect of calcium concentration on the ultrastructure of rat parathyroid in organ culture. *Lab. Invest.* **13,** 331.

Roth, S. I., and Raisz, L. G. (1966). The course and reversibility of the calcium effect on the ultrastructure of the rat parathyroid gland in organ culture. *Lab. Invest.* **15,** 1187.

Roth, S. I., Au, W. Y. W., Kunin, A. S., Krane, S. M., and Raisz, L. G. (1968). Effect of dietary deficiency in vitamin D, calcium, and phosphorus on the ultrastructure of the rat parathyroid gland. *Am. J. Pathol.* **53,** 631.

Russell, J., Lettieri, D., and Sherwood, L. M. (1983). Direct regulation by calcium of cytoplasmic messenger ribonucleic acid coding for pre-proparathyroid hormone in isolated bovine parathyroid cells. *J. Clin. Invest.* **72,** 1851.

Sage, H. J., Smith, W., and Kirschner, N. (1967). Mechanism of secretion from the adrenal medulla. I. A microquantitative immunologic assay for bovine adrenal catecholamine storage vesical protein and its application to studies of the secretory process. *Mol. Pharmacol.* **3,** 81.

Sand, O., Ozawa, S., and Hove, K. (1981). Electrophysiology of cultured parathyroid cells from the goat. *Acta Physiol. Scand.* **113,** 45.

Sauer, R. T., Niall, H. D., Hogan, M. L., Keutmann, H. T., O'Riordan, J. L. H., and Potts, J. T., Jr. (1974). The amino acid sequence of porcine parathyroid hormone. *Biochemistry* **13,** 1994.

Saxe, A. W., Chen, S. L., Marx, S., and Brennan, M. F. (1982). *In vitro* studies of parathyroid hormone release: Effect of cimetidine. *Surgery* **92,** 793.

Schimke, R. T., Sweeney, E. W., and Berlin, C. M. (1965). The roles of synthesis and degradation in the control of rat liver tryptophan pyrrolase. *J. Biol. Chem.* **240,** 322.

Segre, G. V. (1979). Heterogeneity and metabolism of parathyroid hormone. *In* "Endocrinology" (L. DeGroot, ed.), Vol. 2, p. 613. Grune & Stratton, New York.

Segre, G. V., D'Amour, P., and Potts, J. T., Jr. (1976). Metabolism of diodinated parathyroid hormone in the rat. *Endocrinology* **99,** 1645.

Sethi, R., Kukreja, S. C., Bowser, N. E., Hargis, G. K., and Williams, G. A. (1981). Effect of secretin on parathyroid hormone and calcitonin secretion. *J. Clin. Endocrinol. Metab.* **53,** 153.

Setoguti, T., Inoue, Y., and Kato, K. (1981). Electron-microscopic studies on the relationship between the frequency of parathyroid storage granules and serum calcium levels in the rat. *Cell Tissue Res.* **219,** 457.

Settleman, J., Fonseca, R., Nolan, and Angeletti, R. H. (1985a). Relationship of multiple forms of chromogranin. *J. Biol. Chem.* **260,** 1645–1651.

Settleman, J., Nolan, and Angeletti, R. H. (1985b). Chromogranin, an integral membrane protein. *J. Biol. Chem.* **260,** 1641–1644.

Shannon, W. A., Jr., and Roth, S. I. (1974). An ultrastructural study of acid phosphatase activity in normal, adenomatous and hyperplastic (chief cell type) human parathyroid glands. *Am. J. Pathol.* **77,** 493.

Sherwood, L. M., Mayer, G. P., Ramberg, C. F., Jr., Kronfeld, D. S., Aurbach, G. D., and Potts, J. T., Jr. (1968). Regulation of parathyroid hormone secretion: Proportional control by calcium, lack of effect of phosphate. *Endocrinology* **83,** 1043.

Sherwood, L. M., Herrman, I., and Bassett, C. A. (1970). Parathyroid hormone secretion *in vitro:* Regulation by calcium and magnesium ions. *Nature (London)* **225,** 1056.

Shoback, D., Thatcher, J., Leombruno, R., and Brown, E. (1983). Effects of extracellular Ca^{2+} and Mg^{2+} on cytosolic Ca^{2+} and PTH release in dispersed bovine parathyroid cells. *Endocrinology* **113,** 424–426.

Shoback, D. M., Thatcher, J., Leombruno, R., and Brown, E. M. (1984). Relationship between parathyroid hormone secretion and cytosolic calcium concentration in dispersed bovine parathyroid cells. *Proc. Natl. Acad. Sci. U.S.A.* **81,** 3113–3117.

Silver, J., Russell, J., and Sherwood, L. M. (1985). Regulation by vitamin D metabolites of messenger ribonucleic acid for preproparathyroid hormone in isolated bovine parathyroid cells. *Proc. Natl. Acad. Sci. U.S.A.* **82,** 4270.

Silverman, R. and Yalow, R. S. (1973). Heterogeneity of parathyroid hormone. Clin. and physiologic implications. *J. Clin. Invest.* **52,** 1958.

Smith, R. E., and Farquhar, M. G. (1966). Lysosome function in the regulation of the secretory process in cells of the anterior pituitary gland. *J. Cell Biol.* **31,** 319.

Smith, R. E., and Van Frank, R. M. (1975). The use of amino acid derivatives of 4-methoxy-β-napthylamine for the assay and subcellular localization of tissue proteinases. *In* "Lysosomes in Biology and Pathology" (J. T. Dingle and R. T. Dean, eds.), Vol. 4, p. 193. North-Holland Publ., Amsterdam.

Somogyi, P., Hodgson, A. J., DePotter, R. W., Fischer-Colbrie, R., Schober, M., Winkler, H., and Chubb, I. W. (1984). Chromogranin immunoreactivity in the central nervous system. Immunochemical characterisation, distribution and relationship to catecholamine and enkephalin pathways. *Brain Res. Rev.* **8,** 193–230.

Steiner, D. F., Docherty, K., and Carroll, R. (1984). Golgi/granule processing of peptide hormone and neuropeptide precursors: A minireview. *J. Cell Biochem.* **24,** 121.

Struck, D. K., and Lennarz, W. (1980). "The Biochemistry of Glycoproteins and Proteoglycans" (W. Lennarz, ed.), pp. 35–83. Plenum, New York.

Takatsuki, K., Schneider, A. B., Shin, K. Y., and Sherwood, L. M. (1981). Extraction, purification and partial characterization of bovine parathyroid secretory protein. *J. Biol. Chem.* **256,** 2342.

Takatsuki, K., Takano, T., Yoneda, M., Uchikawa, A., and Tomita, A. (1982). *Abstr. Asia Oceania Congr. Endocrinol. 7th, Tokyo* p. 17.

Talmage, R. V., Cooper, C. W., and Toverud, S. V. (1983). The physiological significance of calcitonin. *In* "Bone and Mineral Research Annual I" (W. A. Peck, ed.), p. 74. Excerpta Medica, Amsterdam.

Targovnik, J. H., Rodman, J. S., and Sherwood, L. M. (1971). Regulation of parathyroid hormone secretion *in vitro:* Quantitative aspects of calcium and magnesium ion control. *Endocrinology* **88,** 1477.

Tregear, G. W., van Rietschoten, J., Green, E., Keutmann, H. T., Niall, H. D., Reit, B., Parsons, J. A., and Potts, J. T., Jr. (1973). Bovine parathyroid hormone: Minimum chain length of synthetic peptide required for biological activity. *Endocrinology* **93,** 1349.

Vasicek, T. J., McDevitt, B. E., Freeman, M. W., Fennick, B. J., Hendy, G. N., Potts, J. T., Jr., Rich, A., and Kronenberg, H. M. (1983). Nucleotide sequence of the human parathyroid hormone gene. *Proc. Natl. Acad. Sci. U.S.A.* **80,** 2127.

Wallfelt, C., Larson, R., Johansson, H., Rastad, J., Akerstrom, G., Ljunghall, S., and Gylfe, E. (1985). Stimulus–secretion coupling of parathyroid hormone release: studies of ^{45}Ca and ^{86}Rb fluxes. *Acta Physiol. Scand.* **124,** 239–245.

Walter, P., and Blobel, G. (1980). Purification of a membrane-associated protein complex required for protein translocation across the endoplasmic reticulum. *Proc. Natl. Acad. Sci. U.S.A.* **77,** 7112.

Walter, P., and Blobel, G. (1981a). Translocation of proteins across the endoplasmic reticulum. II. Signal recognition protein (SRP) mediates the selective binding to microsomal membraines of *in vitro*-assembled polysomes synthesizing secretory protein. *J. Cell Biol.* **91,** 551.

Walter, P., and Blobel, G. (1981b). Translocation of proteins across the endoplasmic reticulum. III. Signal recognition protein (SRP) causes signal sequence-dependent and site-specific arrest of chain elongation that is released by microsomal membranes. *J. Cell Biol.* **91,** 557.

Walter, P., and Blobel, G. (1982). Signal recognition particle contains a 7S RNA essential for protein translocation across the endoplasmic reticulum. *Nature (London)* **299,** 691.

Walter, P., Ibrahim, I., and Blobel, G. (1981). Translocation of proteins across the endoplasmic reticulum. I. Signal recognition protein (SRP) binds to *in vitro*-assembled polysomes synthesizing secretory protein. *J. Cell. Biol.* **91,** 545.

Weaver, C. A., Gordon, D. F., and Kemper, B. (1982). Nucleotide sequence of bovine parathyroid hormone messenger RNA. *Mol. Cell. Endocrinol.* **28,** 411.

Williams, G. A., Hargis, G. K., Bowser, E. N., Henderson, W., and Martinez, N. (1973). Evidence for a role of adenosine 3′,5′-monophosphate in parathyroid hormone release. *Endocrinology* **92,** 687.

Wilson, B. S., and Lloyd, R. V. (1984). Detection of chromogranin in neuroendocrine cells with a monoclonal antibody. *Am. J. Pathol.* **115,** 458–468.

Winkler, H. (1976). The composition of adrenal chromaffin granules: An assessment of controversial results. *Neuroscience* **1,** 65.

Winkler, H. (1977). The biogenesis of adrenal chromaffin granules. *Neuroscience* **2,** 657.

Winkler, H., and Carmichael, S. W. (1982). The chromaffin granule. *In* "The Secretory Granule" (A. M. Poisner and J. M. Trifaro, eds.), p. 3. Elsevier, Amsterdam.

Winkler, H., and Westhead, E. (1980). The molecular organization of adrenal chromaffin granules. *Neuroscience* **5,** 1803–1823.

Zull, J. E., and Chuang, J. (1985). Characterization of parathyroid hormone fragments produced by cathepsin D. *J. Biol. Chem.* **260,** 1608.

Zull, J. E., and Lev, N. B. (1980). A theoretical study of the structure of parathyroid hormone. *Proc. Natl. Acad. Sci. U.S.A.* **77,** 3971.

Index

E

F

G

S

T

U

V

W